The Trouble with Medical Journals

Richard Smith

The Trouble with Medical Journals

Richard Smith

Former editor of the *BMJ*

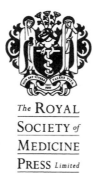

The ROYAL
SOCIETY *of*
MEDICINE
PRESS *Limited*

© 2006 Royal Society of Medicine Ltd

Published by the Royal Society of Medicine Press Ltd
1 Wimpole Street, London W1G 0AE, UK
Tel: +44 (0)20 7290 2921
Fax: +44 (0)20 7290 2929
E-mail: publishing@rsm.ac.uk
Website: www.rsmpress.co.uk

British Library Cataloguing in Publication Data
A catalogue record for this book is available from the British Library

ISBN 1-85315-673-6

Distribution in Europe and Rest of World:

Marston Book Services Ltd
PO Box 269
Abingdon
Oxon OX14 4YN, UK
Tel: +44 (0)1235 465500
Fax: +44 (0)1235 465555

Distribution in the USA and Canada:

Royal Society of Medicine Press Ltd
c/o BookMasters, Inc.
30 Amberwood Parkway
Ashland, Ohio 44805, USA
Tel: +1 800 247 6553 / +1 800 266 5564
Fax: +1 419 281 6883
Email: order@bookmasters.com

Distribution in Australia and New Zealand:

Elsevier Australia
30 52 Smidmore Street
Marrikville NSW 2204, Australia
Tel: +61 2 9517 8999
Fax: +61 2 9517 2249
E-mail: service@elsevier.com.au

Typeset by Phoenix Photosetting, Chatham, Kent
Printed and bound by Bell & Bain, Glasgow

To Chicken (the woman not the bird), Florence (the girl not the city), and Venice, three of the loves of my life.

Moment

Clear moments are so short.
There is much more darkness. More
Ocean than firm land. More
Shadow than form.

Adam Zagajewski
Translated from Polish by Renata Gorczynski
From 'Tremor: Selected Poems' by Adam Zagajewski.
Translated © 1985 Farrar, Straus and Giroux, LLC.
Reprinted by permission of Farrar, Straus and Giroux, LLC.

'When one wanted to arrive overnight at the incomparable, the fabulous, the like-nothing-else-in-the-world, where was it one went?'

Thomas Mann

'Solitude gives birth to the original in us, to beauty unfamiliar and perilous—to poetry. But also, it gives birth to the opposite: to the perverse, the illicit, the absurd.'

Thomas Mann

'To spend one's morning in still, productive analysis of the clustered shadows of the Basilica, one's afternoons anywhere in church or campo, on canal or lagoon, and one's evenings in the starlight gossip at Florian's, feeling the sea-breeze throb languidly between the two great pillars of the Piazzetta and over the low black domes of the church—this, I consider, is to be as happy as is consistent with the preservation of reason.'

Henry James

Acknowledgements and thanks

My thanks to Lin, Freddie, James and Florence Smith for letting me disappear to Venice for eight weeks, to the staff of the BMJ Publishing Group Ltd, the British Medical Association, and in particular Sir Anthony Grabham, Stella Dutton, Kamran Abbasi, Tony Delamothe and Jane Smith for the same, to Stephen Lock for teaching me most of what I know about medical journals and letting me quote his splenetic letter, to Silvia Marsoni, Alvise Marsoni and Selina Marsoni for renting me the beautiful Palazzo Van Axel, to Elide Smaniotto for keeping me in order, being so kind, and tolerating my almost complete lack of Italian (could I really be a professore?), to Alessandro Liberati for being both an inspiration and an intermediary, to Giampaolo and Giulia Velo for constant support and for having me at their home at Bassano del Grappa, to Sandy McCall Smith for inviting me to write the book and for being unwise enough to say 'I'm sure that you could just sit down and write it,' to Joseph Brodsky for being a comfortable ghostly presence (he stayed in the same palazzo in Venice) and tolerating a hack rather than a scrittore, Silvia Bonnacorso, Vikki Entwistle, Magne Nylenna, Gaby Shockley, Finola O'Sullivan, Richard Barling, and Silvio Garattini. Arthur Smith (known to me as Brian) read a few chapters, for which I thank him, but he couldn't be bothered with the whole thing, which I understand. I thank especially Lucy Gardner for her intelligent editing and Beth Kilcoyne and Jane Smith for reading the whole manuscript and making suggestions, some of which I followed. Needless to say, all the mistakes, indulgences, vulgarities, and excesses are mine.

Contents

Section 1: Introduction

Section 2: The nature of medical journals

Section 3: The processes of publishing medical research

Section 4: Problems in publishing medical research

Section 5: Important relationships of medical journals

Section 6: Ethical accountability of researchers and journals

Section 7: The future

Section 1: Introduction

1. **Introduction: medical journals are probably a force for good but need considerable reform**

► 1

Introduction: medical journals are probably a force for good but need considerable reform

Medical journals, which many imagine to be as dull as telephone directories and twice as obscure, influence the lives of everybody—and not always for the better. Not only do they affect what doctors do with individual patients and the actions taken by public health authorities on whole populations, but also they influence how we think about birth, death, pain and sickness. It may therefore make sense for you—the thoughtful but not necessarily expert reader—to pay attention to the ways of medical journals, particularly as many of those ways are deficient and need reform. That is the thesis of this book. I hope that I convince you—intriguing, even fascinating, and sometimes amusing you as we go.

Perhaps you are currently wondering whether your child should have the vaccine against measles, mumps and rubella (MMR). For many parents in many countries this has become a very difficult decision—mainly because of a short, dubious, article published in the *Lancet*.[1] Many parents worry that the vaccine may cause their child to develop autism. Or maybe you are a middle-aged male thinking whether or not you should have yourself tested for prostate specific antigen (PSA) to see if you have cancer of the prostate. You may be perplexed by the emotion that suffuses the debate on the value of this test. Medical journals have provided the information that fuels the debate. Or perhaps you are constantly exhausted, suffering from a condition that many patients call myalgic encephalomyelitis and most doctors chronic fatigue syndrome. You look for help from your doctor, but she tells you that her medical journal tells her the condition does not exist. You are furious. How can this be?

Or maybe you are in circumstances that don't seem to be to do with illness. You are a woman who has lost interest in sex. You're not sure why. One friend says that you may have 'female sexual dysfunction' and should think about medical treatment.[2] Another friend says that she has read in the papers that the *BMJ* (the journal formerly known as the *British Medical Journal*) says that 'female sexual dysfunction' is a condition 'invented' by drug companies to create new markets.[3] You wonder if you 'have a problem' and whether or not you need 'to do something'. You're also approaching the menopause and find yourself receiving very confusing, even contradictory, advice on whether or not you should take hormone replacement therapy. The medical journals have published many papers on hormone replacement therapy, most of them until recently suggesting that women will benefit substantially from taking the treatment. But now there has been a rush of papers suggesting that the treatment may increase the risk of heart disease and breast cancer and not improve quality of life. The tens of millions of women who have taken the treatment are understandably confused: have they been helped or poisoned?

I could go on, but I want to begin to illustrate how medical journals are mixed up in reflections and debates that are important to you. I will enlarge on this theme in other chapters, particularly chapter 2, but you will, I hope, begin to see why you might be interested in what otherwise looks like an arcane subject.

My qualification to write the book is that I have given much of my life to medical journals in general and particularly to the *BMJ*. After training in medicine in Edinburgh and practising briefly in Scotland and New Zealand I joined the *BMJ* in 1979. For 10 years I worked simply as an assistant editor, reading manuscripts, writing and commissioning. During this time I also worked for six years as a television doctor on breakfast television, an experience that taught me much about the craziness and difficulties of the mass media. In 1989, at the instigation of Stephen Lock, my predecessor as editor of the *BMJ*, I went for a year to the Stanford Business School in California.

Soon after returning I was appointed as the editor-in-chief of the *BMJ* and chief executive of the BMJ Publishing Group, positions I held until I left in the summer of 2004. At the *BMJ* I worked roughly half of my time as an editor and half as the chief executive of the publishing group, which grew substantially during those years. I was responsible not only for the *BMJ* in its myriad forms, but also for nearly 30 journals intended for medical specialists, a books programme and various other publishing ventures, including one aimed at the public. When I woke at night during those 20 years, as I often did, it was more often to fret about the journal and the business than it was to think about my family. I write this with some shame, but it illustrates how deeply I was invested in this whole enterprise. My contention in this book is that there is a great deal about medical journals that is ethically sound but also much that is ethically doubtful.

I was asked to write this book by Sandy McCall Smith, professor of medical law at Edinburgh University, editor of a series on medicine, law, and ethics for Cambridge University Press, and chairman of the *BMJ*'s ethics committee (as well as much else, including being a best selling novelist). I replied that I'd love to but could never find the time. 'I think,' he responded, 'that you could probably just sit down and write it.' That was a loaded phrase that lodged in my brain.

Slowly but ineluctably the idea of writing the book combined with an idea that had come to me about five years earlier—the idea that I would love to be in Venice not as a tourist but as somebody with a job to do. I don't speak Italian and so couldn't work in a cappuccino bar, but I could write a book. So there I was in February 2003 in a huge room in Palazzo Venier-Sanudo-van Axel-Barozzi, built in 1473 and within touching distance of Santa Maria dei Miracoli, which John Ruskin thought one of the finest buildings in Venice.

While writing the book in Ruskin's 'the ghost on the sands', I fed on a daily diet of Bellini, Carpaccio, Titian, Tintoretto and Veronese. Maybe some of the voluptuousness of their paintings reflected itself in overambitious prose, but one painting fits particularly with this book. It is Carpaccio's picture 'St Augustine in his Study' in the Scuola di San Giorgio degli Schiavoni. Carpaccio has the unusual ability to paint exquisite paintings that make you not only gasp with their beauty but also laugh. St Augustine, who is squeezed into the right hand side of the picture, is having a vision of the death of St Jerome. I identify with the study, the vision and the apparatus surrounding St Augustine—not a computer with internet access but an astrolabe, sheet music, archeological fragments and shells. I was in a not dissimilar room struggling with a vision of what my book would say. It might conclude that medical journals are lost and corrupt. But I'm most attracted to the small dog that occupies the middle of the picture and looks up at St Augustine thinking, 'What on earth is he up to now?' Not only my dog but also my family and staff often wonder that about me, and this book is written for that dog—and I hope that he or she will understand.

The flat that I lived in was once inhabited by Joseph Brodsky, who now lies in the cemetery of San Michele, less than a mile from the flat. The owner of the flat explained to Signora Elida who looked after the palazzo that I was a 'scrittore like Brodsky'. I felt very silly.

I don't expect—as did Brodsky—to win the Nobel prize for literature for this book, but I would like to produce a book that anybody might read, enjoy and end by thinking: 'I'm glad I read that. I understand just a little more about the world.' The most obvious audience for the book is one interested in what is now called 'publication ethics', but we are an inbred coterie. The next audience is anybody who reads medical and scientific journals. They are counted in millions and I should perhaps have been content with them. But I wanted to try and reach further because the journals deal in issues—birth, death, pain, sickness and sexuality—that affect us all and are perhaps not thought about as deeply as they might be. Richard Horton—a friend, the editor of the *Lancet*, and perhaps touched by the same hubris as me—said that I needed to convince the world that the discourse around health and disease was as important as the discourses around politics, business and the arts. I wanted to try and write a book for everybody because I'm suspicious of experts. After millennia of being a mysterious priesthood, medicine is discovering that better outcomes are to be had by treating patients as partners not supplicants. I'm suspicious too of ideas that are supposed to be so profound and complex that they cannot be expressed in language that everybody can understand. There may be such ideas, but I don't know any.

So I am setting out with the intention of writing this book in language that can be understood by anybody. I will define any technical terms it would be clumsy to try and avoid defining. The book will include many stories and examples, and I will try to avoid being too abstract. Philosophers may enjoy abstraction, but doctors, I've discovered the hard way, do not. In this I judge that the broader public is more akin to doctors than philosophers. Popular newspapers contain few abstractions. I will provide evidence and data to support my statements. The data will be presented in as straightforward a way as I can manage. This talk of evidence and data may suggest that I am writing 'truth'. I will not consciously be writing 'untruth', but I am sufficiently postmodern not to believe that there is one truth. There are many truths. As I've already shown, I plan to write in an unashamedly personal way. My justification is that I've been personally involved in much of what I will be describing. Plus I'm more of an editor than an ethicist—and by exploiting my strengths I hope to write a more useful book. Somebody else can write a book that is less subjective and stronger on ethics and law. Indeed, a distinguished group, many of them friends, already has.[4]

I want the book to be as international as possible. Science has always been universal and medicine is a branch of science. Much of it is, however, culturally bound. Psychiatry in China is very different from psychiatry in Britain, which in its turn is surprisingly different from psychiatry in Germany or the United States. Some major medical journals—particularly the *BMJ*, *JAMA* (formerly the *Journal of the American Medical Association*), the *Lancet*, *Annals of Internal Medicine* and the *New England Journal of Medicine* (often known as 'the big five')—have long been international in that the scientific studies submitted to them and their subscribers come from all over the world. They have, however, been dominated by the countries they come from and have been particularly poor at reaching out to the developing world, the home of most sickness and premature death. Chapter 15 discusses how medical journals are trying to stop failing the developing world. I will strive for an international scope, but the book will, I know, feel British to some. Globalization is still in some ways an aspiration and national identity is not easily discarded.

Before travelling to Venice to write this book I re-read *Death in Venice*. I have no intention of dying in Venice, but nor did Ashenbach. I see no signs of the plague in Venice, but I do see the public being deceived about medical information in the way that Venetians were deceived about the extent of the danger presented by the plague. This thus seems a good place to reflect ethically on medical journals. There seems much to be proud of but also much that is wrong. It occurs to me that this is probably true of most human activities observed closely with an eye that is knowledgeable but attempts to be dispassionate.

Once I had finished the first draft of my book I sent it to Cambridge University Press, recognizing that I had written a distinctly non-academic book. The press wanted to make the book more academic—partly by removing my stories. I decided that I'd try and find another publisher, and I'm very grateful to RSM Press for agreeing to publish the book. I'm grateful as well to Sandy McCall Smith, who rang me between talks to the Palm Beach Literary Society to say that I'd done exactly the right thing to write the book as I wanted.

Scientific journals began in the 17th century with the French *Journal des Savants* and the British *Philosophical Transactions of the Royal Society*. The journals complemented scientific meetings, which had until then been the main way of communicating science. The history of journals since then has been one in which each new discipline eventually grew tired of simply being part of a larger whole and so started its own publication. General medical journals began at the end of the 18th century and specialist medical journals at the beginning of the 20th century. Later in that century came subspecialty journals, and the growth in scientific and medical journals was exponential until a decade or so ago when the whole venture hit the economic buffers.

Some societies and some commercial publishers have grown rich from their journals, earning profit margins of 40%. These were 'must have' journals, quasi-monopolies. New paper journals ceased to appear in such large numbers a decade or so ago because the traditional business model—of selling subscriptions primarily to institutions—would no longer work so well.

The exponential increase in journals may, however, return because new electronic journals can be started with minimal funds. These journals are about the fundamental business of disseminating science rather than making societies or publishers rich. The final chapter, chapter 22, considers the ethical implications of four different but plausible futures for medical publishing.

Some journals have always been about more than publishing science, and chapter 3 asks who and what medical journals are for. Most medical communities have had some sort of journal and journals provide a forum for them to debate an issue in depth. I've always been interested in the question of whether journals can lead or just simply reflect what is happening in their communities. This is a question that has interested scholars in the new discipline of 'media studies', but in reference to the mass media rather than medical journals. I reflect on some of their studies in chapter 4 and my tentative conclusion is that journals can, indeed, lead—but if they are to do so then they cannot be more than a whisker ahead of those they are attempting to lead.

Chapter 5 examines the values that underpin journals, almost always implicitly. Medical journals might be expected to have the values of medicine, science and journalism—and these values conflict. The values of both science and journalism, for example, might favour publication of a weak study with a conclusion that could cause a 'scare' among the public—because publication and debate are fundamental values to both, whereas medical values, which put a strong emphasis on 'doing no harm', might favour waiting until stronger evidence emerged.

The science that underpins medicine is presented in journals and most journals can point to landmark studies that have changed medicine. The *BMJ*, for example, published some of the first studies in anaesthesia, on the cause of malaria, and linking cigarettes to lung cancer. It also published the first randomized controlled trial, which for reasons that I explain in chapter 6 was scientifically a major development. The journals might also be said to have become 'more scientific' over the years in that the rigour of the methods of the studies they publish has improved.

Yet medical journals often contain poor science. Basic scientists who work in biology and chemistry are often scornful of the mostly applied science that appears in medical journals. The journals have, for example, published many reports of treatments applied to single cases and of series of cases, which rarely allow confident conclusions because it is impossible without 'controls' to know what would have happened without the treatment. Journals have also been part of what might be called an 'unscientific' method of encouraging treatments that seem to make anatomical, physiological or biochemical sense but without insisting that they be properly evaluated in practice.

The history of medicine is littered with treatments that seemed to make sense but which ultimately did more harm than good. Sir Arbuthnot Lane, who was mercilessly parodied in George Bernard Shaw's *The Doctor's Dilemma*, removed the colons of Londoners who were severely fatigued and rich enough to meet his high fees. The operation was supposedly removing toxins. One-tenth of his patients were killed by the operation. I belong to a generation who had their tonsils removed to no benefit, while my wife when having our first child in 1982 was given an enema and had her pubic hair shaved, procedures which are unpleasant and of no benefit.

Medicine itself probably deserves most criticism for its unscientific behaviour, but the journals are the major link between science and practice. Journals have been severely criticized in recent years for publishing studies that are scientifically weak (in that their conclusions are not supported by their methods and data) and irrelevant to practitioners (and so patients).[5-8]

Peer review—asking peers of the authors of scientific studies to review the studies critically before publication—is the process that is supposed to ensure the scientific quality of journals. It is a sacred process—and the phrase 'peer reviewed journal' is supposed to guarantee quality. But clearly peer review is deficient. Despite being central to the scientific process, it was itself largely unstudied until various pioneers— including Stephen Lock, my predecessor as editor of the *BMJ*, and Drummond Rennie, deputy editor of *JAMA*—urged that it could and should be studied. Our studies so far have shown that it is slow, expensive, ineffective, something of a lottery, prone to bias and abuse, and hopeless at spotting errors and fraud. As Rennie says, 'If it were a drug it would never get onto the market.' Nevertheless, no journal would dare to abandon peer review. Editors are convinced—even though we are finding it hard to prove—that peer review is invaluable. I will discuss peer review further in chapter 7.

Medical journals differ from scientific journals in that they are mainly read not by scientists but by practising doctors. 'But aren't doctors scientists?' you might ask. We are in that when we were medical students our heads were filled with anatomy, biochemistry, physiology and (if we are under 40) molecular biology, but such teaching does not a scientist make. Most doctors feel uncomfortable describing themselves as scientists. Most are not even trained to appraise critically a scientific article.

Why then do we send them journals filled with increasingly complex science, most of which depends on statistical methods that they do not understand? It is, I think, a historical hangover and we have lots of data to show that doctors spend little time reading the original research in journals. They are sensible not to do so. The average doctor spends not much more than an hour a week on professional reading. It thus doesn't make sense for him or her to spend most of that time reading one complex study. Doctors sensibly should read synoptic, educational material, and mostly that's what doctors do. Often they read this material not in journals but in what are condescendingly known as 'throwaways', newspapers that use journalists to summarize complex material and which are free because they are funded by pharmaceutical advertising.

Journals have long recognized that they are unlikely to flourish if they publish only scientific studies. Increasingly they publish reviews that update practitioners on new developments, educational material, news, reviews of books, articles that are more journalism than science, letters and obituaries. Slowly they have begun to look less like traditional scientific journals and more like popular magazines with shorter articles, brief summaries and graphics.

They try to be useful tools to doctors in their practice, but they have only limited success. Doctors suffer from what Muir Gray, a public health doctor and director of

Britain's National Electronic Library of Health, calls 'the information paradox': they are overwhelmed with material of limited relevance and quality but can't find answers to the many questions that arise when they meet with patients and which thus go unanswered. Journals are not good at getting doctors to change and improve their practice. Words on paper rarely lead directly to change.

What journals can do is to make people think, set agendas, encourage debate, draw doctors' attention to new things that may be important and even legitimize subjects. In short, they are very like newspapers and Robbie Fox, the great editor of the *Lancet* in the 20th century, liked to call his journal a newspaper.

Should journals then abandon publishing science? In the end science might abandon them and be posted on publicly available websites rather than appear in journals, but it is unlikely that the journals will abandon science first (although I can think of at least one American journal of family practice that has done so). Most of a journal's kudos comes from the science it publishes, and it is the science rather than the rest of the material that attracts worldwide media attention and causes subscribers (mostly institutions) to purchase the journals. Some of the scientific studies that journals publish are hugely important, and the science gives journals an authority and legitimacy that separates them from the (usually much more readable) 'throwaways'.

Despite my criticisms of journals I still believe that a good journal can be a major asset to a medical community. It can move medicine forward, less through providing a clear direction of travel but more through highlighting the deficiencies of the present and providing a hundred ideas on how to do better. Most medical communities—be they national or specialist—have journals, and at least some members of those that don't (some Italian doctors, for example) pine for a good journal.

But do journals benefit patients? Medical journals have been intended for doctors not patients. Any benefit to patients would come from improvements in their doctors. Now with the arrival of the internet patients can access the same information as doctors, and sometimes the patient is better informed than the doctor. This is a new world for both doctors and patients, but there is growing evidence that doctors and patients taking decisions together—rather than doctors taking decisions on behalf of patients—leads to patients doing better and being more satisfied. Even if patients have not been readers of medical journals, they have certainly featured in their pages. As recently as 10 years ago journals might publish pictures of patients naked without them knowing a thing about it. Now we are moving into a world where we have patients on editorial boards and even patient editors. Chapter 13 describes how journals are trying to move from a world where patients were objects to one where they are partners, but journals are here, I judge, lagging behind the practice of medicine.

Abuse of patients has been one ethical failing of journals, but section 4 describes others. Chapter 11 deals with the failure of medical journals to manage conflicts of interest. Until very recently journals did not ask authors and reviewers about conflicts of interest and so did not declare them to readers. But most authors in medical journals do have financial conflicts of interest, particularly in their relations with pharmaceutical companies. These undeclared conflicts of interest can have profound effects on the studies authors undertake and the conclusions they reach. On some major issues—like whether passive smoking (exposure to other people's smoke) is harmful or whether new contraceptive pills are more likely to cause clots in the legs and lungs than earlier pills—studies linked to the manufacturers reach completely different conclusions from those that are not. So journals have to do a better job at managing conflict of interest. This doesn't mean getting rid of conflicts of interest because such conflicts are inevitable and all pervasive.

Most journals also face an ethical problem in being so closely associated with pharmaceutical companies. These companies are important in that almost all the new drugs of the past 50 years have been discovered by them, and those drugs have transformed medicine. But the interests of pharmaceutical companies and doctors, patients and so journals (as they should put doctors and patients first) are not always the same. A company might want patients to take its drug even though another drug might be better. Companies will push drug rather than non-drug treatments, even though for many conditions—for example, diabetes—non-drug treatments are often more important. Some journals have been captured by pharmaceutical companies in that they have come to depend on them. Many, including some of the most prestigious journals, publish mostly trials that are funded by the industry. They depend on income from pharmaceutical advertising and sales of reprints (a company might pay over $1m for reprints of one study, which it funded in the first place). Journals should not attempt to separate themselves from pharmaceutical companies, but the relationship should be ethically more sound. This relationship is discussed in chapter 16.

Some would also argue that journals have an unhealthy relationship with the mass media. Journals might, indeed, be degenerating into a branch of show business. Our competitors, I told my staff, were not just the *New England Journal of Medicine* and the *Lancet* but Hollywood films and Manchester United. I meant that we were part of the 'attention economy' and that we competed all the time with rich pleasures for the attention of doctors. I didn't mean that we should abandon our fundamental principles and seek publicity at any price, but there is no doubt that coverage in the mass media is good for journals in both prestige and business terms. All the major journals put out press releases (and some in the United States video clips) and are disappointed if an issue receives no coverage. Sometimes, even often, there will be global coverage. But are journals debasing themselves in pursuit of publicity? I will explore the relationship between journals and the mass media in chapter 14.

Sometimes journals receive coverage in the media that makes them squirm, particularly when they are exposed as having published research that is fraudulent. Fraud in science is as old as science itself—because science is a human activity. But fraud was not high on anybody's agenda until about 20 years ago. As recently as five years ago I heard a fellow of the Royal Society (a position in British science one step short of a Nobel prize) argue that fraud was exceedingly rare, didn't happen with 'proper scientists', had never harmed anybody and didn't matter because science was self-correcting. It's now impossible to take this position in public and there are increasing examples of fraud. In one phone call in December 2002 I had to tell the editor of the *Lancet* that I had compelling evidence that two major trials he had published were fraudulent.

Some countries—particularly the United States and the Nordic countries—have mounted a coherent, national, legally based response to scientific fraud, but most countries, including Britain, have not. Medical editors in Britain have created the Committee on Publication Ethics (COPE), a sort of self-help group for responding to fraud—or as it is better called research misconduct. (Fraud is a severe word that is excessive for much of the comparatively minor forms of misconduct that seem to be common—and has connotations of financial fraud.) COPE started in 1997 and has now dealt with about 250 cases. For some editors it has caused a transformation in how they deal with misconduct. Whereas editors were inclined to look the other way, especially as most of the problems arose in studies they had no intention of publishing, many now feel an obligation to act. This transformation is similar to what has happened in medicine itself, where regulatory bodies will discipline doctors who fail to act on signals of clinical, research or financial misconduct.

But I still feel that editors are at the beginning of responding to research misconduct. Many editors are not sensitized to the problem. Most of COPE's cases come from a few journals, and it's impossible to believe that those journals have many problems while others have none. But even when editors do decide that they need to respond to problems they are often unclear what action to take. And when universities or other employers are alerted to the possibility of misconduct they either will not or cannot take action. I worry that journals are polluted by misconduct and that editors are not responding adequately. I will discuss research misconduct in chapter 8, and to show that I have not forgotten a form of misconduct that editors are most inclined to forget—editorial misconduct—I've devoted the whole of chapter 12 to the subject. Some say that editors are as unaccountable as kings.

Chapter 9 deals with the difficult question of authorship of scientific research. Jane Austen wrote every word of her novels and was indisputably the author. But conducting scientific research often depends on large teams of people with different skills. Deciding who should be listed as an author is not simple and too often the decision is made on the basis of power. The powerful are included, even when they have done nothing, and the weak are excluded, even those who have done most of the work. This unethical behaviour becomes a major problem if the study proves to be fraudulent, as has happened many times. For authorship implies not just credit, which authors love, but also accountability, about which they are much less enthusiastic. Senior authors suddenly say that they cannot be held responsible for a corrupted study because they had nothing to do with it. Such a position does not impress. One radical but rational response to the problem of authorship is to abandon the idea within science. Instead, we should go for contributorship, where the contribution of everybody is simply described, rather as with film credits.

One form of misconduct that seems minor at first thought is publishing the same study—or large parts of it—more than once. This is irritating but surely not serious. In chapter 10 I will try to convince you that this problem is, indeed, serious for patients and the public. It so happens that studies that find a treatment, often a drug, to be effective tend to be published more than once, whereas those studies that find that the treatment does not work are often not published at all. The result is a systematic bias in medical information that makes some treatments seem much more effective than they actually are. Patients are then mistreated.

Many of these ethical problems I'm introducing—weak science, an inadequate response to conflicts of interest, too cosy a relationship with the pharmaceutical industry, research misconduct—could be said to be problems of medicine itself rather than simply journals. The two are inextricably entwined, which is why the author who wrote a history of the *BMJ* called it *The Mirror of Medicine*.[9] But the last ethical problem I want to introduce is more a problem that is squarely the responsibility of journals rather than medicine. It is the problem of journals exploiting—let's say ripping off—the academic community.

'All publishing is theft', the BMA's librarian used to joke—before he left to join the world's largest scientific publishers, Reed Elsevier, and so giving a bitter twist to his joke. As somebody who was something to do with publishing I was offended. But more to the point I didn't understand. Now I do. Most medical journals comprise almost entirely research articles. These articles are written by the researchers and submitted to the journals for free. Consider the value in a major trial published in a medical journal. Such trials can costs millions of pounds to conduct. Almost all of the value is in the trial itself. (By 'value' I mean the unique contribution that customers are willing to pay for.) Most of these trials are conducted by academics and many are funded with public money. The journals conduct peer review, but I have already argued that this is a process that adds little value. What's more the peer review is usually done by academics without pay. Indeed, many journals are edited by unpaid academics. Often it is academics, again unpaid, who edit the studies before they are published. The journals are then sold to academic libraries—and often at huge prices. An annual subscription to some journals may be over $20,000. Publishers— sometimes commercial companies, although often medical or scientific organizations—make substantial profits, but without adding much value. Indeed, publishers may subtract value by 'Balkanizing' the scientific literature, severely limiting accessibility.

Robert Maxwell, a publisher of newspapers and journals who became famous for stealing his employees' pension fund, got rich through publishing scientific journals. The ethics of the business of scientific publishing are highly suspect and I will discuss them in chapter 17.

Section 6 of the book considers attempts to raise the probity of research and increase the accountability of editors. Chapter 18 looks at how descriptions of highly unethical medical research conducted after the Second World War led to the creation of research ethics committees (or institutional review boards in the United States). Across the globe these committees are now proving to be overworked, under-resourced and insufficiently skilled. Radical reform is needed. Medical journals have also been poor at ensuring the ethical acceptability of what they publish—often failing to ensure that research has had approval from research ethics committees. But journals sometimes identity failings in the research ethics committees, and chapter 18 discusses how the committees and journals might work more creatively together.

Chapter 19 looks at the ethical competence and accountability of journals themselves. The *Lancet* took the bold step of introducing an ombudsman to consider complaints against authors. The experiment seems to have been a success but has not been widely copied. The *BMJ* introduced an ethics committee of its own, and almost immediately we wondered how we managed for 160 years without one. But these are small experiments. Much more needs to be done to improve the ethical accountability of editors and journals.

Medical journals, just like any other publications, are covered by the laws of libel. In Britain these are strict and the *BMJ* was involved in one of the longest running libel cases in British legal history. Chapter 20 describes that case and discusses how the law of libel has to balance injury to individuals against freedom of speech. British law is tipped towards the individual, American law towards freedom of speech. Unsurprisingly, I would like British law to move in the American direction.

Chapter 21 examines the case—put most forcefully by Sir Richard Peto, one of Britain's most distinguished medical researchers—that concern with ethical issues in publishing medical research is causing more harm than good. The problem, he argues, is minor, but clamour around the problem is making research much harder to do. The result is that the public is harmed rather than benefited. I agree with some—but by no means all—of his analysis.

So you can see why I was pensive in my palazzo. I'm proud to have been part of such an energetic, exciting and, I hope, ultimately useful enterprise as the publishing of journals, but I'm concerned that much of what journals do is ethically weak. The rest of this book will explore those concerns, searching always for possible means to do better.

Section 2: The nature of medical journals

2. Why bother with medical journals and whether they are honest?

3. What and who are medical journals for?

4. Can medical journals lead or must they follow?

5. What are and what should be the values of medical journals?

▶2

Why bother with medical journals and whether they are honest?

Stephen Lock, my predecessor as editor of the *BMJ*, taught me always to remember that journals would soon 'be wrapping up next week's fish and chips'. Something we expected to cause excitement often, he noted, had all the impact of 'a doughnut in the North Sea'. Journals rarely cause change directly, but I want in this chapter to try and convince you that journals can have profound effects. They might do this through anything they publish, but I'm particularly interested in cases where the journals may have behaved poorly.

Any such debate today tends to begin with the case of the *Lancet* and the measles, mumps and rubella (German measles) vaccine (MMR).[1] Public health doctors froth at the mouth when telling this story. For them it illustrates the waywardness of journals and their ability to create havoc and cause extensive harm.

The *Lancet* in February 1998 published an article by Andrew Wakefield and others that suggested that there might be a link between children being given the MMR vaccine and developing a strange bowel condition and autism. The paper described 12 children who had the bowel condition and a developmental disorder, which in nine cases was diagnosed as autism. In eight cases the parents associated the child developing the condition with having been given the MMR vaccine. What the paper didn't make clear, but an accompanying editorial did, was that these children were referred to Wakefield and others because they were known to be interested in a possible link between MMR and bowel disease.[10]

Wakefield and others concluded that they had not proved a link between the vaccine and the syndrome of bowel disease and autism, and the accompanying editorial said the same. The editorial—which I've heard an editor of a paediatric journal call 'incomprehensible'— predicted, however, that the paper might cause what journalists love to call a 'scare'. 'Vaccine safety concerns such as that reported by Wakefield and colleagues may,' the editorial said, 'snowball into societal tragedies when the media and the public confuse association with causality and shun immunization. This painful history was shared by the UK (among others) over pertussis in the 1970s after another similar case series was widely publicized, and it is likely to be repeated all too easily over MMR. This would be tragic because passion would then conquer reason and the facts again in the UK.'[10]

To many the fact that the authors had identified 12 children with both a strange bowel disease and developmental disorder, and that nine of them became ill soon after being given an MMR, may seem like strong evidence of harm from the vaccine. But it isn't. Let me try and explain why.

Oddly, I want to start by explaining a famous scam. You write a letter to 10,000 people offering free advice on investing in shares. You pick many different shares and by chance some will rise. You ignore all the people to whom you gave poor advice and write to the 'winners' offering further advice. Again by chance some will 'win'. Once you have done this three or four times you write to the handful of people who have 'won' repeatedly asking them for money to invest. You then abscond with their money. To the 'winners' you seem to have remarkable predictive powers. They know nothing of the nearly 10,000 who received poor advice.

Hundreds of thousands of children every year are vaccinated with MMR. Similarly hundreds of thousands have rashes, tens of thousands have fits and thousands will develop behavioural disorders. Inevitably therefore many children will by chance experience problems they would have experienced anyway within hours and days of being vaccinated. To the parents—just like the 'winners' in the scam—it is hard to believe that what has happened to their child is the result of chance.

Such parents may search the internet for information and stand a high chance of encountering a group like that of Wakefield and others who are interested in the problem. It thus isn't so strange that the group managed to collect a series of patients. The difficulty of working out whether or not vaccination might be causing the autism is further complicated by something epidemiologists call 'recall bias'. If you know that A may be associated with B and then experience A, you are much more likely to remember that B happened to you than somebody who hasn't experienced A.

When I was editor of the *BMJ*, for example, we caused a great fuss in France, which depends heavily on nuclear power, by publishing a study—by French researchers funded by the French government—suggesting that walking on a beach near a nuclear reprocessing plant might make people more likely to develop leukaemia.[11] The study asked questions of people who had leukaemia and controls who didn't. There was already a suspicion that these plants might cause leukaemia. The fact that those who had the disease were more likely to report having been on the beach might thus be because they really had been there more often or because they were more likely than the controls to remember that they had.

The alternative explanations of the findings of Wakefield and others do not mean that MMR and autism are not associated, but they do mean that the evidence is weak— too weak, many say, to deserve publication in the *Lancet*, a journal that has space for less than 10% of all the studies submitted to it. Did the *Lancet* publish because it relished the thought of the massive media coverage that would follow publication? That is the suspicion of many.

Extensive media coverage did follow and has continued to follow, and immunization rates have dropped. Some parts of the media—including interestingly the satirical magazine *Private Eye*—have taken up the cause of linking MMR and autism. They smell a conspiracy by the medical establishment. Between the time when I wrote the first draft of this chapter and came to revise it, Melanie Philips ('a top *Mail* writer') published a much hyped series of articles in the *Daily Mail* based on three month's study of the problem. She has no doubt that MMR causes autism, that epidemiology is hopeless and that the 'pro-MMR' researchers all have impossible conflicts of interest.

The Medical Research Council investigated Wakefield's work and found it severely wanting. He has lost the funding for his research and has become something of a pariah among doctors. Now he has moved to America, funded by wealthy people who believe strongly in his work, and sparked anxiety about the MMR vaccine there.

This long running story took another twist in 2004 when it emerged that Wakefield had failed to declare a conflict of interest. He was being paid to see if there was any evidence to support possible legal action by a group of parents who claimed their children were damaged by the MMR vaccine. Richard Horton, the editor of the *Lancet*, conducted a rapid examination of the evidence and declared that he would not have published the paper if he had known of the conflict of interest.[12] Subsequently 10 of the 13 authors of the original study retracted the interpretation that MMR and autism might be linked, something that the original study did not state anyway.[13]

Many studies have been published that do not support a link between MMR and autism. Those who have autism are not more likely than others to have had the vaccine. The introduction of the vaccine was not followed by a surge of cases of autism (although interpretation of these studies is complicated by the fact that autism has been increasing, probably because it is more often diagnosed rather than it is increasing in reality). These studies have been published in all the major journals, including the *Lancet*. But it is hard, even impossible, to prove a negative. One black swan will show that some swans are black, but 10,000 white swans do not prove that there are no black swans.

The battle has gone to the highest in the land with the prime minister being questioned on whether or not his baby son had been given the vaccine. He said that it was a private matter but that his government continued to recommend that all children receive MMR. The fact that he wouldn't answer was seen by some of the media as an admission that his son hadn't received the vaccine and that the government had 'secret knowledge' that the vaccine was harmful. Row upon row of prominent figures in healthcare—chief medical officers, chief nursing officers and presidents of medical and nursing colleges—have lined up to say that there is no evidence that the vaccine causes autism, but immunization rates have gone down in several countries. There have as a result been outbreaks of measles, and sometimes measles causes severe and lasting damage to the brain. The view of those in public health is that a great deal of damage has been done by the *Lancet* publishing the original study.

A sideline in the debate has been whether parents should be allowed to ask for their children to be given the vaccines separately rather than all together in the MMR vaccine. The thinking, which has no evidence to support it but 'feels right' to many, is that a baby's immune system cannot cope with three vaccines at once. The government is in difficulty here. If it allows parents a choice (and patient and parental choice is politically fashionable) then it seems to be admitting that there are problems with MMR. I wrote an editorial arguing that doctors had learnt to go along with what they see as the irrational choices of individual patients—so why shouldn't public health authorities do the same for populations?[14] I also pointed out that there is evidence that excessive reassurance is counterproductive. This editorial caused consternation among some doctors but had no discernible impact on government policy or immunization rates.

And was it the *Lancet* that caused this problem? Wakefield and others would have got their work published somewhere (authors always can, another failing of journals), and maybe it wasn't the study that caused the problem. The idea that MMR might be dangerous was already abroad, and the history of people being anxious about vaccination goes right back to when Edward Jenner first used vaccination—against smallpox—at the end of the 18th century. It could have been that there would have been a decline in rates of MMR vaccination even if the *Lancet* hadn't published the paper. Public health people don't accept this. They pin the blame on the *Lancet*. It gave its valuable imprimatur to the work, created the problem and did itself much harm in the process.

I'm often asked if I would have published the paper. People expect me to say, 'Of course not', but I usually demur. First, it's easy to be wise with hindsight. Second, I know that choices on publication are inevitably somewhat arbitrary. All journals, including the *BMJ*, publish studies that turn out to be nonsense. Third, the articles in the *Lancet* were cautious even if much of the subsequent media coverage was not. Fourth, there is a trade off between what's scientifically exciting and clinically useful. If it had turned out (or does turn out) that MMR and autism are linked, the *Lancet* would have got a 'first', something that is important not only to journalists but also to scientists. The *Lancet* has traditionally been concerned with the scientifically new and exciting. It's one of the reasons people read the *Lancet*. The *BMJ*, in contrast, is more concerned with studies that have a direct clinical or public health message, making it, some say, much duller.

I'm not sure whether the *Lancet* did the right thing or not, but I am sure that this case illustrates powerfully that what journals publish and the ethical issues that arise in making those decisions can have a broad impact on peoples' lives. Many people must have worried whether or not to have their children vaccinated and whether or not a problem with their child, perhaps even autism, might have been caused by MMR.

Some extremists would say that the *Lancet* has blood on its hands. I too have been accused by a knight of the realm and a fellow of the Royal Society, Sir Richard Peto, of 'killing hundreds of thousands'. The *BMJ* was about to publish a major paper from Peto and colleagues showing the power of aspirin and similar drugs in preventing deaths from cardiovascular disease.[15] Peto is convinced that far more patients should be taking aspirin and that many are dying unnecessarily young because they are not taking the drug. He has very strong evidence to support his view, but we were about to accompany his paper with a commentary that was sceptical.[16] It was through publishing this commentary that I would kill hundreds of thousands because doctors would be given a reason, an excuse, not to put their patients on aspirin. I can't say that I have hundreds of thousands of deaths on my conscience, but it shows that somebody of his huge intelligence rates the power of journals higher than I do.

(In the same interchange Peto said that he had looked at the principles of the Committee on Publications Ethics [COPE], which I helped to found [and which is discussed in chapter 8], and discovered that I'd broken every one of them. That gives me another qualification for writing this book.)

My second example also comes from the *Lancet*, and the editor of the *Lancet* before

Richard Horton, Robin Fox, says that when he dies they will find 'Bristol Cancer Help Centre study' written on his heart.[17,18] This is why.

The Bristol Cancer Help Centre offered complementary or alternative therapy to patients with cancer. It was praised by the Prince of Wales, and there was naturally discussion over whether or not its treatments were effective. Britain's two cancer charities—the Imperial Cancer Research Fund and the Cancer Research Campaign (as they were then called)—funded a study to find out. This study was undertaken in the late 1980s and published in the *Lancet* in 1990.[17] It was a time when the mutual suspicion between orthodox and complementary practitioners was not as strong as it was in earlier times but was stronger than now. The Bristol centre and the patients visiting it cooperated with the trial.

Heather Goodare, a singer and now a friend of mine, was a participant in the trial. She had had breast cancer and found the advice and support offered by the Bristol centre very helpful. She provided information with enthusiasm—and so was both devastated and angry when she switched on the television news one night and heard the researchers announce that those who visited the Bristol centre were likely to die sooner than those who didn't. She was devastated because what seemed to her a good experience might be reducing her chances of surviving. She was angry because she expected to hear the results of the trial directly from the researchers, not through the television news. But, as is often the case, that terrible experience led to much that was good, for her, patients in general and journals.

The study compared what happened to 334 women with breast cancer who went to the Bristol centre with what happened to 461 women with breast cancer attending a specialist cancer hospital or two district general hospitals. The authors found that the women attending the centre were roughly twice as likely to die as those simply attending traditional hospitals. (It's important to point out that the women attending the Bristol centre were also cared for by traditional hospitals.)

Making a comparison like this is hard because the two sets of women will be different in many ways—in age, social class and backgrounds, types of cancer, and the extent and seriousness of their cancers. The women will also be different in ways that are not easily measured—like personality and attitude. Furthermore, the information was gathered from hospital notes, which are not a reliable source of information: important information is often missing or wrong. Statisticians can attempt to compensate for the differences in the two groups and the missing information, but the conclusions will at best be tentative. Any differences found may be due to the women being different rather than differences in their treatments.

Unfortunately those who presented the conclusions at the press conference were far from tentative. I wasn't there, but the *BMJ* editor who went said that those giving the press conference positively delighted in the bad results for the Bristol centre. Complementary medicine had been shown not just to be useless but also dangerous. The results reverberated around the world, hitting the mass media before the *Lancet*'s usual embargo of 12.01 am on a Friday morning. The *BMJ*'s report on the study has, I must confess, been described by Heather Goodare as 'particularly lurid'.[19,20] The women who had participated willingly in the study were forgotten in the rush for publicity.

Once the results were fully published they could be critically appraised, and it soon became clear that there were severe deficiencies. Sir Walter Bodmer, Director of Research at the Imperial Cancer Research Fund, wrote to the *Lancet* in 1990 to say, 'Our own evaluation is that the study's results can be explained by the fact that women going to Bristol had more severe disease than control women.'[21]

But harm had already been done. After publication of the study the number of patients attending the Bristol centre fell dramatically and the centre nearly went into receivership. Furthermore, one of the study's authors, Professor Tim McElwain from London University, killed himself two months after the study was published. We can't know what part the study played in McElwain's suicide, but the study and his suicide are forever yoked together.

Many of the women who felt abused by the study formed themselves into an action group, the Bristol Study Support Group. One of their targets was the *Lancet*. They wanted the study 'retracted' from the scientific literature. Retraction is a process that indicates that the results of a study cannot be believed—although, ironically, retracted studies continue to be cited by other researchers.[22] Retraction is usually, however, reserved for studies that are proved to be fraudulent. The potential problem with retracting studies that are 'wrong' is that given enough time almost everything might have to be retracted. Better, many would say, for them just to be forgotten. Neither the *Lancet* nor the cancer charities thought that there had been any fraud in the Bristol study. Gordon McVie, scientific director of the Cancer Research Campaign, said: 'Our view is that the researchers made an honest scientific mistake during their analysis of their findings.'[23]

The authors did not want their study retracted, and the *Lancet* felt unable to do so. The journal did respond, however, by raising its standards of statistical review.

The support group suspected that the results had not arisen from simply 'an honest scientific mistake'. They wanted the original data to be re-analysed by somebody independent of the authors and the charities, but this has never happened. Ethical arguments over who owns data are intense. Many take the view that they belong in some sense to the patients and also that they are a public good, not least because their collection is often funded with public money. Lots of researchers believe, however, that the data belong to them—because they have done the arduous work of collecting them—and are anxious about them being misused by others. There is also an element of competition.

But researchers should be willing, or even obliged, to hand over data when there are anxieties about possible misconduct. The *BMJ* and some other journals write into their guidance to authors that a condition of submission is that authors must be willing to make their data available.

Because the support group got so little satisfaction from the *Lancet* and the cancer charities they compiled a dossier and took it to the Charity Commission, the body in Britain that oversees charities. The commission eventually censured both charities for inadequacies in their mechanisms for supervising and evaluating research.[24] But the main good that came out of this episode was an added impetus to involving patients much more in the process of research. It is becoming normal to keep participants in trials informed of how the trial is progressing and to present the results to them first.

Even more importantly patients are increasingly involved in the planning, designing and performing of research. The guineapigs are taking over the experiments. I discuss the often tense relationship between medical journals and patients further in chapter 13.

A study that some call 'the *BMJ*'s MMR paper' was concerned not with a clinical but rather with a health policy matter.[25] It was a comparison by three authors based in California (although one is English) of the costs and effectiveness of Britain's National Health Service (NHS) and Kaiser-Permanente, a California-based health maintenance organization. (A health maintenance organization provides complete healthcare for a fixed annual sum.) Comparisons between healthcare systems are difficult and this study was unusual in that it was a 'broad brush' study. Its general conclusion was that the costs of the two systems were of a similar order but that on many measures—time to wait to see a doctor or to have an operation, immunization rates—Kaiser performed considerably better. This was counterintuitive. The NHS has been widely regarded, particularly by people in Britain, as highly efficient, and the American system in general as profligate (although Kaiser is a particular and unusual part of it). One message was that the problem with the NHS was not just money.

Just like the MMR study, this study received wide media coverage and the British government was very interested in it, but it was upsetting to the many supporters of the NHS. Severe criticisms of the study flowed in from the moment it was published.[26,27] The method for adjusting for purchasing power was ridiculous. The assertion that the populations served by the two healthcare systems were similar was misleading. There were, critics said, many problems with the study, and the *BMJ* had made a bad mistake in publishing it. Some critics suggested to me that the study was fraudulent. The study would push the government towards making changes that would be damaging to the NHS.[27] Ultimately the harm to healthcare in Britain (and perhaps other countries that were misled by the study) might be more severe than the harm caused by the MMR paper.

I'm unconvinced and unrepentant, but I do believe that the study could have profound consequences. Indeed, the NHS has been studying Kaiser hard, and one study that has resulted supports some of the conclusions of the earlier study.[28] Those who love a conspiracy theory were excited by me leaving the *BMJ* and joining an American healthcare company that was trying to establish a business in Britain. Had I published the paper in order to further my own interests? So here is another example of a journal perhaps having an influence on the lives of many in ethically questionable circumstances.

JAMA—formerly the *Journal of the American Medical Association*—has had its share of dramatic and ethically dubious publications, with one culminating in the firing of the editor. George Lundberg was fired not for publishing but for speeding up publication of a paper that showed that many American students did not think of oral sex as sex.[29] This undramatic finding gained notoriety because of the impeachment of President Clinton, where one of the issues was what exactly had happened between him and Monica Lewinsky in the Oval Office. I discuss this episode in chapter 12 on editorial misconduct.

But an equally controversial episode occurred a decade earlier when *JAMA* published an account of a tired junior doctor killing a 20-year-old patient who was terminally ill with ovarian cancer.[30] The paper—which provoked a huge and stormy debate within the journal, the mass media and the journal's owner, the American Medical Association—is remarkable for its brevity and bluntness. The 500-word piece, which was anonymous, is a first person account of a doctor killing a patient, whom he had never previously met. Called 'in the middle of the night', he (or perhaps she) encounters a patient with 'unrelenting vomiting' and 'severe air hunger' who 'had not eaten or slept for two days'. It was, the author wrote, 'a gallows scene, a cruel mockery of her youth and unfulfilled potential. Her only words to me were, "Let's get this over with."' The doctor draws up some morphine, 'enough, I thought, to do the job'. After the injection 'with clocklike certainty' the patient stopped breathing. 'It's over, Debbie', is both the last line and the title.

JAMA received some 150 letters, which were four to one against the physician's actions and three to one against *JAMA* for publishing the piece.[31] Euthanasia is a subject that generates great emotion. In Britain it has taken over from abortion as the subject most likely to produce a hate-filled postbag. Doctors' organizations—including the British Medical Association (BMA)—tend to be strongly against euthanasia, whereas doctors themselves are much more ambivalent. Most doctors (including me in my limited clinical experience) have given injections to make patients more comfortable, knowing that a 'side-effect' will be the death of the patient. Euthanasia is thus a tricky subject for medical journals owned by medical associations. An editorial I published encouraging continuing debate—rather than supporting euthanasia—led to several letters to the BMA hierarchy calling for me to be fired.[32] Almost 10 years later we published an editorial that argued the case for euthanasia[33]—but not long after publishing an editorial that argued exactly the opposite.[34] The *New England Journal of Medicine*—owned by the Massachusetts Medical Society—has been bolder in its support of euthanasia.[35]

But more relevant to this book than the question of whether or not euthanasia should be supported is the question of whether or not *JAMA* should have published the article as it did. The article described a criminal act. Can it be right for editors to publish accounts by (admittedly untried) criminals of their acts? George Lundberg argued that both the First Amendment of the Constitution of the United States (which says that congress will not pass a law 'abridging the freedom of speech, or of the press') and Illinois state law (*JAMA* is published in Chicago) supported his position. His position was legally challenged—but without success. Lundberg recognized that *JAMA* was 'in conflict with another powerful ethical obligation, that of a physician reporting another physician suspected of wrongdoing'. He then argued that the journal didn't know 'whether this is a clear case of wrongdoing' and that it 'may effectively be hearsay'. This raises the possibility—widely believed by many that the whole thing was a hoax.[30]

If *JAMA* believed that the piece was a hoax then presumably it would not have published it. If it didn't believe it was a hoax, then the author was describing intentionally killing a patient. How could it be hearsay?

Debate also raged over how *JAMA* published the piece. There was no editorial comment and no disclaimer. Didn't this mean that *JAMA* approved of euthanasia?

Mightn't it also mean that the American Medical Association, also approved? Lundberg—correctly to my mind—pointed out that the act of publication does not imply editorial support. Most journals are full of contradictory views. By definition, they can't all be editorially supported. The *BMJ* has carried many letters arguing that I am an idiot. That argument doesn't always have my editorial support. As the journal doesn't automatically agree with what it publishes it follows that neither do the owners.

But shouldn't *JAMA* have published the piece with some ethical commentaries? Many thought so, but Lundberg said that *JAMA* decided not to in order 'to avoid stultifying debate'. That seems reasonable to me. So long as the correspondence columns are open to all it makes sense to publish short dramatic pieces that stimulate debate. Balancing every comment every time makes for a dull journal. I've many times experienced how short, purple pieces with little supporting evidence promote debate in a way that well thought out, balanced and thoroughly referenced articles do not. Journals need both types of articles.

I assume that at least George Lundberg knew the identity of the author of 'It's over, Debbie', but the *BMJ* published a letter where we did not know the identity of the author. Your first reaction will probably be that this is unsupportable. How could we possibly know if the piece was genuine (although the same can be said of pieces that are signed)? We published such a letter—embedded in an editorial—because we were able to check the broad facts.[37] The letter concerned cheating at medical school and is worth republishing here:

'Dear Sir,
I am a graduating student of Royal Free and University College London Medical School. During the finals of clinical exams I was witness to one of the most ugly scenes in my short but eventful life. One of my colleagues had in a brazen attempt to obfuscate the examiners made use of her *Oxford Clinical Handbook* during her long case. Unfortunately (or fortunately) for her, she was caught red handed. The deed was not looked on kindly by the authorities, especially when she attempted to extricate herself by claiming she had also done this in a previous examination and not been caught thereby (or so she believed) justifying her act. . . My colleagues and I were convinced that she would receive her comeuppance.

After meeting the disciplinary board, however, she was allowed to pass her exams without further ado. Fair play and honesty, two virtues I have always believed in, have been made monkeys of again. In future perhaps we should all do as she did. After all, look where it's got her.'

The examining committee, the subdean told us, had decided to let her graduate but had held back distinctions she might have won. We wrote that we understood why the committee had done what it did, but we thought it right that we should publish the story and point out mistakes that the committee had made. 'The problem with cheating,' our editorial said, 'is that it destroys trust. Somebody who can cheat can also lie. Suddenly everything is uncertain.'[37] The biggest mistake of the committee was that it hadn't explained its actions to the rest of the students. The committee had also failed to consider the broader context—of medicine in Britain 'being in the dock' after a series of scandals and failures.

But did we do the right thing to publish? Wasn't this tittle tattle? Weren't we after sensation? Mightn't we damage the student? Many readers thought so, as they made clear in over 100 letters to the editor.[38] We were undermining British medicine when it needed building up. But more readers thought that we had done the right thing, agreeing with us that justice didn't just have to be done, it had to be seen to be done. One unexpected consequence was that we uncovered several other examples of cheating at medical school. Two students who had just graduated wrote and told us that they were bothered by the fact that they—and many others in their class—knew the content of an exam paper in advance. We encouraged them to tell their medical school, which they did.

This article didn't stimulate anything like the media storm of 'It's over, Debbie', but there was international coverage. Medical journals in the two cases have acted questionably to raise issues—euthanasia and the trustworthiness of doctors—that matter to the world at large.

The *Lancet*—yet again—provides a still more dramatic example of raising an issue that matters to the world by deciding to publish some very weak—some would say meaningless—research on the effects of genetically modified foods.[39] The production and sale of such foods has prompted huge controversy in some, but not all, countries. There was considerable public anxiety about genetically modified foods in Germany long before it appeared in Britain, but anxiety swept through Britain a few years ago. Currently, there is much less anxiety in the United States, where genetically modified foods are common, but the government in Zimbabwe is so concerned about the safety of the foods that it prefers to allow people to go hungry rather than eat the foods.

The arguments over genetically modified foods are interesting in that the scientific establishment doesn't think that there is any need for anxiety, whereas much of the public is unconvinced by the reassurances from both the scientists and the government. The public remembers too clearly the same parties insisting that there was no risk to humans from 'mad cow disease'. The public makes its own judgements on risk and it may often be more right than the experts. In a sense there are no experts on risk—because risk is a combination of the likelihood of something happening (which experts are usually better equipped to calculate) and the 'dreadfulness' of that event. There are no standard measures of 'dreadfulness,' but the public must be the ultimate judge.

The *Lancet* stepped into the emerging controversy over genetically modified foods by publishing some research that showed changes in the intestines of rats fed genetically modified potatoes.[39] This research had been trailed on television some 18 months earlier, and some of the media suggested that the scientific establishment was refusing to accept the results and was suppressing them. The *Lancet* published the results primarily to get them out into the open rather than because it believed that the results showed that genetically modified foods were unsafe. Indeed, it simultaneously published a commentary that said that: 'The results are difficult to interpret and do not allow the conclusion that the genetic modification of potatoes accounts for adverse effects in animals.'[40] This is clearly so. It's always hard to know what animal research means for humans (which is why the *BMJ* virtually never publishes animal research), and the meaning of the changes in the rats' guts is impossible to interpret. There were too few animals in the study and no controls, making it impossible to know what would have happened to animals fed a similar diet that lacked the genetically modified potatoes.

The study was sent to six reviewers by the *Lancet* and some recommended rejection.[41] The authors revised the paper three times before it was published. Nevertheless, this is a study that probably would not have made it into the *Lancet* in normal circumstances. The *Lancet* does have a tradition of publishing research that may be scientifically intriguing but that doesn't allow conclusions that would matter to practising doctors, but this was a study on rats that was scientifically very weak. Was the *Lancet* yet again indulging its taste for sensation and publicity or was it acting responsibly by peer reviewing and putting on the public record research that had been widely discussed but seen by few? I like to believe the latter, although I don't think that we would have published the research in the *BMJ*—just because it was too far removed from our sort of research.

Can it ever be right consciously to publish scientifically weak studies? (Journals regularly do so unconsciously.) Many seem to believe that a journal should publish only research that crosses its particular line of scientific worthiness. Top journals should publish only top research. Otherwise, a 'stamp of approval' may be given to an unworthy study. It's a belief based on the false idea that peer review is an exact process that strictly ranks scientific studies. But it isn't. As I discuss in chapter 7, peer review is a flawed and inevitably subjective process. It also has to consider many factors at once, including originality, clinical importance, scientific importance and validity. A journal may appropriately choose to publish a clinically important but scientifically weak study—if no better evidence is available. Similarly, there are circumstances where journals might publish very weak studies together with commentaries pointing out their weaknesses. One such set of circumstances is where the research is widely discussed but has been seen by few.

Many of the ethical difficulties of medical journals arise in their relationship with pharmaceutical companies (as I discuss in chapter 16). The study funded by industry that has caused the greatest difficulties in recent times is the VIGOR (Vioxx Gastrointestinal Outcomes Research) study, which was published in the *New England Journal of Medicine* in 2000.[42] The study was a trial in which over 8000 patients were randomized to receive either naproxen, a long-established non-steroidal anti-inflammatory drug, or rofecoxib, a Cox-2 inhibitor that the manufacturers, Merck, hoped would have fewer gastrointestinal side-effects. There were sound theoretical grounds for expecting that this would be the case. The primary endpoint of the trial was gastrointestinal side-effects, and sure enough the patients given naproxen experienced 121 side-effects compared with 56 in the patients taking rofecoxib. This was a marvellous result for Merck and contributed to huge sales of rofecoxib. Merck reportedly bought a million reprints of the article from the *New England Journal of Medicine* to use in promoting the drug. (My estimate would be that this must have meant several hundred thousand dollars of profit for the journal.)

The trial also showed an increase in myocardial infarction in the patients given rofecoxib (0.4%) compared with those given naproxen (0.1%). This was an unexpected result and the difference was interpreted to be caused by naproxen having a protective effect. In September 2004 Merck withdrew the drug from the market when it became clear that rofecoxib did have serious cardiovascular side-effects.

It subsequently emerged that the VIGOR article 'did not accurately represent the safety data available to the authors when the article was being reviewed for publication'.[43,44] These data showed that there were 47 confirmed serious thromboembolic events in the patients given rofecoxib and 20 in those given naproxen—so wiping out the gastrointestinal benefits from rofecoxib. There were also three extra cases of myocardial infarction in the patients on rofecoxib that were not declared. If all of these data had been included in the original report then the interpretation that naproxen was protective rather than rofecoxib harmful would have been much less convincing.

The *New England Journal of Medicine* published an expression of concern in December 2005 and then reaffirmed it in March 2006 after giving the authors a chance to explain themselves.[43,44] But is the *New England Journal of Medicine* blameless in all this? It published the expression of concern at the end of 2005 because the problems with the study had emerged as evidence was gathered for a court case against Merck brought by patients who allege that they have been damaged by rofecoxib. The lawyers discovered that changes had been made in the submitted manuscript. The full data were, however, given to the Food and Drugs Administration (FDA) at about the same time that the article was published—and the data were on the FDA website. Shouldn't the journal have picked up on these data and published a correction? Even if they didn't at the time, shouldn't they have done so as doubts began to be published about the safety of rofecoxib? And wasn't it poor practice that only percentages of cardiovascular side-effects were given in the original report? Could it be that the editorial standards of the journal were conflicted in some way by the huge profits made from reprints of the original article?

In all my 25 years at the *BMJ* we were not involved in such dramatic happenings as the three cases I've described from the *Lancet*, the one from *JAMA* and the one from the *New England Journal of Medicine*. These are all cases where there has been worldwide impact from the studies accompanied by questions about the ethical behaviour of the journals. Neither the Kaiser study nor the cheating editorial had the same impact, but I want to tell just a few further stories from the *BMJ* to build my case that the wider world should be interested in the ethical behaviour of journals.

I thought this a few years ago as I spent most of a day traipsing from one television studio to another giving an account of a paper we had published on female sexual dysfunction.[3] This was an unusual paper in that it was not research by scientists but rather research by an investigative journalist, Ray Moynihan. He argued in his paper that drug companies were playing a central part in defining sexual problems in women as a 'disease' with the implication that they might best be treated with drugs. The companies were, argued Moynihan, 'disease mongering'. I found myself in some of my many interviews suggesting that 'because drug companies were having problems creating new drugs they were turning their hands to creating new diseases'.

This story was covered by media right across the world and there can be little doubt that it got such wide coverage because it was published by 'a prestigious medical journal' (as journalists love to call journals when they want added weight for their stories). But should journals be publishing papers that use the methods of investigative journalism rather than the methods of epidemiology or molecular biology? Most editors of medical journals would probably answer no and certainly most journals don't publish such pieces (although interestingly both *Nature* and *Science*, the two leading science journals, do—and it is these parts of their journals that are the best read, because everybody can understand them).

The paper on female sexual dysfunction was interesting in that it potentially affected the lives of most adults. Sex is a complex process and often unsatisfactory. Moynihan's article described studies (funded by the drug industry and the main one published in *JAMA*[45]) that suggested that almost half of American women might have female sexual dysfunction, but they might be defined as dysfunctional if they sometimes didn't want sex, didn't enjoy it or found it uncomfortable. Should this be thought of as a disease? Should women seek treatment if they don't want sex? Some of those who joined the debate said 'Why not?' Develop a female equivalent of Viagra and women can benefit from it as men have benefited from Viagra. Others drew analogies between sex and dancing: you need medical help to improve your dancing if you break your leg, but otherwise doctors and drugs have nothing to offer to improve your dancing. There were feminists on both sides of the argument.

The debate will rage on, but this is an example of medical journals—and drug companies—intruding into the lives of many. The *BMJ* did something similar when we ran an exercise on our website to identify 'non-diseases'.[46] Over a hundred conditions were suggested and we then asked readers to vote for their top non-diseases. This caused outrage among some who argued that it was a cheap publicity stunt that mocked the suffering of many. I responded by arguing that it was primarily an exercise to alert people to the fact that diseases are not 'out there' like animal species waiting to be discovered but rather medical, social and even sometimes political constructs. We also wanted to point out that having your problem defined as a disease may not be the best way to deal with it.

One group who were particularly upset by this exercise were sufferers from chronic fatigue syndrome or myalgic encephalomyelitis (ME). (Even the name is disputed. Doctors prefer chronic fatigue syndrome and have produced an operational definition of it. Many patients prefer ME. In a spirit of conciliation I'll now use ME.) They are an interesting group of patients who have in some sense been 'at war' with the medical establishment in general and medical journals in particular. They have entered the discourse that goes on in medical journals in a way that not many other patient groups have done. (Another group are those concerned with Munchausen-by-proxy.) Sufferers from ME think that their condition is not taken seriously by most doctors. In particular, they resent the contention of doctors that the problem has a psychological component and is not simply a physical condition (not that any condition, doctors argue, is 'simply physical').

Each year one of the ME organizations gives a prize for 'the worst medical journal'. Usually it is won by the *BMJ*, sometimes tying with the *Lancet*. Some of those interested in ME have made complaints about me to various authorities. They saw the *BMJ* as pushing the line that the problem is psychological, using only advisers whom they despise (many of them psychiatrists), and publishing only research that supports our line. My line was that we don't have a line. We took the best research that we could get and asked people who were recognized experts to write and review for us. We didn't publish research because the results pleased us and we didn't tell any of the experts what to write. Plus anybody could send us electronic letters and we posted all of those that were not obscene, libellous, incomprehensible, wholly unsubstantial or gave information on patients without their written consent. We posted and published on paper many contributions from people who were very critical of what we published on ME.

I am perhaps being disingenuous here. I can see that one view of ME—we might call it the orthodox view—did dominate in the *BMJ* and most (perhaps all) other major journals. The *BMJ* is the establishment. It favours particular methods. It has strong views that some sorts of evidence—for example, well done randomized trials—are superior to other sorts of evidence—for example, case reports. I often said—and repeat in this book—that the '*BMJ* is not in the truth business but the debate business'. I favour a postmodern view of the world, where there are many truths not one, but we didn't practise that view consistently with the *BMJ*. Almost anything might go in electronic letters, but anything did not go in the main body of the journal.

My next example is strange. I read in the *Independent* newspaper of 10 June 2000 the headline '*BMJ* admits "lapses" after article wiped £30m off Scotia shares'.[47] Could a *BMJ* mistake really have such dramatic consequences? The story began with the *BMJ* publishing a very short article that suggested that a new anticancer drug that was being tested might cause skin burns in 40% of patients.[48] The drug—temoporfin (Foscan)—accumulates in malignant tissues and then is activated by light to destroy the tissue. We published the article to alert readers to this possible side-effect. Medical journals face a difficult problem with such reports, which are usually based on a single case or a small series of patients. Journals know that they don't get it right every time. Sometimes they publish reports of effects that turn out not to be 'real' and sometimes they reject reports that do turn out to be 'real.' We do know, however, that case reports in journals are an important means to identify adverse drug effects.

The central medical and scientific question was how common were serious burns. Another important question was whether or not it was the drug itself that had caused the high incidence of burns, the way it was given or some other explanation. But the major question for the shareholders of Scotia, the company that manufactured the drug, was whether or not the drug would get to market and produce a return on their investment.

The medical and scientific questions were not of great interest to general journalists because the drug was not even on the market. This was not a major public health issue. The financial journalists on the newspapers (not regular readers of the *BMJ*) could, however, be prompted to take an interest and this is what happened. Credit Suisse First Boston, market analysts, put out a release describing the *BMJ* article and wondering 'what this report means for the approval, partnering and commercialization of Foscan'. 'First impression,' it continued, 'is that this is highly negative.' The release also said: 'We have long been skeptical about the commercial value of Foscan.' The share price of Scotia fell from 150p to 120p. Its highest price in the previous year was 230p, although it reached 800p in 1996 and dipped below 100p in early 1999. Share prices in biotech companies fluctuate greatly. Crucially the share price needed to reach 340p by March 2002 for a £50m bond issue to convert into shares.

Scotia responded by pointing out that the burns seemed to be much more common in this series of patients than in other series.[49] It questioned how the drug had been given and threatened to sue the authors. The story was covered on the financial pages in seven newspapers.

The *BMJ* had not been blameless in all this. We failed to require the authors to include in the article the manufacturer's data on the frequency of the side-effect. We did, however, post the information on our website the day after publication and we published letters from the company within a few days. Another problem was that the article did not include any statement on conflicts of interest from the authors. We failed to send them our standard form. The company tried hard to suggest that it was our 'lapses' that caused the problem rather than the fact that the drug had been associated with so many severe burns. After this episode the drug was denied a licence in both Europe and the United States, but later both jurisdictions did grant a licence.

This was in retrospect a storm in a teacup, but it generated great excitement at the time and at least suggested that medical journals could be so powerful as to wipe £30m off a company's value with 150 words—that is, £200,000 a word. There are other examples of where publications in journals have had very dramatic effects on share prices, leading some to suggest that studies that might affect share prices, which are almost always to do with drugs, should be published in the *Stock Exchange Bulletin* rather than in a medical journal.

After I returned from Venice and before I left the *BMJ* I was embroiled in two of the biggest controversies of my time at the *BMJ*. One links to the previous story as it concerns an obituary of David Horrobin, the founder of Scotia.[50] The obituary said: 'The products [of Scotia] contained evening primrose oil, which may go down in history as the remedy for which there is no disease, and David Horrobin, Scotia's former chief executive, may prove to be the greatest snake oil salesman of his age.' It continued: 'He often wrote about ethics, but his—or his company's—research ethics were considered dubious.' The obituary also made the point that Horrobin was unusually clever, charming, creative and charismatic, but Horrobin's many friends were appalled. We received more than a hundred electronic letters condemning the obituary, and a complaint was made to the Press Complaints Commission. The complaint got as far as an adjudication which happens with only about 1.5% of the 2000 complaints made each year. The commission decided that no further action was necessary—partly because we had apologized to the family for the distress we had caused (not for publishing the obituary).

This episode does not support my case that medical journals can have strong effects on people's lives—because it doesn't concern the public health. But the case does raise important ethical questions? Can it be acceptable to speak ill of the dead? Is it fair to publish a defamatory piece a few days after somebody is dead when a libel action is no longer possible—because under English law you cannot libel the dead? If such a piece is to be published should it include evidence to support its assertions?

My other post-Venetian controversy was more directly relevant to this chapter. The *BMJ* published a study suggesting that passive smoking did not kill.[51] The results did not please the antismoking lobby, of which the *BMJ* is a part, but the biggest problem with the study was that the authors were connected to the tobacco industry. The BMA, owners of the *BMJ*, put out a press release condemning the study as 'flawed', and the American Cancer Society, which some 40 years ago had started the study that was reported, said the same. Hundreds of rapid responses flooded into the *BMJ*'s website, most of them furious that the *BMJ* had published the study but some delighted that the *BMJ* had not bowed to 'political correctness'.

The study reported on what had happened to more than 100,000 adults from California who were first studied in 1959. It found that those people who did not smoke but were married to partners who did were not more likely to die of coronary artery disease, lung cancer or chronic obstructive lung disease (all diseases caused by smoking) than those who were married to partners who did not. The main flaw in the study, according to critics, was that most of the population smoked most of the time in the late 1950s and the early 1960s, meaning that almost everybody was exposed to lots of smoke. But strengths of the study are its large size, its long follow up, and the fact that the outcome was death. The weakness of the study may also in some ways be a strength. A worry about studies conducted after the link between smoking and disease became fully apparent—in the early 1960s—is that the middle classes stopped smoking in large numbers. So people who lived with smokers were likely to be poorer, less well educated and of lower social class—possibly explaining their excess mortality compared with people living with others who did not smoke.

I must not be too defensive here—because it is certainly conventional wisdom, supported by many studies (many of them published in the *BMJ*), that passive smoking increases premature mortality by about one-third. Nevertheless, the editors and reviewers who reviewed the controversial paper thought that it was asking a question that wasn't completely resolved. The study then made it through our peer review system. And we had already decided that we would publish studies linked with the tobacco industry—so there was no reason not to publish.[52]

Some American journals have adopted policies of refusing to publish studies funded by the tobacco industry. Their argument is that the industry is thoroughly untrustworthy and deliberately tries to obfuscate the scientific record. Furthermore, publication in an academic journal gives the mendacious industry respectability that is undeserved. We decided that it was to go too far to assume that every study funded by the industry was a lie, and that it would be antiscience to suppress systematically one source of research. We may be wrong and may have damaged public health by publishing the California study.

I could tell many more stories, but I hope that even the most sceptical reader will be convinced that medical journals can have extensive effects on ordinary people and that it is worth paying attention to their ethical behaviour.

▶3

What and who are medical journals for?

Medical journals have existed for 200 years, but will they continue? The answer must be that they will if they do something that people value and that isn't done more effectively or more cheaply by some other means. This iron law of economics applies to everything. So what do journals do that people value and who are their customers?

Scientific journals exist primarily to disseminate and record science, but many medical journals, although they include science, have been about more than simply recording science. Around 40 medical journals were begun in Britain between 1640 and the end of the 18th century.[53] None survives. Journals are like restaurants (or any small business): many start, few survive long term. Another 100 journals began in Britain between 1801 and 1840, and one of these—the *Lancet*, which began in 1823—does survive. The *Lancet* has always been a fascinating, energetic journal, reflecting its aggressive, combative, crusading and controversial founder, Thomas Wakley.[54] At the prompting of his radical friend William Cobbett, he started the *Lancet* as a 28-year-old general practitioner with a mission to 'inform and reform'. That formula persists today, and perhaps the current editor, Richard Horton, who became editor at 33, is closer in spirit to Wakley than any other *Lancet* editor has been.

Wakley from the beginning produced the *Lancet* for 'the profession at large' rather than 'the eminent few'. Doctors outside the main cities in Britain were, he observed on the first page of the first issue, 'almost without the means of ascertaining its [medicine's] progress'. An important feature of his journal was reports on lectures given by prominent doctors in London. The doctors charged for these lectures and objected to them being reproduced in the *Lancet* without permission. There were many legal actions. Wakley also provided medical news, case descriptions and non-medical articles that would entertain and instruct the general public as well as medical practitioners. So there was little or no science, entertainment was a specific aim, and the journal was aimed at the public as well as doctors.

But Wakley's other aim—and perhaps his primary aim—was reform, and in wildly intemperate language he attacked nepotism, incompetence, quackery and corruption, all of which were rife in early 19th century British medicine (and perhaps still are). Libel actions were 'plenty as blackberries', but Wakley had hit on a formula that was commercially acceptable. We can easily imagine a provincial but progressive practitioner—like George Eliot's creation Dr Lydgate in *Middlemarch*—reading the *Lancet* not only to find out what was new and to improve his knowledge but also to be amused and excited by Wakley's latest attack on the establishment.

Eliot does not tell us whether Lydgate read the *Lancet*, but the traditional, and incompetent, doctors suspect him of doing so.

'Hang your reforms!' said Mr Chichely. 'There's no greater humbug in the world. You never hear of a reform, but it means some trick to put in new men. I hope you are not one of the *Lancet*'s men, Mr Lydgate—wanting to take the coronership out of the hands of the legal profession: your words appear to point that way.'

'I disapprove of Wakley,' interposed Dr Sprague, 'no man more: he is an ill-intentioned fellow, who would sacrifice the respectability of the profession, which everybody knows depends on the London Colleges, for the sake of getting some notoriety for himself. There are men who don't mind about being kicked blue if they can only get talked about.'

(I've heard almost exactly those words said about Richard Horton.)

The *BMJ*, which doesn't merit a mention in *Middlemarch*, got off to a much duller start.[9] It was founded in 1840 as the journal of the Provincial and Medical Surgical Association, which was formed by Charles Hastings, a Worcester doctor, and eventually became the British Medical Association (BMA).[55] The first issue of the *Provincial Medical and Surgical Journal* was 16 pages long and the longest items were the editor's introductory address and a report of the annual meeting and dinner of the association's eastern branch. What could be more boring?

The editors announced that the aims of the journal were the same as those of the association—the promotion of the medical profession. There were clinical papers, case notes, a summary of a medical reform bill and some book reviews. At least one of these was lively: Charles Waller's *Practical Treastise on the Function and Diseases of the Unimpregnated Womb* was described as '200 scanty pages of commonplace professional twaddle'. The editors also took a swing at the *Lancet* by boasting that they had 'received as many advertisements (in proportion to the quantity of letter press) for our first number, as the most popular Medical Journal of the present day after 17 years of existence'. This was empty boasting: advertisers are always attracted by novelty—at least briefly.

(Anybody who would like to read this fascinating material for themselves will soon be able to do so courtesy of the National Library of Medicine in Washington. It is digitizing the whole of the *BMJ* and many other journals. Stephen Lock, my predecessor, told me, however, that the only thing that was interesting in old *BMJ*s was the advertisements—and they are not being digitized.)

The *BMJ* thus shared the aim of the *Lancet* in wanting to inform practitioners, and it was in some ways a development of the *Midland Medical and Surgical Reporter*, which recorded pathological observations made in provincial hospitals and other aspects of medicine and medical practice in the Midlands. But even with its role of informing it can be seen that its bill of fare was less attractive than that of the *Lancet*, which was including up to the minute lectures from leading practitioners. In addition, the *BMJ* lacked the reforming zeal of Wakley's *Lancet*. A description of the annual dinner of the eastern branch would not make such good reading as an attack on the wickedness of a leading London practitioner. It's not surprising that while the *Lancet* flourished commercially the *BMJ* struggled for most of its first 25 years.

The *Lancet* is highly unusual in not being linked to a medical organization. All the other 'big five' medical journals are owned by medical organizations. The *Annals of Internal Medicine* is owned by the American College of Physicians, the *BMJ* by the BMA, *JAMA* by the American Medical Association, and the *New England Journal of Medicine* by the Massachusetts Medical Society. Journals owned by associations can degenerate to being simply mouthpieces of the association, suppressing anything that for whatever reason doesn't suit the aims of the association. Journals tend to fight with their owners and my (wholly biased) judgement is that journals flourish when they are most independent of their owners.

One issue that seems to be constantly debated in medical journals is how political they should be.[56] 'Politics' says *Chambers Dictionary* is 'the art or science of government, the management of a political party, political affairs or opinions, manœuvring and intriguing, policy making, as opposed to administration, the civil rather than the military aspects of government.' Rudolf Virchow, a great 19th century doctor and editor, famously said that medicine was 'a social science, and politics nothing but medicine on a grand scale'. For him and many others—including Wakley and Ernest Hart, the leading 19th century editor of the *BMJ*—it made no sense to think of an 'apolitical' medical journal. There is also the argument that being 'apolitical' is in itself a political position—usually one that supports the status quo.

Nevertheless, a great many readers of medical journals object strongly to them being political. Tony Delamothe, deputy editor of the *BMJ*, wrote an editorial asking 'How political should a general medical journal be?' and quoted a correspondent who wrote in response to a letter describing the pattern of injuries suffered by Palestinians in the Israeli occupied territories, 'I am terribly sorry to learn that...the *British Medical Journal* has become a politically motivated journal... I hope that this would be the first and last political letter published in this journal.'[57] I can't help observing that if the correspondent imagined this letter in 2002 to be the first political letter to appear in the *BMJ* he'd either never read the journal before or had a very strange idea of what constituted a political letter.

Another correspondent wrote in response to Delamothe's editorial:[58]

'The problem with medical journals entering into politics is that it subjects them to the accusation of bias...You may disagree with your government's stance on [the coming war in] Iraq, but that disagreement has no place in a medical journal... Cataloguing the health effects of weapons of mass destruction or debating (honestly and fairly) the merits and demerits of smallpox vaccine are appropriate for the pages of the journal. It isn't appropriate, however, for you to use your influential position to trumpet your own political biases. Continuing to do so only discredits the journal. How will we know you haven't rejected papers simply because their findings disagree with your politics?'

In the 19th century it probably seemed impossible to separate medicine from politics. Life expectancy improved dramatically in the industrial world towards the end of the century not because of medical practice but because of improvements in sanitation and housing, reductions in poverty, better nutrition, the spread of education and other social developments. These are still the major influences on health and it wasn't until antibiotics, other drugs and modern surgery were developed in the middle of the 20th century that medicine began to have some appreciable effect on how long people lived. It then began to be possible to imagine a general medical journal that would not be political. It would restrict itself to physiology, pathology and therapeutics. It wouldn't stray into public health and the wider determinants of health.

When discussing the damage to health caused by tobacco, for example, this apolitical journal would restrict itself to material describing the effect of tobacco on the body and the steps that individual doctors might take to stop individual patients smoking. There would be no discussion of the price or promotion of tobacco or the malignant activities of the tobacco industry: these are clearly political issues. The journal would not even consider the availability of smoking cessation services or whether nicotine replacement therapy should be available on prescription, both issues that have been the cause of intense political argument in Britain recently. I wonder whether or not such a journal—where the editor watches with an eagle eye to exclude any political material—is even theoretically possible. Can medicine and politics be separated? I don't think they can, but even if they could I can't see the point. Any journal that wants to have any influence on health and medicine will have to deal with the political.

The real question is not whether a journal should be political but rather, as Delamothe asked, how political should it be? We at the *BMJ* were somewhat taken aback by the extensive coverage that the *Lancet* gave to the attacks on New York and Washington on 11 September 2001. This was clearly a major geopolitical event and there were many deaths. We carried news stories and first person accounts of being caught up in the attacks. The *Lancet*, in contrast, carried nine articles, several having what seemed to us tenuous links to health or medicine. Much of its coverage was similar to that in newspapers and the weekly news magazines.

This seemed to us a step too far. We felt the need to maintain a link with 'health'. Thus we joined the debate on whether or not there should be an attack on Iraq but always within the context of what the casualties might be. Yet we published a piece that argued that the main reason behind the war was the need of the United States to gain access to cheap oil.[59] The link to health was the possible effects of this on global warming with its undoubted consequences for health. The author of this piece—Ian Roberts, a professor of health policy—also pointed out that many journals that tried to be 'apolitical' were publishing a great deal on bioterrorism. This meant, argued Roberts, that they were being political because bioterrorism was a minor influence on health but a major part of the argument for going to war.[60]

When we published Delamothe's editorial we held a vote on our website in which we asked readers how much space we should devote to political issues. In all 366 people answered and in comparison with current coverage, 45% wanted more or much more coverage, 31% the same and 22% less or much less.

The possible functions of journals are thus informing, reforming, disseminating science, educating, providing a forum for a community to debate the issues of the day, entertaining and making money. I believe that a good journal will do all of these things, trying always to maintain a balance. Some journals do perform all the functions, but most don't. Many current journals, particularly specialist ones, are primarily concerned with disseminating science, informing in a small way (with occasional editorials) and making money. They don't see it as their business to reform and the idea that they might entertain they find silly. Medical journals, they believe, should be serious. Unfortunately, many—even if they don't intend to be—are pompous. They fail to understand that humour well used is not only entertaining but also a powerful tool for informing, reforming and educating.

Many also imagine that journals are about changing what doctors do, bringing their practice up to the minute. That's what I thought myself when I first joined the *BMJ* and many, including journal editors, believe that journals are a major engine—perhaps *the* major engine—of change and improvement. But it isn't like that at all. We have overwhelming evidence that there is a substantial gap between what the published evidence suggests is best practice and what doctors and other healthcare workers do. The influential Institute of Medicine in the United States labelled the gap 'a chasm'—and there is no reason to think that it is worse in the United States than in any other country.[61]

Why don't medical journals change practice? The main reason is that change is hard, involves many factors, and can rarely be achieved by words on paper alone.[62] Sending practitioners written guidelines changes little.[62,63] Other interventions are needed in addition—for example, one to one meetings, feedback on performance, organizational change or sessions with people called in the jargon of marketing 'opinion leaders'.[64] And guidelines give specific information on what actions to take with patients with specific problems. Journals, in contrast, contain a hotchpotch of different sorts of information, little of which is 'actionable'. Even when the information seems to give a clear message on the best actions to take it would probably be unwise for a doctor immediately to take that action. Much of the evidence in medical journals is in evolution. It's undigested. Much is shot down. Publication is not the end of the peer review process but a part of it.

David Slawson and Allan Shaughnessy, two American doctors who have taken a great interest in trying to help doctors through the jungle of medical information, have described a formula that helps assess the utility of information in various sources available to doctors:[8]

$$\text{Utility} = \frac{\text{Relevance} \times \text{Validity}}{\text{Work to access}}$$

If we consider the original research in journals we can see that any given study is likely to be of limited relevance to any particular doctor. Some studies have high validity, but many do not. And the work to access the information in original research is high: it takes a long time to read research and critically appraising it is difficult and needs special skills that many doctors lack. So the usefulness of individual studies to a particular doctor at a particular time is low, but their usefulness overall may not be low. They need to be systematically combined with other studies.

Many studies have shown that when doctors have questions that they need answering they mostly go to colleagues, even though they may say that they use journals.[65] Colleagues can give answers that are directly relevant. They are easy to access and (with luck) will provide valid answers.

After listening to a Ugandan PhD student describe the characteristics that made information useful to health workers in rural Uganda, I added 'interactivity' to the top of Slawson and Shaughnessy's formula. This explains still further why doctors go to colleagues for information: they can discuss (an old fashioned word for interact) the question with them and get the answer clear in a way that can't be done with a journal article. David Slawson says that 'interactivity' is simply a function of 'relevance' and 'work to access', not something independent. I'm unconvinced.

The thinking behind this formula has led various people, including the BMJ Publishing Group when I was there, to try and come up with 'knowledge tools' that will be more useful to doctors than journals. The BMJ Publishing Group has, for example, produced something called *Clinical Evidence*, a compendium of regularly updated, evidence-based (jargon for valid) answers to clinical questions on treatment commonly asked by doctors and patients.[66] *Clinical Evidence* has been made available to all healthcare workers in Britain, 500,000 doctors in the United States and 300,000 doctors in Italy. It's available not only in English but in Spanish, Italian, Russian, French, German and Japanese.

For a while I found myself wondering why we needed the *BMJ* and other journals when we had knowledge tools like *Clinical Evidence*. But it goes back to Wakley's original formula of informing, reforming, debating and entertaining. At the *BMJ* we went as far—inspired by my days at the Stanford Business School—as developing a 'mission statement'.[67] The journal had survived 150 years without one, but I believe it to be a useful exercise to define together what you are trying to do. How, otherwise, could you know if you were succeeding? Increasingly journals—along with hospitals, practices and many other medical institutions—have mission statements.

I thought that it would be useful to include our mission statement here. Such a statement should last for decades and every word in the statement should matter—but the thinking is often clear to those who devise it and less clear to those who read it. So I will explain the thinking behind the statement.

'To publish rigorous, accessible and entertaining material that will help doctors and medical students in their daily practice, lifelong learning, and career development. In addition, to be at the forefront of the international debate on health.

To produce sufficient surplus to develop the primary mission and in good years to invest in the rest of the group and contribute to the activities of the BMA.'

Publish means more than putting words and pictures on paper. It certainly includes putting words and pictures on screens but also creating talks, videos and meetings. If journals have a future then it is likely to be multimedia.

Rigorous: we might have chosen the word 'scientific', but the *BMJ* includes much material that is not scientific—and we wanted our news, views and even humour to be rigorous.

Accessible means not only readable but also easy to find and understand and attractive to look at.

Entertaining: we wanted reading the *BMJ* to be a pleasure, not a chore.

Material: we wanted constantly to broaden the range of things we published. We long ago moved beyond simply publishing research papers, but the journal has a long way to go with publishing more than words and pictures. Some journals are now beginning to include podcasts on their websites.

Help: if we could be helpful we would prosper. Sometimes we 'preach at', but we try not to do so too often. Being helpful certainly includes 'bringing new and possibly uncomfortable material to the attention of doctors', and it probably includes providing leadership.

Doctors and medical students: this means doctors and medical students everywhere, not just in Britain. We knew that the *BMJ* is read by many people who are neither doctors nor medical students, and we were pleased that they enjoyed the *BMJ*—but we thought it important to focus on doctors and medical students. By concentrating on helping them we would, we hope, help others.

In their daily practice: we aspired to be helpful to doctors and medical students every day, by providing information that would help them not only with clinical problems but also with issues like ethics, the law, science, education, communication, critical appraisal, improvement methods, management, statistics, economics and the many other subjects that modern doctors and medical students have to understand. The *BMJ* could not be in the business of teaching specialist skills to specialist groups because most of our readers do not belong to that specialist group, but we wanted to help doctors and medical students with the skills, both clinical and otherwise, that are important to them all.

Lifelong learning: to continue to learn throughout their careers matters greatly to doctors and their patients. The *BMJ* wanted to help them do this not only by providing material on medicine and science but also by providing material on learning and teaching.

Career development: many doctors and medical students are confused about their careers and the skills needed to develop them. The *BMJ* aimed to be an unequalled source of advice for doctors and medical students everywhere.

To be at the forefront of the international debate on health: The *BMJ* had ever since its beginning been international, but the World Wide Web and the dozen or so local editions of the *BMJ* offered unprecedented means of reaching out beyond Britain. The *BMJ* was concerned not just with medicine and healthcare but also with health. We might have chosen the word 'lead' instead of 'be at the forefront of', but that seemed too pretentious a step.

Debate is a crucial word for the *BMJ*. We wanted to be a place where almost every view can be expressed and follow the teachings of John Milton, the great British poet. 'Give me,' he wrote, 'the liberty to know, to utter, and to argue freely according to conscience, above all liberties. Truth was never put to the worse in a free and open encounter…It is not impossible that she [truth] may have more shapes than one…If it come to prohibiting, there is not ought more likely to be prohibited than truth itself, whose first appearance to our eyes bleared and dimmed with prejudice and custom is more unsightly and implausible than many errors…Where there is much desire to learn there of necessity will be much arguing, much writing, many opinions; for opinion in good men is but knowledge in the making.'[68]

I found this guidance of Milton's more useful than any other in my time as editor of the *BMJ*. There were many circumstances in which people were infuriated by what they read in the *BMJ* and wanted the words retracted and the author punished. Milton's quote was useful to me then not only because I had it ringing in my ears but also because I sent it to the critics. Usually it shut them up.

To produce sufficient surplus to develop the primary mission and in good years to invest in the rest of the group and contribute to the activities of the BMA: the *BMJ*, like every other organization, has to think about finance. Members of the BMA tend to think that much of their subscription to the BMA comes to the *BMJ*—because the *BMJ* is what they see every week. In fact none of it does. Money flows from the BMJ Publishing Group to the BMA—over £9m in 2003. The *BMJ* itself is also profitable, with income from subscriptions, advertising and several other sources. Our financial mission was to be able to invest to develop the *BMJ* itself and also, when profits were good, to invest in the rest of the publishing group and in the activities of the BMA.

The BMA has now made clear, however, that it expects profits from the BMJ Publishing Group—and it is right that the owners should set the mission of the journal. They will destroy a journal if they interfere with day-to-day editorial decisions, but it's surely right that the owners should set the mission, approve the strategy for achieving it and monitor progress with the strategy. I will return to this theme in chapter 12 on editorial independence, but nobody from the BMA told me what they wanted from either the *BMJ* or the BMJ Publishing Group. My predecessor simply told me, 'make sure the journal comes out on time and don't introduce American spelling'.

Partly because our mission statement was hard to remember, the *BMJ* also had a vision of what we would like to be:

'To be the world's most influential and widely read medical journal.'

We didn't want to be the world's richest, biggest, most profitable or even most scientific journal; we simply wanted to be the world's most influential and widely read medical journal. One snag with influence is that it's hard to measure, but we kept trying to develop a score—without success.

While it's important for an organization or journal to know what it is trying to do, it's equally important for it to identify its customers—and I'm using the word in the broad sense of not just people who hand over money for what the organization or journal has to sell but also all those people who have to be satisfied if it is going to flourish. Another word is 'stakeholders'. So, who are medical journals for?

The *BMJ*'s mission statement mentioned doctors and medical students. These were the people at whom we aimed the *BMJ*, and we mean doctors and medical students everywhere. This would not have been the case when the *Provincial Medical and Surgical Journal* began. At some point—probably in the later part of the 19th century—the *BMJ* aspired to become an international journal. But perhaps initially it was 'a showcase of British medicine'. I wanted it to be truly international, gathering material from everywhere. But we knew we had a long way to go. To many we were irredeemably (but sometimes attractively) British. Furthermore, some British doctors wanted us to stay firmly British and resented us publishing material that they did not see as directly relevant to them.

Other journals also aspire to be global, but none succeeds completely. Many journals, however, are very much national or regional. They distinguish themselves by understanding the issues of that country or region in a way that no international journal can match.

The mission statement of the BMJ Publishing Group (as opposed to the journal alone) mentioned groups other than doctors—'members, other health professionals, the scientific community and the public'. By members we meant members of the BMA and members of organizations with which we co-own journals, like, for example, the British Cardiac Society. Many journals are sent to members of medical organizations as part of their membership fee and those publications may put the needs of the members of that organization first.

Most journals are read predominantly by particular professional groups. Doctors read medical journals. Nurses read nursing journals. Health managers read newspapers, the *Economist* and perhaps the *Harvard Business Review*, but don't really read anything that looks like a medical journal. There are some health professionals who read across the divide, but they are rare. Many people have observed that one of the barriers to improvement in healthcare is the professional tribalism. Wouldn't it be marvellous if somebody could create a journal that crossed these professional divisions? Nobody has succeeded.

Wakley set out to create a journal that could be read by the public. He failed, but it was a bold idea. We live in a world where there is increasing evidence that health will be improved if doctors and patients work together as partners rather than in the traditional role with doctors as authority figures making decisions on behalf of patients.[69,70] This logic suggests that there should be publications that are aimed at both health professionals and patients. But then, as I've just written, nobody has yet succeeded in producing a publication for all those within healthcare let alone patients as well.

Those in health publishing have looked enviously at the *Economist*. It is a publication that started at about the same time as the *BMJ* and has broken out of the ghetto of its discipline. It's also become a major international force with its readership numbered in millions, including United States presidents and other world leaders. Why couldn't a medical publication do the same? Many have dreamt of a medical equivalent of the *Economist*—called perhaps 'Health'—but it is just a dream. Economics, like it or not, drives the world. Everything—war, politics, even football— can be legitimately and insightfully analysed using economic thinking.

But doesn't health similarly encompass everything? The World Health Organization (WHO) famously defined health as complete physical, mental and social wellbeing— prompting one wag to suggest that it was thus achieved only at the point of mutual orgasm. Disraeli said that the health of its people should be the first concern of a government. Now the WHO's Commission on Macroeconomics and Health, a commission mostly of financiers not health experts, has said that investment in health hastens economic development more than any other investment: health is not a benefit that comes from development but an engine of development.[71]

Despite all this, those of us interested in health do not have a means to comment on the world in a way that brings fresh and exciting understanding in the same sense that economics can. We may deal with the eternals of birth, death, pain and sickness, but we are mostly preaching to each other. Some members of the public stumble into medical journals, particularly through the World Wide Web. Some like what they find enough to keep visiting, and some of the most positive comments I ever received about the *BMJ* came from non-doctors—usually husbands, wives or children of doctors. They have perhaps a sense of discovering a secret garden, but if the garden is thrown open to the public nobody is much interested. Perhaps the next breakthrough in medical journalism and editing will be to find a way to make health one of the great discourses along with politics, business, the environment and the arts. I think it could be done.

Scientists or researchers are customers of medical journals, but more perhaps as authors than readers. Brian Haynes, a physician from Canada with a great interest in information in healthcare, classifies journals as 'researcher to researcher', 'researcher to clinician' and 'clinician to clinician'. A journal like *Nature Medicine* is a 'researcher to researcher' journal. The only practising doctors who read it are those few who are also involved in research in basic science. I've hardly met an ordinary doctor who reads *Nature Medicine*. Many specialist journals are 'researcher to clinician' journals and they can be the great unread journals if they are not careful. Journals like *Clinical Medicine* or the *Postgraduate Medical Journal* are 'clinician to clinician' journals and usually of low status. The major medical journals might best be described as 'researcher and clinician to researcher and clinician' journals and the mix can be uneasy. Basic scientists are often scornful of medical journals, judging them to be scientifically weak and containing too much of what they dismiss as 'soft science'— science with its roots in the social rather than biological sciences.

Journals live with a constant tension between the needs of authors and readers, and traditionally they were much more concerned with authors. Some journals, often highly profitable ones, have been 'sausage machines' for processing authors' studies. Authors got the credit for having their papers published. Librarians got copies to add to their collections. Publishers got paid well for their journals. Everybody was happy and nobody was much bothered that nobody read the journals. Half the journals in the BMA library are not photocopied once in a year. Half of the articles published in journals are never cited, not even once. The joke is that publishers are like mustard makers—they make their money from material that is never used. I once saw a senior manager from Reed Elsevier, the biggest science publisher, describe the 27 strategic relationships of publishers. The 27th was 'readers', which she described as 'the great unknown'. The company had decided that it wanted to know more about them, but I found it astonishing (until I reflected further) that a publisher could be so large and profitable without having bothered to think about readers.

Nevertheless, authors are essential to journals. Little of what appears in most journals is written by the editors. Most of the material comes from authors who submit their valuable material for free and then traditionally hand over copyright to the journals and publishers. A journal like the *BMJ* receives 6000 submissions a year and publishes less than 10%. This might make it blasé about authors and the *BMJ* had a rather brutal triage system that left some authors feeling almost abused. But there is great competition among journals for the best papers and authors. Franz Ingelfinger, the great editor of the *New England Journal of Medicine*, made the journal pre-eminent by banging on the doors of all the major researchers in Boston and persuading them to submit their best studies to the journal. The *Lancet* has had something it calls 'Project Capture' to attract to the *Lancet* studies that might otherwise be published in the *New England Journal of Medicine*.

So pleasing authors is important but not at the expense of readers. Authors usually want longer papers with more data, more references, more explanation and more reflection on what the study might mean (often nothing in reality, but the moon to the authors). Readers, in contrast, want papers that are shorter and sweeter. One of the important talents of an editor has been to balance the needs of both authors and readers, but the arrival of the electronic world potentially means that both can be fully satisfied. Long versions of studies can be published on the web and shorter versions on paper. The *BMJ* calls this systems ELPS—'electronic long, paper short'.[72] Eventually the short version might be a piece written by journalists rather than the authors.

The owners of journal are clearly important stakeholders, and the relationship between owners and editors is often fraught. In the past five years the editor of one major American journal, *JAMA*, has been fired, and the editor of another, the *New England Journal of Medicine*, did not have his contract renewed. A few years before that the editors of the third major American journal, the *Annals of Internal Medicine*, left the journal after a dispute with the chief executive of the American College of Physicians, the owners of the journal. George Lundberg, the fired editor of *JAMA*, told me sometime before he was fired that the remarkable thing was that he hadn't been fired already. Many of the editors of *JAMA* have been fired and the man who fired George was himself subsequently fired. Not only the editor but also the deputy editor of the *Canadian Medical Association Journal* were fired early in 2006. Editors in many other countries, including Australia and Ireland, have been fired, but, as far as I can tell, no editor of the *BMJ* has been fired—although there was a major dispute between the BMA and the journal in the middle of the 20th century, as is described in chapter 12.

Editors are usually fired because of disputes over politics or money. With *JAMA* it's often been politics. The American Medical Association (AMA), the owner of *JAMA*, is a right wing, Republican organization comprised mainly of older doctors who hanker after the days of 'fee for service' medicine (when doctors were paid for what they did and 'managed care' had not been invented). Only about 30% of American doctors belong to the AMA. Yet the editors of *JAMA* are trying to produce a journal that will appeal to all doctors and not just to doctors in the United States. It's inevitable that tensions will arise. The *BMJ* doesn't have the same problem because 80% of doctors (and 60% of medical students) belong to the BMA, its owner, making it a broad church.

The problem for the *New England Journal of Medicine* is more money. The Massachusetts Medical Society has grown very fat on the huge profits of the journal and needs the money badly. It is keen to increase the profits of the journal by exploiting the brand, thus creating tension with the editors, who see themselves as responsible for upholding the quality of the journal and therefore the brand. Bud Relman, one of the editors of the journal, used to joke that the society would like to create 'New England Journal fried chicken' if it could be profitable. Because the society needs the profits of the journal it is also likely to be wary of developments that might make the journal less profitable.

The BMJ began to have this problem. The BMJ Publishing Group has become steadily more profitable, whereas the BMA has seen a growing gap between its income from members' subscriptions and expenditure on professional activities. Once a journal is viewed by its owner as a 'money machine' there is lots of scope for tension.

Advertisers are the final group of stakeholders I want to discuss. Some journals are dependent on advertisers and the advertisers are mainly the pharmaceutical industry. Because the industry has not in most countries been allowed to advertise directly to the public it has concentrated its advertising spend on journals. Most countries have medical newspapers that are sent free to doctors funded by pharmaceutical advertising. With these newspapers advertisers come first and editorial staff second. Editorial material will be cut if advertising is cut, and editors have quickly to produce more material if extra advertising is forthcoming. Most journals have other sources of income, usually subscriptions from institutions, and so are less dependent on advertising. They thus tend to have policies of editorial matters first and advertising matters second. Editors are willing to publish material that they know will offend advertisers, and the journals are not willing to place advertisements beside particular articles at the request of authors.

Many journals are, however, becoming more dependent on advertising and pressure then increases to please advertisers. Increasingly journals are willing to tell advertisers what they are going to publish and then to sell advertising space beside particular articles. Readers might then see a study showing advantages for a drug side by side with advertisements for that drug. The next step—which effectively destroys the independence and value of a journal—is to publish studies that support the advertisers' products and to decline those that don't. 'Freedom of the press in Britain,' said Hannen Swaffer, 'is freedom to print such of the proprietor's prejudices as the advertisers don't object to.'

Medical journals have many functions and diverse customers. They seem to be good at stirring up debate but poor at affecting change. Traditionally they have been more concerned with authors than readers, but their future—if they have a future—lies in being more concerned with readers.

▶4

Can medical journals lead or must they follow?*

For Thomas Wakley, the founder of the *Lancet*, an important function of his journal was to reform medicine, which he saw as full of incompetence, quackery, corruption and nepotism. He wanted to reform as well as inform. But can journals reform? Can they lead? Are medical journals important for leadership in medicine? Or is this grandiosity on the part of editors? Aren't journals there to follow, reflect and comment rather than to lead? These are the questions I want to explore in this brief chapter.

I never used the word leadership until I spent a year at the Stanford Business School in 1989–90 and discovered that people studied leadership. It is a word that wasn't used in Britain until recently. Doctors certainly didn't use it. But now leadership is seen as something central to the reform of the National Health Service (NHS). There are programmes to train leaders, particularly clinical leaders, throughout the NHS.

There is no simple definition of leadership, which is one source of confusion in research into the subject, but a working definition is that leaders have two main tasks—to set a path, goal or vision for the people who are being led, and to motivate people to pursue and eventually achieve the goal. For Mahatma Gandhi, one of the great leaders of the 20th century, the goal was to free India from the British. For Winston Churchill it was to defeat Germany in the Second World War. For Iain Chalmers, one of the founders of the Cochrane Collaboration and one of the leaders of medicine, the goal is to organize medical information and to create a medicine practised on evidence not tradition. All of these are goals that can be achieved only through effective leadership of large numbers.

But could editors or editorial teams have such specific goals? Some do. *Tobacco Control*, a journal within the BMJ Publishing Group, has one aim—the reduction and perhaps even eradication of the damage caused by tobacco. The goal is clear and the journal provides material (both research and advocacy) for those who share its aims. It is read by all those who might be regarded as leaders in the antismoking movement, and it provides a forum for them to debate with and motivate each other. It does seem to me that the journal and its editor, Simon Chapman, are leaders. Something similar might be said of another journal the BMJ Publishing Group publishes, *Injury Prevention*. Its goal is the reduction of injuries everywhere and in all age groups. This is a more diffuse goal than that of *Tobacco Control* and involves many different groups, many of whom do not read and have never even heard of *Injury Prevention*.

* A shortened, somewhat different, and illustrated version of this chapter has been published in *Med J Aust* 2005;**183**:665–8.

And when it comes to general medical journals they inevitably have diffuse goals and must cover a huge intellectual territory. It would be wrong for such a journal to become too obsessed with too narrow a goal, but can it provide leadership on particular themes? Some years ago I asked various editors if they could provide me with examples of where journals had shown leadership.

George Lundberg, who was then editor of *JAMA*, thought that *JAMA* had led on promoting a tobacco-free society, preventing nuclear war, drawing attention to the plight of the uninsured in America, promoting the control of violence and encouraging research into peer review. (In chapter 3 I discussed how political journals should be: four of these five issues are political in the broadest sense. They are far from clinical.) The *New England Journal of Medicine* had led, said Lundberg, by describing and deploring the industrialization of medicine, encouraging health reform and drawing attention to the importance of conflict of interest. The *BMJ* had led on fighting tobacco, calling for a ban on boxing (this was actually the BMA not the *BMJ*) and improving the standard of statistics in medical journals. The *Lancet* had led with reducing the risk of nuclear war and encouraging the internationalization of medicine. The *Canadian Medical Association Journal* had shown leadership by publishing a highly influential series of articles on critical appraisal of scientific papers.

Suzanne and Bob Fletcher, former editors of the *Annals of Internal Medicine*, agreed that the *New England Journal of Medicine* had led with its articles on the industrialization of medicine. *JAMA* had led on the prevention of disease and the promotion of social justice. The *Annals of Internal Medicine* had led on health services reform and the promotion of clinical guidelines.

Laurel Thomas, former editor of the *Medical Journal of Australia*, thought that her journal had led with antismoking campaigns, promoting reform of the World Medical Association, AIDS awareness, aboriginal health and traffic safety.

Magne Nylenna, who was then editor of the *Norwegian Medical Journal*, thought the *Lancet* had led on nuclear war, the *BMJ* on smoking, and his own journal on promoting medical education, particularly in the campaign to start a new medical school in Tromsø.

The most interesting response came from Stephen Lock, my mentor and predecessor as editor of the *BMJ*. He wrote:

'There are no examples of where medical journals have led. Nor is it the journal's role—which is to provide a forum for debate and to publish checked data. In fact, despite what editors say, I doubt whether any publication has done much leading—for instance, the Socialist landslide in [the British general election in] 1945 was probably due to the WEA [Worker's Education Association] influence in the forces during the war rather than the *Daily Mirror*, while Ernest Hart's [great editor of the *BMJ* in the 19th century, see below] successes owed more to the BMA Parliamentary Bills Committee, and his numerous social contacts, than to the *BMJ* and even Robbie Fox's [great *Lancet* editor of the 20th century] often cited role in the introduction of the NHS was secondary to Moran's [Lord Moran, Churchill's doctor] leadership at the RCP [Royal College of

Physicians] and in the Lord's [House of Lords] debate. Think of the contemporary issues—AIDS, health reform in the USA and the current NHS debate—and you'll realize how little influence the journals are having, can have, or should have.'

Stephen, as always, put his case powerfully, and there is much truth in what he says—but I want to continue to explore the question. One advantage of having asked those editors about examples of leadership nearly 10 years ago is that it's now possible to take a longer-term look at whether they were examples of leadership. I will define leadership as effecting a change that wouldn't otherwise have happened.

Ironically the best two examples of leadership from the list involve Stephen himself. Stephen together with Drummond Rennie from *JAMA* and John Bailar, statistical adviser to the *New England Journal of Medicine*, played a central part in prompting the study of peer review. This process, which is fundamental to all of science not only in deciding which papers to publish but also in the giving of research grants, was largely unstudied until these three urged that it should be. There have now been five international congresses on peer review (organized by Rennie and *JAMA*) and a body of research has been completed.[73] This has happened almost entirely within biomedicine, but its results are beginning to percolate to other areas of science. I cannot see that this would have happened without the leadership of Lock, Rennie, Bailar and their journals.

Similarly the work to improve the quality of statistical reporting was led by Lock and the *BMJ* together with other journals. The *Lancet* published an important series on statistics by Austen Bradford Hill, the *BMJ* published a series called 'Statistics at Square One' (which later as a book sold over 100,000 copies), and Lock and other editors involved statisticians in the peer review process. Many studies showed that the standard of statistics in medical journals was woeful and it's now better (although still far from perfect). This has an importance way beyond journals themselves. Bad statistics means false conclusions. Doctors and patients were thus being misled.

These two examples of leadership are of course to do with journals themselves. It is easier for journals to reform themselves and closely related activities than to reform the broader world. Another subject close to the journals where another journal—this time the *New England Journal of Medicine*—has shown leadership is over conflict of interest.[74] It led the way in encouraging journals, and medicine in the broad, to consider this important issue, although, as I will discuss in chapter 11, the state of play is still that most authors have conflicts of interest but much of the time don't declare them.

Journals have also been important in campaigning against smoking and nuclear war. All the major journals have published on these subjects, but they have been far from alone. Many medical bodies have been prominent in campaigning against the dangers of tobacco and International Physicians for the Prevention of Nuclear War won the Nobel Peace Prize for its work.

History can help us with trying to answer the question on whether or not journals can lead, and rather than considering Wakley this time, as I did extensively in chapter 3, I want to examine the work of Ernest Hart, editor of the *BMJ* from 1867 to 1898, and the closest the *BMJ* has come to a figure as important as Wakley.[9] Hart was a major public figure in a way that no *BMJ* editor had been before or has been since. He was highly controversial, believing (like Wakley) that: 'An editor needs, and must have, enemies; he can't do without them. Woe be unto the journalist of whom all men say good things.'

Hart tried to lead on many issues, but two of his most prominent campaigns were against 'baby farming'—giving infants (often bastards) over to carers for money, knowing that the carers often neglected and even murdered them—and 'secret remedies'—medicines that did not declare their constituents.

Baby farming was first raised in the *BMJ* in 1865, two years before Hart became editor.[9] In his first year as editor the journal carried a story on the inquest on four children who had all died under the care of the same 'nurse'. The journal also published several leading articles on the subject. In 1868 Hart put an advertisement in a newspaper as a father-to-be, offering money for adoption. He received 333 replies and identified Mrs X, who had seven malnourished infants living in her care in dreadful squalor. In the previous two years she had registered seven deaths of infants under one year. Articles in the journal led to questions in parliament. More cases were reported in 1870 and Hart formed with others the Infant Life Protection Society. He was also appointed chairman of the BMA's Parliamentary Bills Committee in 1872. A bill was drafted and enacted in 1872. It proved to be a weak bill and a much stronger bill was passed in 1877.

The problem was not solved. In 1896 Mrs Dyer of Reading was executed for strangling her charges and throwing them into the Thames. The *BMJ* published a six-part series on 'baby farming and its evils'. The child protection movement grew enormously at this time and the National Society for the Prevention of Cruelty to Children was founded in 1889. The problem still persists at the beginning of the 21st century—indeed, the week that I wrote the first draft of this chapter the first *BMJ* editorial described a failure of the authorities to prevent the killing of a child.[75]

Ernest Hart and the *BMJ* didn't defeat baby farming on their own, and Lock argued in his quote above that it was less Hart's role as editor and more his chairmanship of the BMA Parliamentary Committee and his social contacts that led to the change. But Peter Bartrip in his history of the *BMJ* concludes: 'The Journal did not singlehandedly cause the Infant Life Protection Act to be passed, but it undoubtedly exerted a powerful influence.'[9] We can probably never separate out the role of the journal from broader influences, but, as I argue below, journals seem to be good at putting issues onto the professional and public agenda.

At the end of the 19th century proprietary medicines that contained poisons and addictive substances were freely available. In 1890 the *BMJ* published a leading article that proposed a ban on any proprietary medicine unless all the ingredients were listed.[9] In 1891 the BMA Parliamentary Committee, which was still chaired by Hart, demanded prosecutions. It conducted analyses of the medicines and sent them to the government. Prosecutions followed.

This campaign was continued by Hart's successor, Dawson Williams, and in 1903 the journal published the constituents of remedies, beginning with treatments for epilepsy. 'With one exception they are weak preparations of well known drugs supplied at considerably more than the usual cost, and administered without the adjustment of dose to the needs of the particular patient, which is, after all, the most essential part in the treatment of epilepsy by bromide salts. The exception contains an old fashioned herb once praised by the superstitious, but abandoned time and again even by them.'[9]

These analyses were gathered together and published in 1909 in a book called *Secret remedies: what they cost and what they contain*. Despite newspapers, which were profiting from advertisements for the remedies, refusing to advertise or review the book it sold out in one month: by 1910 some 62,000 copies had been sold. A parliamentary committee was appointed to consider the problem, but then the war interrupted activities. It was another 20 years before quack remedies were brought under legal control. Again the *BMJ* played a prominent part in this process, although many other groups participated.

This question of whether journals lead or follow is similar to the question of whether the mass media lead or follow, and some in the discipline of 'media studies' have addressed exactly this question. The story of Watergate is often cited as a classic case of the media leading people on what to think. It was in June 1972 that five men broke into the campaign headquarters of the Democrat party. The incident received extensive publicity from the *Washington Post*, but initially there was little public interest. Yet the press kept on and by April 1973 over 90% of the American population knew the word 'Watergate'. In 1974 President Nixon was forced from office.

Did the media depose the president? Clearly they didn't do so alone, but they played a crucial role. Maxwell McCombs and Donald Shaw, two pioneers in media studies, have developed the theory of 'agenda setting'.[76,77] This means that: 'We judge as important what the media judge as important.' Bernard Cohen, a political scientist from the University of Wisconsin, puts it this way: 'The press may not be successful much of the time in telling people what to think, but it is stunningly successful in telling its readers what to think about.' This chimes with a saying of Hugh Clegg, editor of the *BMJ* from 1947 to 1965, 'A subject that needs reform should be kept before the public until it demands reform.'

McCombs and Shaw analysed the 1968 presidential race between Richard Nixon and Hubert Humphrey to see if they could work out whether the media were leading or reflecting public opinion.[76] They looked at nine print and broadcast media used by Chapel Hill residents and ranked stories by position and length. They considered five major issues: foreign policy, law and order, fiscal policy, public welfare and civil rights. They then looked at how undecided voters ranked these issues and found that they ranked them exactly the same as the media.

But which came first, the media agenda or the voters' agenda? There have been many subsequent studies and the general finding is that the media interest comes first.[77] Later work suggests that agenda setting works best when people are interested in a subject but very uncertain about what to think.[77] For example, I own a dog and hence I am interested in animal experimentation, but I am very uncertain about what the risks and benefits might be.

Nobody, as far as I know, has conducted any studies like this with medical journals, but it might be that the findings can be generalized from the mass media to general medical journals. If so, journals can put issues on the agenda and do have some influence on how people think about them—a limited form of leadership.

Another insight into leadership can be gained from studying campaigns. Many campaigns fail, but some succeed spectacularly. Why? The Institute for Healthcare Improvement in the United States is running a campaign to reduce unnecessary deaths in hospital, many the result of medical error. The campaign is called 'The 100,000 Lives Campaign', and its slogan is 'Some is not a number, soon is not a time'. Before launching the campaign the institute studied political campaigns—and identified six essential features: platform, measurement, communication, field, funds and values. The start is a clear, scientifically sound, highly developed *platform* or message. *Measurement* is essential to know if the campaign is succeeding, and *communication* must be constant, two way and involve many different media. Impact will depend on signing up many people and institutions (creating a *field* force), and The 100,000 Lives Campaign has signed up some 2000 hospitals. *Funds* are essential, but so are explicit *values*; the values of The 100,000 Lives Campaign include 'all in' but 'staying on message'.

I don't know of a medical journal that has campaigned so carefully, and perhaps a more important question than 'Whether journals can lead?' is 'What must they do to make change happen?'

Studies on leadership emphasize five characteristics of leadership and I want to end this chapter by seeing if journals have displayed them and shown leadership.

The first characteristic is that leaders set a *vision*. The *BMJ* did this with wanting to abolish baby farming and secret remedies. The vision was clear and understandable, as it is with wanting to get rid of smoking. But often it's much harder to paint a clear vision, especially when the aim is to create rather than abolish something. Abolition we can all grasp, but to convey a compelling vision of something entirely new is hard. Stephen Lock and Drummond Rennie had a vision of the processes that lead to journals being based on evidence, but what is the aim, for example, with healthcare reform? In the United States it might be 'universal coverage', but what is the vision for the majority of countries that already have universal coverage?

The second job of leaders is to *motivate* people to want to achieve the vision. This is difficult for journals. They do not want to commit the cardinal sin of boring their readers, but they have to keep returning to the subject. They must come at it in different ways. The *BMJ* kept on with the subjects of baby farming and quack medicines for more than 20 years, finding different ways to cover the subjects. Some journals struggle now to remind readers of the gross inequalities in the world, but they have to avoid 'compassion fatigue' by finding new ways to present the subject.

Third, leaders *inspire trust*. Journals try hard to achieve trust, but at the same time they must show all sides of debates. The *BMJ* asked doctors in Britain whom they trusted, and they replied that they trusted journals much more than they trusted the government or the NHS. Trust may come not from sticking relentlessly to a point of view but from being open and truthful, even when what is being published undermines your traditional message. Trust is, of course, one of the main arguments for editorial independence. Readers trust that editors have a fair peer review process and are independently making decisions on what to put before their readers. If there is any hint that hidden political or business processes are influencing those decisions, then trust can be lost. And trust takes years to build but can be destroyed in an instant.

Fourth, leaders *empower* and journals can do this by providing information on which their readers and others can take action. This was the case with both baby farming and particularly with the quack medicines where the analyses were useful to both individuals and organizations. *Tobacco Control* is doing this now by providing its readers with a constant flow of information that is useful ammunition in the battle to prevent the enormous harm from tobacco.

Finally, leaders *work with others*—other media and other organizations. Again this happened with both baby farming and quack remedies. The *BMJ* in 2003 planned a campaign to refresh and promote academic medicine worldwide. We realized that if we were to have the faintest hope of success we would need to work with as many other organizations as we could muster. We did so and yet the campaign achieved very little.

I must confess that most of my conscious attempts to achieve change through the *BMJ* failed. We were part of the Rationing Agenda Group which argued for open debate on the inevitability of rationing healthcare. England and Wales do now have the National Institute for Health and Clinical Excellence which makes semi-transparent decisions on which treatments will be available within the NHS—but it refuses to use the word rationing. The *BMJ* participated in the development of the Tavistock Principles, which was an ethical code for everybody in healthcare not just individual professions. After a flurry of activity the principles were forgotten.

These campaigns may have failed because the leaders were too far ahead of those they were trying to lead: they were proposing action on subjects that seemed unimportant to those who might have followed. The research in Chapel Hill suggested that the media could be only slightly ahead of their readers. Leaders must somehow create their visions from a deep understanding of the thinking of those they would lead. The vision can then be compelling.

My cautious conclusion is that journals can lead, in limited ways. And perhaps—as both Thomas Wakley and Ernest Hart clearly believed—they have a duty to do so. It may be hubris, but I believe that medical journals can lead—less by achieving precise reform but more by putting issues firmly on the agenda. I also have a hypothesis that journals are most likely to achieve real change when they concentrate on subjects that are close to them and work together. Thus real progress has been made with studying peer review and improving statistics in medical journals, subjects close to journals and where they have worked together. Where journals worked together on subjects that were not close to them—like ageing and emergent diseases—they have made little progress. Similarly, if a journal promotes a change close to the journal but alone it will achieve little. The *BMJ*'s campaign for open peer reviews is perhaps an example. Where journals campaign alone on subjects not close to them they are perhaps bound to fail—as my stories in the previous paragraph illustrate.

In my years at the *BMJ* we tried to lead by promoting evidence-based medicine, encouraging doctors and patients to work in partnership, reminding the rich world constantly of its obligations to the poor world, battling against research misconduct, hastening the flow of information to the developing world, securing the independence of medicine from the pharmaceutical industry, promoting patient safety and emphasizing the importance of a 'good death'. History will attempt to judge if we had any success, but even its judgement will be uncertain.

►5

What are and what should be the values of medical journals?

I don't know of a medical journal that explicitly declares its values, but all journals—just like all organizations—have them. They are simply implicit rather than explicit. As journals flourish in a place where medicine, science, public health, journalism, healthcare and business meet they may pick up values from all of those disciplines. And often those values conflict.

Most medical journals think of themselves primarily as part of medicine, and so they start with the values of medicine—and medicine is the discipline relevant to medical journals which has the deepest ethical roots. The Hippocratic Oath, still valued by many but thought hopelessly outdated by others, is the inevitable starting point for describing the values of medicine. (It is reproduced in Appendix 1.[78]) It begins by emphasizing respect for your teacher and has the feel that your first commitment is not to your patients, as might be expected, but to the rest of the 'tribe'. It happened as well in Hippocrates' time to be an exclusively male tribe.

Respect for your teacher is straight away a problem for journals. Both Thomas Wakley and Ernest Hart, the great 19th century editors of the *Lancet* and *BMJ* respectively, were far from respectful of their teachers. The essence of 'evidence-based medicine', which is transforming medicine, is that you rely not on experts, who are often wrong, but on evidence. 'In God we trust', goes the American joke, 'but all others must bring data'. Being respectful is not a journalistic value. Indeed, journalists are taught to be distrustful of authority. Scientific values too are about testing the old ideas until they break and new ones are needed.

It is of course possible to combine respect for your teachers and the past with the urge to question what you are taught and move inquiry on. That is perhaps a value that is shared by medicine with science and journalism, but the original Hippocratic Oath described a claustrophobic world where the sacred teaching was passed on from master to pupil. Teaching was encouraged but only within the tribe. You teach 'pupils who have signed the covenant and have taken an oath according to the medical law, but no one else'. Some journals have catered for a closed world, where the language is arcane, identical values assumed, and intimate details of patients revealed on the assumption that only members of the tribe will see the material. All of this is anachronistic. Editors of journals cannot assume that their journals will be seen only by their fellow professionals. 'The whole world's watching', chanted American anti-Vietnam demonstrators in the 1960s as they were hauled away by the National Guard. It's true for journals.

Passing on information is central to journals, but 'teaching' implies more: teaching is an active process that involves interaction and change in both the teacher and the pupil. Many journals have not valued education in the broader sense: they have simply not used every means possible to improve the educational value of their material. One of the BMJ Publishing Group's journals, *Heart*, has in recent years placed a heavy emphasis on education. It had always published original research and some review articles, but a few years ago it consciously created an education section. It set educational objectives, created a curriculum, and then provided first class—but not scientifically original—material to cover the curriculum. Quickly that section became the best read part of the journal. Now *Heart* is using the web to provide interactive cases for learning. It has decided that education is a core value. Most journals have not taken such a step.

Healing the sick is of course core to medicine—and to most medical journals. Some journals are, however, more to do with basic science, public health, and health services or policy. David Slawson and Allen Shaughnessy have also observed that many of the articles published in medical journals are not what they have cleverly called 'POEMS' (patient oriented evidence that matters).[8] As a student I often fretted that too much of medicine was for the benefit of doctors rather than patients, and some journals seem to reflect that world.

Louis Lasagna, academic dean of the School of Medicine at Tufts University, wrote an updated version of the Hippocratic Oath that is used in many American medical schools today. (This is reproduced in Appendix 2.[79]) In it he says more on healing the sick, urging the avoidance of 'overtreatment and therapeutic nihilism', and reminding students that 'there is art to medicine as well as science, and that warmth, sympathy, and understanding may outweigh the surgeon's knife or the chemist's drug'. Some journals set great store by this human side of medicine. The *Lancet*, a journal famous for both its radical stance and science, has emphasized the medical humanities, and the BMJ Publishing Group has published a supplement to the *Journal of Medical Ethics* called *Medical Humanities*. The *BMJ* published a piece called 'The inhumanity of medicine', by David Weatherall, probably Britain's most respected doctor, and it produced a huge response.[80]

Lasagna also included in his oath the sentence: 'I will prevent disease whenever I can, for prevention is preferable to cure.'[79] Placing prevention above cure is one of medicine's values that is often poorly observed, but some journals—for example, *Preventive Medicine*—emphasize this value.

The ancient oath talks of keeping the sick (and it's clearly plural) from 'harm and injustice'. This would seem to encourage the social role that has been very important to some journals—for example, the 19th century *BMJ*.[9] Some journals are nervous about straying beyond 'strictly medicine' into 'politics'. I explored this issue in chapter 3 and my conclusion was that it was impossible to avoid being political to some extent—partly because to attempt to be apolitical is in itself a political step.

The modern oath by Lasagna says: 'I will remember that I remain a member of society, with special obligations to all my fellow human beings, those sound of mind and body as well as the infirm.'[79] Doctors in other words cannot forget that they are members of a broader society and that they have 'special obligations'.

The Hippocratic Oath is strongly against euthanasia and abortion. Many countries have legalized abortion, making this part of the Hippocratic Oath particularly anachronistic. But many doctors—especially those who are Roman Catholics or Muslims—remain unhappy with the legalization of abortion. Some journals, particularly those intended for doctors of particular religions, may make it a fundamental value to oppose abortion. But do all journals need to adopt a particular position? Many do not. They publish widely different and often conflicting views. Some may try to avoid the subject.

The ancient Hippocratic Oath puts strong emphasis on confidentiality: 'What I may see or hear in the course of the treatment or even outside of the treatment in regard to the life of men, which on no account one must spread abroad, I will keep to myself, holding such things shameful to be spoken about.' Confidentiality is clearly an important value for medical practice. Patients must be able to tell their doctors everything if an accurate diagnosis is to be made. But confidentiality cannot be absolute. The law in Britain requires doctors to break confidentiality if they suspect child abuse. Clearly, if a doctor diagnoses epilepsy in a pilot of a jumbo jet who refuses to tell his employers, then the doctor must break confidentiality.

Confidentiality is a less clear value for journals to uphold. In fact they have tied themselves in knots. First, there is the confidentiality of patients. Editors and readers of journals used to assume that publishing case reports that didn't give the patient's name was not a breach of confidentiality. They assumed this partly because only doctors read journals, so the information was kept within the 'tribe'. They (I should say we) also underestimated how easy it is for somebody somewhere to recognize the case. I will write more about this in chapter 13, but for now I'll simply say that we moved to requiring written consent from the patient in almost all circumstances.[81] The General Medical Council, the body that regulates British doctors, adopted similarly strict standards. But then when I was at the *BMJ* we concluded that we had overdone it and retreated.[82] There is still uncertainty.

The *BMJ* also tended to adopt confidentiality in its relationships with authors. Thus the journal would not tell a third party whether or not an author had submitted a paper to it. But why did the *BMJ*—and most other journals—adopt such a strict standard? The *BMJ* did so because the editors are mostly doctors and it was easy to extend the rules of confidentiality with patients to the journal's relationship with authors. It avoided having to invent a new code—to think, in other words. But why should information on whether an author has submitted a study be confidential? It's hard to see why and journals may well be moving to a world where studies when submitted are immediately posted on the web. But I can think of at least one good reason why such information shouldn't be confidential. It allows quacks to give information to gullible journalists, saying that they have submitted their studies to the *New England Journal of Medicine*, the *BMJ*, the *Lancet* or any journal. This gives the studies a spurious second-hand respectability that they do not deserve.

Journals have traditionally as well required peer reviewers to keep confidential studies they have been sent to review. There is some logic here in that ideas and data might be stolen if distributed too widely before publication. But ironically the secrecy of the process, with authors routinely not knowing who has reviewed their papers, probably makes it easier for ideas to be stolen. If I knew that Professor Plum had reviewed my study then it would require near pathological aplomb on the part of Plum to submit stolen ideas to another journal.

I suggest that by simply transferring the value of confidentiality from medicine to themselves, journals have created less than optimum values. They need to think through their own values.

I've related the values of the Hippocratic Oath to the values of journals, but the oath was created 2000 years ago—and values change. About 10 years ago the British medical profession was urged by the then chief medical officer, Ken Calman, to consider its 'core values'.[83] This was partly a response to a feeling that medicine was losing its way and doctors becoming disillusioned. The first summit of British medical organizations since the 1960s came up with the following core values: caring, integrity, competence, confidentiality, responsibility and advocacy.[84] These are what the Americans disparagingly call 'motherhood and apple pie'. A particular problem was that the implications and possible contradictions of the values were not thought through. A philosopher friend was scornful that the massed brains of British medicine could manage nothing better.

(An aside that I hope you might find interesting. There was intense debate and a major split over one particular value. The older members of the gathering, the majority, thought that a central value of medicine was to put your patient first, even before your own family. Many older doctors describe, almost with pride, 'never having seen their children grow up'. Younger members disagreed strongly. 'Not only do I think it's wrong, but I wouldn't want to be looked after by doctors who put patients before their families. They would be weird people.' The division continues.)

Although the values proposed by the good and the great of medicine don't seem very valuable, those proposed by Ken Calman, who suggested the meeting, are: a high standard of ethics; continuing professional development; the ability to work in a team; concern with health as well as illness; patient and public focus; concern with clinical standards, outcomes, effectiveness and audit; ability to define outcomes, interest in change and improvement, research and development; and ability to communicate.[83]

I find it interesting that he put 'a high standard of ethics' first. This applies as much to journals as it does to doctors and implies two things, the second of which I have only recently come to understand. The first implication is that ethical problems are not something that crop up once a year when you have to make a dramatic decision on whether or not to switch off the ventilator for somebody rendered brain dead in criminal circumstances. Ethical decisions arise all day every day in both medicine and editing. Most doctors, I think, now understand that ethical issues are ubiquitous. Many editors don't. I was once at a seminar for editors on ethical issues, and Raanan Gillon, who at the time was editor of the *Journal of Medical Ethics* and who was conducting the seminar, began by asking the dozen or so assembled editors to describe ethical problems they'd encountered recently. Almost all said that they hadn't encountered any ethical problems. This was, I must say, at least eight years ago. It might be different now, particularly since the founding of the World Association of Medical Editors and the Committee on Publication Ethics (see chapter 12).[85]

Calman's second implication is that 'high ethical standards' or 'integrity' is not something you have and lose if you fall into wicked ways. You need to work every day at integrity. You are constantly presented with ethical issues where it is far from clear what is the 'right' thing to do. In fact there may be no 'right' thing. You have alternatives, none of which is wholly wrong or wholly right. To flourish in such a morally complex universe you need to be helped with how to think about the problems that confront you and to constantly exercise your ethical muscles. You probably also need help and more than one mind for the problem—together with a transparent process for identifying and addressing ethical problems. That is why the *BMJ* founded an ethics committee and is the reason (apart from an excuse to spend eight weeks in Venice) that I am writing this book.[86]

Calman's second value was continuing professional development, meaning that you are never complete as a professional. You must learn constantly, not least because you are continually presented with new challenges and new circumstances. This is as true for journals and editors as it is for doctors, and yet traditionally many medical journals have been edited by academics who have no training in editing. One day they are professors of cardiology, the next editors of major journals. Nobody would launch into being a cardiologist, inserting a catheter into an artery of the heart, without training. Yet it is routine the other way round. Editors similarly often do not seek training and to improve their craft. Drummond Rennie, the organizer of the congresses on peer review, castigated editors at the end of the last congress for not coming in greater numbers and for neglecting their craft.[87]

The ability to work in a team is another excellent value for editors. One of my favourite sayings is that 'any journal that can't be better than its editor' is doomed. Yet there is a long tradition of editors working alone, like St Jerome translating the bible in his desert cave. Good journals depend on many different ideas, contacts, views and attitudes. Diversity is a virtue, but will be beneficial only if it is combined with effective team work.

'Concern with health as well as illness' and 'patient and public focus' are values that seem essential to good journals, but 'concern with clinical standards, outcomes, effectiveness, and audit' again is an excellent value for journals. All journals would claim to be high quality, but, as I describe in chapter 6, there is lots of evidence of poor quality. There was no tradition of measuring the effectiveness of journals and their processes, and little tradition of audit. Many journals take months to make decisions on whether or not they will publish papers and then months, even years, to publish them. Some papers fall into 'black holes', and the standard of what might be called 'customer service' is generally lousy. Journals have been able to get away with it because they are mostly equally bad.

'Ability to define outcomes, interest in change and improvement, research and development' are values related to what I've already discussed, but I've always been interested that professors of neurology who have learnt to base their neurological opinions and practice on evidence are happy to make strong statements about ways of editing journals with no evidence. The tradition of research into journal processes— what I sometimes pretentiously call 'evidence-based editing and publishing'—is only at the beginning.[88]

'The ability to communicate' would seem like the *sine qua non* value of journals (and in that spirit, and despite horror from the literati, the *BMJ* banned Latin and Greek because many readers didn't understand them and many authors got their classical languages wrong), but many journals have bothered little with the clarity and comprehensibility of what they publish. Many studies have shown that journals have very low readability scores,[89] and Michael O'Donnell, one of British medicine's great medical communicators, can keep an audience laughing for an hour with egregious examples of medical writing.[90,91] He calls doctors' style of writing 'decorated municipal gothic'. It's full of wind and pomposity and designed to make the author look important, not to let the reader understand. Journals also tend to look awful, with pages and pages of unbroken prose.

So far I have discussed the values of medicine and how they may apply to medical journals, but I want now to move on to other relevant values. I was part of a group called the Tavistock Group (after Tavistock Square where we first met) that tried to derive a set of principles that might apply to everybody in healthcare, not just doctors.[92] We observed—following the American ethicist Will Gaylin[93]—that much of the universal disarray in healthcare arises from people trying to solve ethical problems with technical solutions. We also observed that conflicts in values among those in healthcare—particularly doctors and managers—were part of the problem. Doctors with their ancient ethical codes might use those codes more as battle implements than as a means to elucidate a problem. The Tavistock Group, which was predominantly American and British, went through an elaborate process to derive principles for everybody in healthcare. I have to say that they have not been widely adopted, but they are useful for this process of exploring the values of medical journals.

Rights: People have a right to health and healthcare.

Balance: Care of individual patients is central, but the health of populations is also our concern.

Comprehensiveness: In addition to treating illness, we have an obligation to ease suffering, minimize disability, prevent disease and promote health.

Cooperation: Healthcare succeeds only if we cooperate with those we serve, each other and those in other sectors.

Improvement: Improving healthcare is a serious and continuing responsibility.

Safety: Do no harm.

Openness: Being open, honest and trustworthy is vital in healthcare.

Many of these principles overlap with values I've already discussed, but some provide a new twist. The principle that healthcare is a right is uncontroversial almost everywhere apart from America, but one of the leading American journals, the *Annals of Internal Medicine*, has argued that the right to healthcare ought to be incorporated into the American constitution.[94] (As my friend, Ian Morrison, observes, only in

America is carrying a gun a right and healthcare a privilege.) The principle that health might be a right seems at first strange. Isn't it like suggesting a right to be tall or beautiful?

Amartya Sen, Nobel prize winning economist, explained to a meeting organized by the Tavistock Group why it was not absurd to make health a right. He began by explaining how Immanuel Kant distinguished between 'perfect' and 'imperfect' obligations. Perfect obligations impose a duty on particular people and institutions, whereas imperfect obligations do not. In many countries healthcare has become a perfect obligation (for instance, in Britain, where the government has accepted the duty to provide healthcare), although it remains an imperfect obligation in others. But imperfect obligations can move—perhaps through legislation—to become perfect obligations.

By making health a right, Sen argued, we gain people's attention: a debate begins on who might have the duty to try to achieve health for everybody. There is a pressure to begin implementation. And it's important also to make health a human right because the main health determinants are not healthcare but sanitation, nutrition, housing, social justice, employment and the like. Health as a right is a value that many medical journals might like to adopt.

'Do no harm' is a central value of medicine and the Tavistock Group thought that it should adopt the principle for everybody. It is not only doctors who can do harm but also politicians creating new policies and managers implementing new systems. Doctors are sadly familiar with the idea that they can act in what they think is the best interest of patients but do them more harm than good. But this is perhaps a less familiar idea to politicians and managers who deal in words not knives and drugs. Some are perplexed by the principle 'do no harm' because they know that all effective interventions may harm, but the intention behind the principle is not that practitioners should never make an intervention: it is that they should struggle to maximize benefit, minimize harm and reduce error.

Is this a principle that journals should adopt? I think that it would be hard, although many—particularly public health practitioners—would like journals to adopt such a principle. Perhaps if the *Lancet* had done so it would not have published the study that linked the measles, mumps and rubella (MMR) vaccine with autism (see chapter 2). But journals must surely value debate and must have a bias towards publishing rather than not publishing. And because they deal very much with provisional truths, the nature of science, there is a huge uncertainty about what may flow from what they publish. If journals were to become anxious about everything they might publish that might cause harm then they would, I fear, become paralysed.

As I read this previous paragraph, some three months after I first wrote it, I worried that it seemed breathtakingly complacent. After arguing strongly that not only doctors but also politicians and managers should adopt the principle, I suggest that it would be bad for journals. It reads to me now as if I was supporting the idea that editors could be cavalier about doing harm—because of some higher commitment to open debate. The position reads to me now overstated, but rather than simply revise the paragraph I thought that I should keep it to illustrate how I—and I suspect many other editors—are not as bothered by harm as perhaps we should be.

Medical students who come and worked with us at the *BMJ* were often able to publish something within the journal—usually a news story—within days of arriving. I told them that: 'Medical journalism is not like neurosurgery. You can't go guddling around in people's brains a few days after beginning neurosurgery, but you can write a news story in your first week at a medical journal. Most students do.' Maybe this statement betrays the same complacency about harm.

After first writing the overstated paragraph I became embroiled in a controversy over a highly critical obituary that the *BMJ* published, as I discussed in chapter 2.[50,95] It described the dead man, the founder of the pharmaceutical company Scotia, as a 'snake oil salesman'. The family were understandably upset. They were harmed; so, they argued, was the reputation of the dead man. A complaint was made to the Press Complaints Commission, the body that self-regulates the press in Britain, and we apologized for the upset we caused but not for publishing the obituary. Even if it was 'true' (which of course we believed it to be), should we have published such a thing? My conclusion today is that journals must think about harm, and there will be times when they shouldn't publish because of the harm they might cause. Journals have clearly adopted that position in relation to publishing information about patients without their consent.

The problem is to balance 'good' and 'harm'. There is substantial good in the free flow of information, even when particular pieces of information are trivial, caviling and offensive. Hence the high value placed on free speech and the freedom to publish, but editors cannot use the excuse of the substantial good to publish whatever they want regardless of harm—which is what I seemed almost to be arguing. Editors must consider harm, but—unlike doctors—I don't think that we should put it first. The bias towards publishing should come first. Many readers will, I'm sure, not agree.

I again had to consider the issue of harm when *Nature* published a news piece in which AIDS researchers criticized the *BMJ* for posting on its website many rapid responses (electronic letters to the editor) that argued that HIV was not the cause of AIDS.[96] The AIDS researchers argued that the *BMJ* was causing harm by giving respectability to a scientifically ridiculous case that was leading to some authorities— for example, in South Africa—holding back antiretroviral treatments that would save lives. I responded by arguing for free speech and suggesting that most readers of the *BMJ* were well aware of the speciousness of the arguments.[97] The rapid responses appeared on the *BMJ*'s website, not in print where the journal is more selective. I don't believe that any serious harm resulted, but if the critics could have shown me corpses I would probably have thought differently.

The Tavistock principle of being 'open, honest and trustworthy' might be both the most banal and the most profound.[94] Nobody could argue against being open, honest and trustworthy, and yet every day in every healthcare system people fail on all three counts. It's difficult to be open and honest about deficiencies in your hospital or practice, or the bleak fate awaiting a patient. There's always a way to 'soften the blow' or 'be economical with the truth'. You worry that you might lose the trust of patients or the public if you tell the unvarnished truth, yet nothing destroys trust faster than being found to have been deceived.

We live in a world, I believe, where, whether we like it or not, what is not open is assumed to be biased, corrupt or incompetent until proved otherwise. Yet journals are often not very open. Classically their peer review systems are closed in that neither authors nor readers know who have reviewed papers. Journals are also not open about their finances.

I want now to turn to the values of journalism, many of which ought to be fundamental to journals but haven't been. Journalists put great value on being interesting. One of the worst things that you can say about a mass media publication is that it is boring. Medical journals have not worried about being boring. A closely related journalistic value is putting readers first. Without readers a newspaper is nothing. Medical journals, in contrast, have often put authors first. Journalists also see themselves as being on the side of the governed rather than the governors. Medical journals have, in contrast, often been organs of the establishment. Innovation and creativity are important within journalism. A publication should innovate and reward creativity. These have not been fundamental values for medical journals, but I believe they should be.

What about 'getting things right'? I remember once being shocked by a BBC reporter declaring at a press conference, 'It is not my duty to get things right.' How could this be, I wondered? He explained, 'I get things as right as I can, but I know that I often have only part of the story. Sometimes people won't tell me things. They deliberately keep them hidden. And I'm always against the clock. I don't have time to check every fact, speak to everybody involved. I have to get a story out.' All this is true, particularly with electronic media. We would be unlikely to watch CNN if it were to say, 'Something important has probably happened, but we won't be telling you until we've checked every fact and spoken to all parties. We'll hope to bring you a report tomorrow.'

The idea that we can arrive at 'the truth' is anyway an illusion. Ask five people to give you an account of what happened in front of all their eyes 20 minutes ago, and you will have five accounts which will probably conflict. Historians know that truth is unachievable. EH Carr, a great historian, famously argued that history tells you more about the time when it was written than the time that is written about.[98] Most modern historians would agree.

Scientists too would agree. Science deals in provisional truths. The theory of science proposed by Karl Popper is that you propose a falsifiable hypothesis to explain the facts you observe.[99] (The falsifiable part is important: it is unscientific to create hypotheses that cannot be falsified, which is why some fundamentals like 'love' and 'freedom' are not easily investigated by science.) You then try as hard as you can to devise experiments that will show your hypothesis to be false. Until an experiment disproves your hypothesis it stays intact—but as a hypothesis not truth. The expectation of science is that eventually the hypothesis will be found to be false and a more elegant one proposed. An alternative theory of science proposed by Thomas Kuhn is that scientists fit together pieces of data to create a paradigm for explaining the world.[100] New data emerge, and the model of the world is adapted. Eventually the paradigm is so shaky, so patched that it collapses, and a new paradigm emerges. Newtonian physics replaced Aristotelian physics but was in its turn replaced by Einstein's theories.

Science sets great store by evidence, and so should medical journals. Medicine has often not been scientific. Medical grandees have pronounced on methods of diagnosis and the best treatments, and medical journals and ordinary doctors have followed. Increasingly at the *BMJ* we have been concerned with raising the standard of the science we published and avoiding conclusions that are based on poor evidence.

Interestingly the values of scientists, journalists and historians combine to be highly sceptical about claims to be publishing the truth. We at the *BMJ* did not believe that we were publishing truth. But this did not mean that we were consciously publishing untruths. We inclined towards the dictum of CP Scott, the great editor of the *Manchester Guardian*, that 'comment is free, but facts are sacred'.[101] We hoped that the 'facts' that we publish were true. If somebody told us that there were 234 patients in a trial, then we trusted (note the word) the authors that there were. If we were writing pieces ourselves we checked every fact we could. We expected journalists who worked for us to do the same. But—perhaps unlike Scott—I do not believe the world divides neatly into 'facts' and 'comment'. If I say that there are six people in a room that is a verifiable fact. If I say two of them are bad people that is comment. But what if I say two of them were dark skinned? Is this a fact or a comment? I think that it's somewhere between the two. Analyse this chapter and you will find that you cannot put every assertion into two neat boxes, one labelled 'facts' and the other 'comment'.

Journalists and scientists also share a 'publish and be dammed' view of the world. Both exist to publish. A scientist who never publishes is as dead as a journalist who never publishes. For both too it is often important to be the first to publish. Thus both journalistic and scientific ethics support the publication of the paper linking the MMR vaccine with autism (see chapter 2).[1] For the journalist it's a strong story and it would be wrong to keep it from the public. For the scientist it's data, albeit weak data, supporting a potentially important hypothesis.

Public health values, which are understandably utilitarian (the greatest good for the greatest number), would not perhaps support publication—and certainly many public health doctors have condemned the publication. The benefit for the many, their argument goes, is small. The paper contains very weak, possibly (even probably) misleading data supporting a connection between the vaccine and autism. Even if the connection is real it's unlikely to be important in public health terms. But the risks are many. People may be put off having their children vaccinated, and then the infections may return. Herd immunity might be lost.

Great enthusiasts for public health might even be strongly against publishing something that was highly likely to be true and yet which might have negative effects on a population. Consider, for example, the evidence that smoking might be beneficial for some particular conditions—for example, inflammatory bowel disease. This does seem to be the case, although even for an individual with inflammatory bowel disease the overall effect of smoking would probably be harmful because the small benefit to the bowel disease would be outweighed by harmful effects on heart, lung, brain, blood vessels and the many other organs damaged by smoking. The population risk is that this small 'positive' message on smoking might be used by tobacco companies and the public relations firms they employ to confuse the otherwise clear message that smoking is harmful. If even a few people, particularly young people with their lives before them, were to take up smoking (or fail to give up) then the overall harm would be large. The utilitarian public health doctor would see little benefit in publication, particularly in a major journal, and would advise against.

The *BMJ* experienced a storm of protest after publishing a study that suggested that passive smoking may not kill (see chapter 2).[51] The authors had links with the tobacco industry, as the journal declared. Many people were furious, and the BMA, the journal's owners, put out a press release dissociating itself from what it considered to be a flawed study. Some critics were upset that the *BMJ* should publish anything that undermined the case against tobacco, regardless of its 'truth'. Others objected to us publishing anything linked with the tobacco industry—partly because it gave respectability to the industry and partly because nothing linked with the industry could be believed.

The study presented us with an interesting clash of values. We were for health and against both tobacco and the industry. I resigned as an unpaid professor of medical journalism at Nottingham University because it accepted £3.8m from British American Tobacco. How then could I publish a study from the industry? The answer was that we put the scientific importance of publishing completed research above our concern about health. Some American journals have policies of refusing to publish research linked with the tobacco industry, but we decided in 1996 that such a policy was unscientific.[52]

This is back to journals doing harm. For me—and, I suspect, many editors—the idea of suppressing information and debate for some supposed greater good was unacceptable. The channels of information must flow freely and the debate must rage.

And might we in that debate publish information that we thought—or even knew—to be wrong? The answer from me was yes, but this was probably a step too far for many editors. As an editor I published information, particularly letters, with which I strongly disagreed and which in some sense I thought to be 'wrong'. I put a higher value on free speech and debate than on the value of 'truth'—partly because, as I've explained above, I think truth to be very slippery. It was obviously true to many that the sun went round the earth, and Galileo Galilei was put before the inquisition for suggesting otherwise. John Milton, whom I've already quoted, said that, 'If it come to prohibiting, there is not ought more likely to be prohibited than truth itself.'

This putting a very high value on debate and free speech came to the fore in intense discussions we had over 'rapid responses' (electronic letters) to the *BMJ*. We adopted a policy of posting within 24 hours all responses that were not obscene, libellous, incomprehensible, wholly insubstantial or included information on patients without accompanying consent. We posted around 20 a day and many were poorly written, inconsequential, ungrammatical, rude or plain bonkers. They also provided an excellent forum for mavericks and those with highly unpopular views. They were like a cross between the letters pages of *The Times*, conversations in a pub, questions after a lecture, and Speakers' Corner, a place in London where anybody can climb onto a soap box and say whatever he or she wants. They were also very international. Rapidly increasing numbers of people in the developing world had access to the web, and we were also quite happy to post responses in Italian–English or even in Italian (although responses in foreign languages were rarely sent).

For me—an irrepressible lover of free speech—these responses were a marvel of nature. In their sum they provide as rich a debate on health and medicine as was to be had anywhere. But even those with the strongest stomachs got bothered by them at time, particularly when people were rude, promoted crazy—even dangerous—ideas, or sent us a dozen responses every week. Twice we debated at our editorial board whether we should raise the bar and be more selective. Both times the board voted against, the last time unanimously.

One editorial aphorism that I value perhaps more than any other is that of the great pathologist and thinker Rudolf Virchow, 'Anybody,' he said, 'is free to make a fool of himself in my journal.' But after I left the journal the editorial team decided that it would raise the bar for rapid responses.[102] The weeds were choking the flowers.

So journals do have values, even if they rarely make them explicit. Different journals and different editors of the same journals will have different values, which must be a good thing and will add to the rich mix that will, I believe (and this is a value that a strictly religious person would not accept), lead to greater wisdom. But there are—and this may be overly bold—some values that should apply to all journals. Here's my list.

- Be interesting—don't be boring
- Set high store by debate
- Raise the quality of medical science
- Check facts
- Promote team work
- Improve
- Innovate
- Communicate clearly
- Promote high standards of ethics
- Be concerned with health and illness not just disease
- Encourage a public and patient focus
- Engage in research and audit
- Be open
- Celebrate creativity

Appendix 1 Hippocratic Oath—Classical version

I swear by Apollo Physician and
Asclepius and Hygieia and Panaceia
and all the gods and goddesses,
making them my witnesses, that I will
fulfill according to my ability and
judgment this oath and this covenant:

To hold him who has taught me this art
as equal to my parents and to live my

life in partnership with him, and if he is
in need of money to give him a share
of mine, and to regard his offspring as
equal to my brothers in male lineage
and to teach them this art—if they
desire to learn it—without fee and
covenant; to give a share of precepts and oral
instruction and all
the other learning to my sons and to the sons of him
who has
instructed me and to pupils who have signed the
covenant and
have taken an oath according to the medical law,
but no one else.

I will apply dietetic measures for the benefit of the
sick according
to my ability and judgment; I will keep them from
harm and
injustice.

I will neither give a deadly drug to anybody who
asked for it, nor
will I make a suggestion to this effect. Similarly I
will not give to a
woman an abortive remedy. In purity and holiness I
will guard my
life and my art.

I will not use the knife, not even on sufferers from
stone, but will
withdraw in favor of such men as are engaged in
this work.

Whatever houses I may visit, I will come for the
benefit of the sick,
remaining free of all intentional injustice, of all
mischief and in
particular of sexual relations with both female and
male persons,
be they free or slaves.

What I may see or hear in the course of the
treatment or even
outside of the treatment in regard to the life of men,

which on no
account one must spread abroad, I will keep to
myself, holding
such things shameful to be spoken about.

If I fulfill this oath and do not violate it, may it be
granted to me to
enjoy life and art, being honored with fame among
all men for all
time to come; if I transgress it and swear falsely,
may the opposite
of all this be my lot.

Translation from the Greek by Ludwig Edelstein: Edelstein L. *The Hippocratic Oath: text, translation, and interpretation*. Baltimore: Johns Hopkins Press, 1943.

Appendix 2   Hippocratic Oath—Modern version

I swear to fulfill, to the
best of my ability and
judgment, this covenant:

I will respect the
hard-won scientific gains
of those physicians in
whose steps I walk, and
gladly share such
knowledge as is mine
with those who are to
follow.

I will apply, for the benefit of the sick, all measures which are
required, avoiding those twin traps of overtreatment and
therapeutic nihilism.

I will remember that there is art to medicine as well as science,
and that warmth, sympathy, and understanding may outweigh the
surgeon's knife or the chemist's drug.

I will not be ashamed to say 'I know not,' nor will I fail to call in my
colleagues when the skills of another are needed for a patient's
recovery.

I will respect the privacy of my patients, for their problems are not disclosed to me that the world may know. Most especially must I tread with care in matters of life and death. If it is given me to save a life, all thanks. But it may also be within my power to take a life; this awesome responsibility must be faced with great humbleness and awareness of my own frailty. Above all, I must not play at God.

I will remember that I do not treat a fever chart, a cancerous growth, but a sick human being, whose illness may affect the person's family and economic stability. My responsibility includes these related problems, if I am to care adequately for the sick.

I will prevent disease whenever I can, for prevention is preferable to cure.

I will remember that I remain a member of society, with special obligations to all my fellow human beings, those sound of mind and body as well as the infirm.

If I do not violate this oath, may I enjoy life and art, respected while I live and remembered with affection thereafter. May I always act so as to preserve the finest traditions of my calling and may I long experience the joy of healing those who seek my help.

Written in 1964 by Louis Lasagna, Academic Dean of the School of Medicine at Tufts University, and used in many medical schools today.

Section 3: The processes of publishing medical research

6. The complexities and confusions of medical science

7. Peer review: a flawed process at the heart of science and journals

▶6

The complexities and confusions of medical science

'You open the papers one day and read that alcohol's bad for you. Two days later there's another report saying it makes you live longer. Do these scientists know what they're doing?' You must have heard such sentences. Scientists are sometimes inclined to blame the media, but the reality is that the study of health and disease is hard, incremental and full of false signals. I think it's important in a book like this to provide some insights into how difficult many of the studies published are both to do and to interpret. I don't want to provide a crash course in clinical epidemiology, but I will illustrate the difficulties by discussing how you can determine whether or not a treatment works together with some of the traps that you see commonly in medical journals.

This isn't an easy chapter. I've tried to write this book so that people can read it without too much effort, and Beth Kilcoyne, a writer and actress, who read the whole book in draft, told me that she could read the book easily—apart from this chapter. She found it turgid and was left wondering at the end 'Why bother publishing anything?' In my anxiety to make clear to readers the complexities and confusions of medical science I'd clearly gone too far. Progress in medicine may not be straightforward, but it has been dramatic in the past 60 years—and publishing research is central to making progress. It may be that most research papers disappear within a few years, but the same is true of literature: only a few great works survive for centuries. So publishing in medical journals is important, and I've tried in response to Beth's criticism to lighten this chapter. I don't, however, think that there is anything in the chapter that cannot be understood by anybody, and I hope that it doesn't sound patronizing if I suggest that it may be worth the effort of reading the chapter slowly and carefully.

I've chosen to use the example of trying to determine whether a treatment works because it is important to both patients and doctors. In addition, assessing evidence on whether or not a treatment is effective is simpler than working out whether or not a diagnostic test works, what the prognosis might be of a disease or what the adverse effects of a treatment might be. Nevertheless, the history of medicine is largely a history of ineffective and often dangerous treatments. 'The role of the doctor,' joked Voltaire, 'is to amuse the patient while nature takes its course.' It may for millennia have been acceptable to treat a patient based on a plausible theory or simple experience, but increasingly it isn't. New drugs must undergo rigorous testing in order to get onto the market, and slowly but surely surgical treatments are also being regulated.

The simplest way to see if a treatment works is to give it to a patient and see what happens. The resulting publication is called a case report and was for many years the mainstay of medical journals. But you don't need to be much of a scientist to see the limitations of such evidence. What would have happened if the patient hadn't been given the treatment? How do I know as a reader whether or not the reported patient is like my patient and whether or not what happened to that patient would happen to my patient?

And what about the 'placebo effect'? We know that whatever you do to patients about one-third of them will improve. There is also evidence that the more severe the intervention—for example, an operation rather than a pill—the more powerful will be the beneficial effect. (A friend of mine has applied for a licence for a drug called 'placebo'. There is overwhelming evidence from many trials showing that it works in any condition and has a powerful effect, more powerful than the many drugs that actually have rather limited effects.) New drugs are routinely tested against placebos, but using placebos in surgical trials is difficult: it means, for example, making incisions in patients' skins so that they think that they have had a full operation but actually not performing the operation. Ideally, new surgical treatments should be tested against such sham operations—and when they are, they are shown to be less effective than previously thought.

Then there is a powerful statistical force called 'regression to the mean (the average)'.[103] If you find somebody with, for example, high blood pressure, it is highly likely that the next time you measure his blood pressure it will be lower. Blood pressure like most biological variables (cholesterol, mood, heart rate) swings around, and if you measure the variable when it happens to be especially high or low—and so far from the mean—then the chances are that it will be closer to the mean the next time. The treatment might then seem to be working when in reality it is doing nothing. Much of the seeming effectiveness of antidepressants may result from regression to the mean. Patients are treated when particularly depressed and inevitably seem to improve as their mood returns towards the mean. Doctors and other readers of medical journals consistently underestimate the power of regression to the mean.

The next test for a treatment after giving it to a single patient is to give it to a group of patients—a series or a cohort in the jargon of medical journals. Reports on series of patients are still the staple diet of surgical journals, which is why surgical research has been compared unkindly to comic opera: such studies are not scientifically serious—and as such are a poor basis for surgical practice.[104] The problems that apply to case reports also apply to case series plus there is much room for manipulation, either conscious or unconscious.

The best way for a surgeon to get good results is to operate on people who don't need an operation in the first place. The way to get bad results is to operate on very sick people. This is one of the fundamental problems of 'league tables' of performance of surgeons or hospitals. Those who compile such tables are aware of the problem and so try to 'risk adjust'—statistically manipulate the results to allow for things like the age, sex, social class and degree of sickness of the patients. But this is an inexact science. Sometimes the 'risk adjustment' is overdone, encouraging surgeons to operate on sick patients because they know that their results will 'improve' as a result. Or surgeons may 'game' the process.[105] They might, for example, report patients who have smoked five cigarettes in their lives as smokers and so increase their patients' recorded risk (because smokers have poorer results from operations than non-smokers) and 'improve' the performance of the surgeon after risk adjustment.

Another problem with league tables, in passing, is that we all tend to underestimate the power of chance. We published a study in the *BMJ* in which a statistician calculated the range of results that would by chance alone occur in a year in a group of surgeons doing a small number of operations each year with a high failure rate.[106] The surgeon at the bottom of the list would have results several times worse than the average and many more times worse than the 'best surgeon'. It's hard to believe that such differences could all be due to chance, and yet by definition in this case they were. The following year the results would be completely different. 'The worst' might now be 'the best'. This illustrates the difficulty of us all wanting to be operated on by 'the best surgeon'. Not that we could anyway: she'd be run off her feet and all other surgeons would be unemployed. Plus nobody could ever get trained.

The problems of patient series and risk adjustment have been well illustrated by studies of the benefits of hormone replacement therapy for women at the menopause. It is a major, expensive and time consuming business to do a randomized trial (see below), and so with many treatments we have to make do initially with results from large cohorts of patients. So there are many reports of thousands of women, even tens of thousands, taking hormone replacement therapy. What happens to them is compared with what happens to women who didn't take hormone replacement therapy. (So this is one step up in terms of evidence from a simple series in that a comparison is made with a group not taking the treatment.) The women taking the therapy seem to have fewer deaths from heart disease, which is important because in women as in men heart disease is the most common form of death. So a small reduction in the risk of death can result in many lives being prolonged. This seems like an important benefit and is heavily promoted, not least by the companies which manufactured the treatments. (Although the *BMJ* was also rather carried away some years back with the benefits of the therapy and argued that every woman should take it.)

Unfortunately the women who take the therapy are not the same as those who don't. Women who take the therapy are likely to be better educated, richer, more concerned with their health, less likely to smoke, more likely to exercise and generally healthier. So it's not surprising that they have fewer deaths from heart disease. Statisticians 'risk adjusted' the data and many declared themselves satisfied that the therapy is truly beneficial. Those who are doubtful are denounced (not too strong a word) as naysayers. But when the first results were announced at the end of 2002 from a large randomized trial published in *JAMA* it emerged that the therapy made you more likely to suffer heart disease.[107]

This pattern of studies of a series of patients suggesting benefits from a treatment and randomized trials showing no benefit or even harm is repeated time and time again. I think that I see it happening now with various interventions for dementia. (A month after I wrote this sentence it emerged—from the same large randomized trial— that hormone replacement therapy, which had seemed to protect against dementia, actually made it more likely.[108] I'm not claiming supernatural powers but just illustrating the dangers of drawing premature conclusions from scientifically weak studies.)

These studies of hormone replacement therapy have compared women taking treatment with women not taking treatment. Another way to make a comparison is with patients treated in the past—'a before and after study'. This could potentially be better than a simultaneous comparison because everybody should have been treated with the old treatment in the past and the new now. This might then avoid the problem of the treated patients being fundamentally different from the untreated patients. But unfortunately there will be changes over time—in staff, the processes in the hospital, the weather and dozens of other things. So it is hard to be sure that any benefit you see in the group given the new treatment comes from the treatment rather than something else.

Then there is the problem of the 'Hawthorne effect', which was first noticed in studies conducted in the Hawthorne factory of Western Electric. The studies showed that the minute you started to study people results improved. The very fact of being studied led to improvement. So, if you make a comparison between patients you are studying and results from patients that you simply treated in the past but not as part of a study, then you may see benefits that result simply from the study not from the treatment.

One of the biggest problems of all in assessing the effectiveness of treatments is bias. Bias is a strong word and has overtones of naughtiness, but it simply means that if you think that a treatment may work (even subconsciously) then lo and behold it may seem to work even though in reality it doesn't. Bias might result from you trying harder in other ways with people receiving the treatment, excluding from the treatment patients who may be less likely to benefit, or taking measurements in patients in a different way. Or the patients, detecting your enthusiasm for the treatment and wanting to please you, will try and give you the results you want, telling you perhaps that they feel better when they don't. There are a thousand subtle ways in which bias can arise, and it's important to make clear that it is not dishonesty. Bias is unconscious and pervasive.

That's one reason why the double blind randomized trial—where the doctors, the patients and the researchers do not know who is being treated and who isn't—is so important. Allocating the patients to different groups randomly also means that the problem of patients being different in age, sex, social class, degree of sickness or many other ways that cannot be identified but may be important will also disappear. And it turns out that all the aspects of a trial matter. If patients are not adequately randomized (but allocated to groups alternately or by the first letter of their surname, the day of the week they are admitted to the trial, or whatever) or the trial is not properly double blind, then the results are distorted—usually the weaker the study the more likely it is to show that the treatment works. The bias is towards the positive.

But randomized trials are no panacea. The biggest problem with trials is that they have usually been too small.[109] If a treatment is so powerful that everybody who gets its lives and everybody who doesn't dies (and I don't think that there is such a treatment), then you probably don't need a randomized trial. But with most treatments you need to treat dozens of patients in order to have one fewer death or heart attack or whatever. This means that you need large trials—with perhaps thousands of patients—to be sure whether a treatment works or not. Unfortunately—perhaps because of the inherent over-optimism of doctors or perhaps because of the reluctance of pharmaceutical companies, who fund most trials, to get results that they don't want—most studies have been too small.

There are many other possible problems that can arise with trials and I want to describe just a few more. One problem arises from having many different possible outcomes to a study. You measure not just whether patients live or die but also whether they have heart attacks, strokes or other problems, whether they are admitted to hospital, whether they have time off work and so on. If you measure enough things then you will find differences in some of them between the treated and the untreated that seem too big to be due to chance. They are, in the jargon of medical journals, 'statistically significant'. But they may still be related to chance. You've increased the chance of finding a result that seems not to be due to chance by measuring so many things.

It's again really the trial being too small, as is the next problem of over-analysing the data. A famous saying of statisticians is that 'if you torture the data long enough they will confess'. You do a trial of X against Y. You find no difference in the outcome. So you then look at different groups within the study, and you will find, by definition, groups—perhaps men aged 40 to 50 who smoke—where there are big differences between those treated with X and those treated with Y. It might be that this is a real difference or it might be chance. It's important for readers to know whether you hypothesized that such a group would show a difference before you analysed the results. You perhaps had biological reasons for your hypothesis. If you did the difference might be real. Otherwise, it almost certainly would not be.

Sometimes people will deliberately torture data to produce the result they want. This is misconduct. More often naïve researchers—and there are many such in medicine—play around with the data to produce 'interesting positive results', unaware of the implications of what they are doing. The wide availability of statistical packages for computers makes this very easy to do.

Leonard Leibovici, an Israeli physician, illustrated some of these problems and others in a very tongue-in-cheek way by conducting a trial of what he called 'retroactive intercessory prayer'.[110] He and his team prayed, within a randomized trial, for a group of patients who had been in their hospital four years previously. They found that compared with controls the patients they prayed for did better. This paper was published in the Christmas edition of the *BMJ* and greatly perplexed some readers and journalists. Should it be taken seriously? The authors pointed out that it was human and small minded to think that time flowed in only one direction. God is under no such restrictions. I think that the results can be explained without resorting to the supernatural. It may be that the authors looked at many possible outcomes and reported on only the positive, or it may be, as I explain below, that you have a high chance of coming up with positive results by chance when testing silly hypotheses.

Other sorts of problems that can arise with clinical trials are illustrated by the famous but apocryphal statistical story trial of getting patients to run up Ben Nevis (Britain's highest mountain) as a treatment for heart attack. The fact that the treatment works is illustrated by the 25 patients who completed the treatment all surviving 10 years. But the authors of this important trial (sponsored perhaps by the Scottish Tourist Board) neglected to report the 25 patients who refused the treatment, the 25 lost on the mountain and the 25 who died while running. This story illustrates the importance of keeping results on all patients who enter trials. In the jargon of trials you should conduct 'an intention to treat analysis', which will include all those who refused to take the treatment, didn't take it or who disappeared from the trial. This is the relevant analysis to the doctor and the patient thinking of starting a treatment because many patients will be just like the patients in the trial.

(Reliable evidence suggests that only about one-half of patients take drugs as they are prescribed.[111] I heard Richard Doll, perhaps Britain's pre-eminent doctor researcher of the 20th century and one of those who developed the randomized trial, tell another story that illustrates the difficulty of doing trials. A patient is entered into a double blind randomized cross-over trial [which means at a point unknown to either the doctor or the patient the drug the patient is taking changes]. During the trial the patient asks the doctor: 'Have you changed my treatment?' The doctor explains, yet again, that he wouldn't know. 'But what,' the doctor asks, 'makes you think that I have?' 'Well now when I flush the tablets down the toilet they float. They never used to.')

The outcomes of trials can also be analysed by using results only from those who completed the treatment as described—that is, in the Ben Nevis example, all those who reached the top of the mountain and came back. This is called in the jargon a 'per protocol analysis'. Such an analysis can be useful to the doctor and patient because it provides information on what might happen to the patient if he or she does follow the treatment. It is common that 'intention to treat' analyses will suggest that treatments don't work and 'per protocol' analyses that they do. In such circumstances it may be tempting for the researchers—and particularly the manufacturers of a drug—to report simply the 'per protocol' analysis. Would this be wrong? Until recently it probably would not have been regarded as 'wrong' and was common. Now, however, as standards are rising, it would perhaps be regarded as wrong—'misconduct' in some form—to not present both analyses.

Because another problem with randomized trials is not just how they are done but how they are reported. There is substantial evidence that many trials have been badly reported.[112] They have not given full information on patients, not described the methods of randomization and blinding, not given both 'intention to treat' and 'per protocol' analyses, not given data on adverse effects and failed in many other ways. This is an indictment not only of authors but also of journals, editors and the whole system of peer review. Widespread recognition of these deficiencies in reporting led a group of researchers and editors to develop a standardized form of reporting randomized trials—called CONSORT (Consolidated Standards for Reporting of Trials).[113] Many journals have now adopted these criteria and the reporting of trials seems to have improved as a result—although this conclusion was made from a 'before and after' study comparing trials in journals that adopted CONSORT and those that didn't (not, as readers of this chapter will now know, the best way to decide if the intervention worked).[114]

Randomized trials, despite their problems, have become very important within medicine. Pharmaceutical companies must conduct such trials of their drugs before they can be put on the market. Classically the trials of new drugs have been conducted against placebos. The companies were simply required to show that their drugs were pure, safe and effective (that is, better than placebo). They have not had to show that their new drug is better than treatments already available. But the question that matters to doctors and patients is not whether the new drug is better than a placebo but whether it is better than the existing treatment. Many, including the World Medical Association, have declared it unethical to conduct trials against placebo rather than against the standard treatment.

At the *BMJ*, for example, we would not publish a trial of a new drug against a placebo when there was good evidence (derived from randomized trials) that an existing treatment works. There are many cases, however, where there is no good evidence to support the standard treatment. The standard treatment is simply what doctors have always given.

Increasingly the authorities who make decisions on which drugs will be available are requiring evidence that drugs are not simply pure, safe and effective, but also that they are better in some ways than existing treatments. There are many ways in which they might be better. They could be more effective, have fewer side-effects, be easier to take (perhaps once rather than three times a day) or cheaper. In England and Wales the National Institute for Health and Clinical Excellence (NICE) needs such evidence before advising that a new treatment be made widely available within the National Health Service.

Randomized trials are important to pharmaceutical companies not only for getting their drugs through regulatory authorities but also for the marketing of their drugs. Those who prescribe drugs increasingly want evidence from trials, and a huge trial conducted in many institutions in many countries can itself be a form of marketing— it draws the drug to the attention of a great many doctors and patients. But these trials can cost many millions of dollars to conduct. In such circumstances it can be disastrous for a company to carry out a trial that shows its drug to be inferior to a competitor drug. Not only will the millions spent on the trial be counterproductive but the hundreds of millions spent developing a new drug will be wasted.

Pharmaceutical companies are thus reluctant to conduct trials of their new drug against competitor drugs, the very trials that doctors and patients want. The answer, argues Silvio Garattini, director of the Mario Negri Institute in Milan, and others, may be for public money to be used to conduct such trials. Garattini also points out that companies are clever at conducting trials that will be beneficial for marketing but do not run the risk of damaging their drug. They conduct trials that are big enough to show that their drug is no worse than that of a competitor (a 'non-inferiority' trial in the jargon) but not big enough to run the risk of showing it to be worse.[115] There are many other ways in which companies can be sure of getting the results they want, and these were brilliantly and wittily parodied in an article by Dave Sackett and Andy Oxman, two of the founders of 'evidence-based medicine', in which they describe a research company called HARLOT (How to Achieve positive Results without actually Lying to Overcome the Truth).[116]

Garattini and others mockingly ask that patients entering such trials to sign a consent form saying:

'Draft informed consent for an underpowered "equivalence trial": "Let us treat you with something that at best is the same as what you would have had before, but might also reduce—though this is unlikely—most of the advantages previously attained in your condition. It might even benefit you more than any current therapy, but, should that actually happen, we will not be able to prove it or let you know whether the new treatment may somehow bother or even harm you more than the standard one, as potential side-effects may be too rare for us to be able to measure them in this study.'''[115]

I paraphrase: 'I agree to participate in this trial which I understand to be of no scientific value but will be useful for pharmaceutical companies in marketing their drug.' The influence of pharmaceutical companies over what is published in medical journals is discussed more fully in chapter 16.

Because so many randomized trials are too small researchers have developed a means of combining the results of many small trials into something called a meta-analysis or systematic review. These reviews also have the benefit that they include a wider range of patients than are usually included in any single trial. A common problem with trials is that they do not include elderly patients, patients with more than one condition or many other groups. Doctors are thus left wondering whether or not the results of the trial are relevant to the patients they see. Systematic reviews can thus have advantages over single randomized trials.

But just like every other methodology they have deficiencies. The essence of doing a systematic review is that you ask a question that is important to doctors and patients, gather all evidence on the question, evaluate the quality of that evidence, and then combine—perhaps statistically—the high-quality evidence. This is conceptually straightforward, but there are severe problems with every step.

Often the questions that matter to patients and doctors are different from those answered by researchers. It may thus be that there is no useful evidence.

The next problem is finding all the available evidence, and the all is important. It is easy to be misled if you find just some of the evidence and finding all relevant evidence is hard because there is so much and it is so disorganized. Major databases—like PubMed, which is compiled by the National Library of Medicine in Washington—contain only some of all published evidence, and then finding the relevant evidence within the database is difficult. Furthermore, much of the evidence is not published at all, and unfortunately an important bias is usually introduced by looking only at the evidence that is straightforward to find. This is because evidence that suggests that a treatment works is likely to be published in major journals and so easy to find, whereas the evidence that suggests that a treatment does not work may not be published at all or may be published in more obscure journals that are not included in the major bibliographic databases.

The next problem is to evaluate the quality of the evidence. There are many different methods for doing this, and they often do not select the same studies. This matters as well because often the poorer-quality studies suggest that a treatment works, whereas the higher-quality studies suggest it doesn't. The cut-off point used by the person conducting the review may thus make a difference to the conclusion of the review. Another common problem encountered in such reviews is that there are many studies but all of low quality. The conclusion of the review is thus that we do not know if a treatment works or not. We had intense debates over whether or not we should publish such studies in the *BMJ*, but increasingly we did. Surely patients should be told that there is no good evidence to support a treatment that may be offered to them.

Finally, combining results from very different sorts of trials can be both difficult and misleading. There are sophisticated statistical tests for assessing the heterogeneity of trials, but—just as with risk adjustment—they can never entirely compensate for inadequate data.

So far I have discussed the evidence that might be used to assess whether or not a treatment works, and I hope the reader—whose head may be spinning—will agree that this is no simple task and that the studies published in medical journals are hard to do, hard to interpret and may often mislead. John Ioannidis, a researcher from Greece, has gone as far as to argue in an article that has attracted lots of attention that 'most published research findings are false'.[117] If you spend your time reading medical journals you may more often be misled than informed. You may be wasting your time. You'd be less misinformed if you never read a journal.

I don't want to discuss the problems with every other sort of study, but if readers would like to read more on this subject in language that they will understand I suggest that they read Trish Greenhalgh's book *How to Read a Paper*.[118] (Trish is a friend of mine and the book is published by the BMJ Publishing Group of which I was the chief executive, but I will not benefit financially from increased sales of the book)

Before finishing I do, however, want briefly to discuss the sort of study that associates X with Y—because these are the studies that are most commonly reported in the mass media. X might be alcohol, smoking, exercise, coffee, garlic, sex or a thousand other things, and Y could be death, breast cancer, heart attacks, stroke, depression or many other horrors. Two cartoons tell the story. In the first a newsreader on 'Today's Random Medical News' has behind him three dials indicating that 'smoking, coffee, stress, etc' cause 'heart disease, depression, breast cancer, etc' in 'children, rats, men aged 25 to 40'. In the second cartoon a listener with a spinning head is being told 'Don't eat eggs. . .eat more eggs. . .stay out of the sun. . .don't lie around inside'.

These stories come usually from epidemiological studies in which the researchers examine measurements in a large group of people and look for statistical associations between X and Y. Even if optimally done they do not prove causation. The fact that X and Y have a statistical association is a long way from proving causation. There is probably a fairly strong correlation between cases of autism and the numbers of people using personal computers in that both have climbed in the past 15 years, but there is no reason to think that there is any causal link (or maybe now somebody will suggest it).

Too many small studies and imprecise testing of improbable hypotheses in medical journals lead to an excessive numbers of associations that then spread through the mass media, according to statistician Jonathan Sterne and epidemiologist George Davey Smith.[119] The other part of the problem is that medical journals and researchers have been obsessed with a statistical test (called a *t*-test). It produces something called a *p* (for probability) value. Traditionally if *p* is less than 0.05 (meaning that there is a probability of only 5%, or one in 20, that the finding could have arisen by chance), then the result is taken as positive or 'true'—X and Y are linked. And both authors and the media are then quick to suggest that X causes Y, which, as I've said, doesn't follow even if X and Y are truly linked.

These studies can produce a result called a 'false positive' (when the result suggests a true link but in fact there is no link) and 'false negatives' (when the study says there is no link but in fact there is). (This is true, importantly, of all diagnostic tests. No test is perfect. They all produce false positives and false negatives, providing one reason why the art of diagnosis is so hard.)

Sterne and Davey Smith explain why we are deluged with bogus associations by making a plausible assumption that 10% of hypotheses are true and 90% untrue. Their second assumption is that most studies are too small and that studies reported in medical journals therefore have only a 50% chance of getting the right answer. Lots of evidence supports this assumption. They then consider 1000 studies testing different hypotheses. One hundred (that is, 10%) will be true, but 50% of those will be reported as untrue. From the 900 hypotheses that are untrue 45 will be reported as true because of the use of $p<0.05$ as true. So almost half of the 95 studies reported as 'positive' are false alarms.

Doctor and medical journalist, James le Fanu, has suggested that the answer to the problem would be the closure of all departments of epidemiology.[120]

The problems of doing and interpreting studies on whether or not treatments work and whether or not X and Y might be linked go for every other sort of study published in journals, and journals are publishing an ever wider range of studies. For example, the *BMJ* was publishing steadily more studies that use the methods of the social sciences and economics. We did so because these methods are the best for answering some of the very broad range of questions that arise in healthcare. The methods of social science are, for example, optimal for asking questions like, 'What do doctors and patients think of a subject and how do they behave?' Economic methods clearly must be used for assessing the cost-effectiveness of treatments and healthcare systems have to consider costs not just clinical effectiveness. This, for example, is exactly what NICE does.

We thus need new methods, but each time a journal publishes new methods the editors must try to understand how to assess the quality of studies—and so must readers. Editors are, of course, paid to read studies and assess their quality, and so they work hard at understanding new methods. It does, however, take a long time to understand them—and most editors never achieve complete mastery of the methods, which is why they need reviewers and advisers. Readers, in contrast, are not paid to understand the methods—and most of them never do. Journals provide readers with an increasingly complex diet of research, most of which most of the readers are not able to assess. They have to trust the journals—despite the evidence that journals mostly publish material of limited relevance and low scientific quality.

The problem of complex and unfamiliar methodologies is likely to get much worse, warns Doug Altman, one of the *BMJ*'s statistical advisers. The easy and cheap availability of immense computing power means that highly complex calculations can be easily done. But how can editors and statistical advisers review the validity of such tests when they don't understand them and the results cannot be presented on paper? Salvation might lie, I hope (perhaps naïvely), in electronic publication of studies.

Authors will publish raw data together with the computer programs used to analyse the data. Editors, reviewers and readers might then be able to repeat the analyses for themselves.

You are convinced, I hope, that there is lots of room for error and misunderstanding in what medical journals publish even when everything is done honestly and in good faith. If we add misconduct and manipulation into the mix then the potential for confusion and harm is greatly increased. The answer is not, however, to abandon medical journals—as Beth was led to conclude—but to promote critical reading and debate. Or maybe Beth is right.

7

Peer review: a flawed process at the heart of science and journals

Peer review is at the heart of the processes of not just medical journals but of all science. It is the method by which grants are allocated, papers published, academics promoted and Nobel prizes won. Yet it is hard to define. It has until recently been unstudied. And its defects are easier to identify than its attributes. Yet it shows no sign of going away. Famously, it is compared with democracy: a system full of problems but the least worst we have.

When something is peer reviewed it is in some sense blessed. Even journalists recognize this. When the *BMJ* published the highly controversial paper that I mentioned in chapter 2 that argued that a new 'disease', female sexual dysfunction, was in some ways being created by pharmaceutical companies,[3] a friend, who is a journalist was very excited—not least because reporting it gave him a chance to get sex onto the front page of a highly respectable but somewhat priggish newspaper (the *Financial Times*). 'But,' the news editor wanted to know, 'was this paper peer reviewed?' The implication was that if it had been it was good enough for the front page and if it hadn't been it wasn't. Well, had it been? I'd read it much more carefully than I read many papers and had asked the author, the journalist Ray Moynihan, to revise the paper and produce more evidence. But this wasn't peer review, even though I'm a peer of the author and reviewed the paper. Or was it? (I told my friend that it hadn't been peer reviewed, but it was too late to pull the story from the front page.)

My point is that peer review is impossible to define in operational terms (an operational definition is one whereby if 50 of us looked at the same process we could all agree most of the time whether or not it was peer reviewed). Peer review is thus like poetry, love or justice. But it's something to do with a grant application or a paper being scrutinized by a third party—who is neither the author nor the person making a judgement on whether a grant should be given or a paper published. But who is a peer? Somebody doing exactly the same kind of research? (In which case he or she is probably a direct competitor.) Somebody in the same discipline? Somebody who is an expert on methodology? And what is review? Somebody saying 'The paper looks all right to me', which is sadly what peer review sometimes seems to be. Or somebody pouring all over the paper, asking for raw data, repeating analyses, checking all the references and making detailed suggestions for improvement? Such a review is vanishingly rare.

What is clear is that the forms of peer review are protean. Probably the systems of every journal and every grant giving body are different in at least some detail, and some systems are very different. There may even be some journals using the following classic system. The editor looks at the title of the paper and sends it to two friends whom the editor thinks know something about the subject. If both advise publication the editor sends it to the printers. If both advise against publication the editor rejects the paper. If the reviewers disagree the editor sends it to a third reviewer and does whatever he or she advises. This pastiche—which is not far from systems I've seen used—is little better than tossing a coin—because the level of agreement between reviewers on whether or not a paper should be published is no better than you'd expect by chance.[121]

That's why Robbie Fox, the great 20th century editor of the *Lancet* who was no admirer of peer review, wondered whether or not anybody would notice if he were to swap the piles marked 'publish' and 'reject'. He also joked that the *Lancet* had a system of throwing a pile of papers down the stairs and publishing those that reached the bottom. I was challenged by two of the cleverest researchers in Britain to publish an issue of the *BMJ* comprised only of papers that had failed peer review and to see if anybody noticed. I wrote back 'How do you know I haven't already done it?'

I think that I ought to describe at least one peer review system and I hope you will forgive me if I describe the system the *BMJ* had when I left. (It's since changed.) The old *BMJ* system is obviously the one I know best, but it had features that made it unusual. I'll describe what they were as we go.

One thing that is currently unusual about the *BMJ* peer review process—but will not be for much longer—is that it's conducted on the World Wide Web. Soon, I suspect, all peer review will be conducted on the web. So far the *BMJ* has simply transferred a traditional paper-based system to the web, but even the 'simple transfer' may have had unexpectedly profound effects. For example, I found at the end of my time at the *BMJ* that I didn't know many of the people I was asking to review, whereas a few years before I knew most of them. As one editor put it to me, 'The old guys are gone. They don't like computers.' In the longer term many things will be possible with a web-based system that would be impossible with a paper-based system—for example, conducting the whole process in realtime in full public view. Already authors can interrogate the system to find where their paper is in the system.

The *BMJ* has about 6000 papers submitted a year. In the end it publishes about 8%. Most major general journals have a similarly low acceptance rate. Smaller and specialist journals accept many more, and some journals, I suspect, publish almost everything they receive. Paradoxically, it always seems to me, editors boast about their rejection rates. The editor with the highest rejection rate is like the banker with the tallest skyscraper. Where else do people boast about rejection?

Editorial folklore says that if you persist long enough you can get anything published, no matter how terrible. Stephen Lock, my predecessor, followed up studies rejected by the *BMJ* and found that most were published somewhere.[121] He found too that most authors had ignored any suggestions for changes suggested by reviewers. My friend Drummond Rennie, deputy editor of *JAMA*, has produced one of the greatest (and certainly longest) sentences of medical journalism to illustrate that any paper can get published:

'There seems to be no study too fragmented, no hypothesis too trivial, no literature citation too biased or too egotistical, no design too warped, no methodology too bungled, no presentation of results too inaccurate, too obscure, and too contradictory, no analysis too self-serving, no argument too circular, no conclusions too trifling or too unjustified, and no grammar and syntax too offensive for a paper to end up in print.'[122]

(In admiration of such a sentence one of his readers sent him the whole sentence embroidered.)

There is a 'food chain' with medical journals down which rejected studies pass. Unfortunately the *BMJ* is not at the top, but fortunately it's a long way from the bottom. This is clearly a very inefficient system. Studies may be reviewed many times before they are published. Similarly grant applications may be reviewed many times before they are funded or, worse, rejected. The total time spent reviewing must be huge and must be increasing as the rates at which grants are funded and papers published declines. By 2020, one wag calculated, academics will do nothing but peer review.

The *BMJ* triaged the studies submitted to it, rejecting two-thirds without sending them out for external peer review. We had around a dozen different editors doing this and had a system of duty editors. Our aim was to make an initial decision on a study the day it arrived. We were looking for studies that had an important message for clinical medicine or public health and were original, relevant for our audience and valid—meaning that their conclusions were supported by their evidence and data. I posted an account of how the *BMJ* triaged studies on its website. We began by asking whether the study had anything interesting and new to say. If not, we rejected it. We then had many methodological signals that caused us to reject, including, for example, any survey that had a response rate below 50% (with very rare exceptions) or any study advocating a treatment that was not a randomized trial unless the paper gave compelling reasons why a randomized study was impossible. Sometimes an editor rejected the study alone, but more often two editors looked at a study before rejecting it.

This system may have seemed brutal (and certainly some authors felt so), but the editorial team at that time thought that it had an unanswerable logic. We would waste everybody's time, including the authors', by sending out for review a study that had no chance of making it into the *BMJ*. Authors could send their rejected study to a journal that might publish it without losing a lot of time, and the *BMJ* could make sure that it used the highly valuable time of reviewers on studies that it might publish and that could be improved by their attention. It was sensible for the *BMJ* to spend its resources on papers it was going to publish, not on those it was not. Some will argue that journals ought to be helping authors improve their papers even if they are not going to publish them, and sometimes at the *BMJ* we did that when we wanted to encourage new types of research. We did it many years ago with research in primary care (general practice), and we did it with research on quality improvement, information and learning.

The two-thirds of studies that were rejected without external review were rejected with a ticksheet that included a list of about 40 common reasons for the *BMJ* rejecting studies—the editors ticked the reasons for rejecting that particular study. Authors would naturally prefer a personal letter explaining why the *BMJ* had rejected their study, but this would not be a good way for the journal to use its resources. We thought that the ticksheet was better than just a rejection slip and our research among authors showed that they, grudgingly, agreed. Unsurprisingly, they didn't like rejection in any form.

The one-third of studies that remained after triage were sent to an external reviewer. Usually the *BMJ* had just one reviewer for a paper, although it used two when the editors and the reviewers were learning about a new methodology. So we always sent a paper that used economic methods to an economist as well as to a clinical reviewer, whereas we thought that most of our reviewers were familiar with methods like randomized trials. Using a single reviewer was unusual. Most journals use at least two and some use as many as a dozen.

When I first arrived at the *BMJ* in 1979 we probably didn't use more than a hundred reviewers altogether, and there was no database of reviewers. Initially I would have to ask the senior editors to suggest somebody. We had perhaps two reviewers for the whole of rheumatology and almost all the reviewers were from Britain and over 50. Such a system could have advantages in that you knew and trusted your reviewers, but it had the obvious disadvantage that one or two individuals had undue influence over what was published.

The *BMJ* when I left had a database that included several thousand reviewers from all over the world, most of whom the editors didn't know. Unusually we asked people to volunteer to be reviewers and in this way we have found many hundreds of excellent reviewers. One result that emerges from all studies on who make the best reviewers is that those under 40 do better than those over 40, even after allowing for the fact that younger people often have more time.[73] We graded the reviews produced by reviewers on a four-point scale and generally used only once somebody who got the lowest score. Increasingly we used only people who had repeatedly scored highly for their reviews. We also had data on the time people took to review and we tended to discard those who were always slow.

Our database had detailed information on the particular interests of reviewers. So we would not send a study on rheumatoid arthritis to any rheumatologist but to one who had a particular interest in rheumatoid arthritis, and we would often make a still closer link between the content of the study and the interests of the reviewer.

It's a hard—and largely thankless task—being a reviewer. To review a paper properly takes several hours and the mean time that *BMJ* reviewers spend on a study is over two hours. Some spend as many as 20 hours. The *BMJ* is unusual in paying reviewers, but we paid only £50 to people whose market rate would be more than £100 an hour. Furthermore, most peer review systems are closed in that the names of the reviewers are known only to the editors. So most reviewers receive no public or academic credit for their work. The *BMJ* is again unusual in having a system where the authors know the name of reviewers, but—at the moment—readers do not.

A good review will comment on the originality of the work (preferably with references to related work), discuss the importance of the question being asked, give a detailed account of the strengths and weaknesses of the study, comment on the presentation of the paper and give constructive comments on how it might be improved. Published accounts of the quality of reviews show that perhaps one-fifth are outstanding, one-fifth of little or no use and the rest somewhere in the middle. My impression, not supported by strong data, is that the quality of reviews for medical journals is improving—not least as increasing numbers of doctors are trained in the critical appraisal of studies, statistics and clinical epidemiology.

I didn't when I left the *BMJ* very often see the review that said: 'I'm scanning this at the airport and it looks excellent to me—but then it would be because Joe is a first class researcher.' Nor did I see: 'I wouldn't touch this with a bargepole. That lot at St Domino's can't be trusted.' It would be unwise to sign your name to such reviews, but I saw such reviews in the bad old days—that is, 10 years ago.

If a *BMJ* reviewer gave cogent reasons why a study should not be published, then we rejected the study, sending the authors a copy of the reviewers' comments. It wasn't long ago that many journals and grant giving bodies did not send back the reviewers' comments. They would simply reject without explaining why, fearing that sending reasons would only encourage authors to disagree and appeal—so creating more work.

If the reviewer thought that the paper might be worth publishing or the *BMJ* editor thought it might be, perhaps because the reviewer was uncertain or hadn't given a good opinion, then editors discussed the paper at a weekly meeting. Sometimes the paper was rejected at that point or, if it was still thought publishable, it was sent to one of our pretentiously and ominously named 'hanging committees' (so-called after a committee of the Royal Academy which decides which pictures will be hung in the summer exhibition).

The hanging committee made the final decision on the paper and comprised one or sometimes two editors, two people from a pool comprised mainly of practising doctors (we called them 'hangers') and a statistician. The committee never had more than a dozen papers to consider and everybody was supposed to have read every word of every paper together with the comments of all the reviewers. The committee decided which papers to publish and in particular it gave detailed suggestions on how the papers that were going to be published could be improved. As I will discuss below, the evidence on peer review suggests that the benefit of peer review lies less in deciding which papers to publish or grant proposals to fund and more in improving the papers that are published or the proposals that are funded.

The *BMJ*'s hanging committee was unusual in at least four ways. First, many (probably most) journals simply have one or two editors make decisions without needing to meet. Second, it is unusual to have statisticians and clinicians discuss studies together. Usually, the statistician produces a written report. But we thought that the discussion among clinicians, editors and statisticians was one of the greatest benefits of the process—both for each to understand the others' worlds and for learning. Third, even when journals do have a meeting to decide which papers to publish it is unusual for more than one or two people to have read every word. Usually somebody simply presents the paper to the group. Fourth, the *BMJ*'s decisions on which papers to publish were made not by editors but by 'outsiders', albeit people who came regularly to the journal and were paid by the journal. The idea was that these hangers not only were good at making decisions on the validity of studies but also represented the readers of the *BMJ*. They were, as I've said, mostly practising doctors—in touch with the realities and brutalities of daily practice in a way that *BMJ* editors were not. (Ironically the most common criticism of the *BMJ* was that it didn't publish enough for hospital doctors and yet most of our hangers were hospital doctors.)

Arguments against hanging committees were that they were expensive, inevitably slowed decision-making and were inconsistent, even quixotic, in their decision-making—not least because the membership constantly varied. There was also something odd about editors abrogating their responsibility for their content of the journal. For whatever reason, Fiona Godlee, my successor as editor of the *BMJ*, decided to end the system of hanging committees.

Very few papers were published in the *BMJ* without extensive revision and a common decision of the hanging committee was to reject a paper but offer to see it again if it was heavily revised. We allowed appeals against our decision to reject and many appeals succeeded. We did not, however, allow second appeals. We realized that almost all such appeals ended in tears. Either the authors were fed up with rejection after a long process or we were unhappy because we'd agreed to publish a paper that we didn't really like. If we were the only journal in the world this would have been unacceptable, but luckily for everybody we weren't.

If we rejected a paper without sending it out for external review then we aimed to do so within two weeks—and we mostly succeeded. If the paper was sent out for review, then we aimed for a decision within eight weeks. We met this target about three-quarters of the time, but I have to confess that there were papers where the process became inordinately complex and prolonged. Many might think the system horribly slow, but the *BMJ* had a reputation for being fairly fast compared with many other journals. Nevertheless, I know of at least one journal—*Cardiovascular Research*—that with the arrival of a new editor went from taking months to make decisions to making every decision within three weeks. Old systems can be reinvented.

Like various other journals the *BMJ* had a fast track system, whereby we made a decision and published within four weeks—compared with the usual two months to make a decision and another three months to publish. There is something silly about fast tracking in that the time between a study being conceived and submitted is usually several years and then the time between publication of a paper and doctors changing their practice is also years. So why bother with shortening this process of nearly a decade by four months? The answer is in an attempt to attract the best studies. I don't think that the *BMJ* succeeded, but it has seemed to work better for the *Lancet*, which did it first.

Chris Martyn, an associate editor of the *BMJ* and the editor of the *Quarterly Journal of Medicine* (which to everybody's delight is published monthly), has written a witty essay arguing the case for slow tracking.[123] The short-term gain from fast tracking is quickly obliterated as everybody does it, and most human activities—particularly cooking and making love—benefit from slowness not speed. The same might well be true of peer review, and the most recent example of a spectacular failure of peer review—*Science*'s publication of the fraudulent stem cell research study[124]—was associated with the journal reviewing the paper in half the time it usually took.[125]

I ought to make clear that I do not regard publication as the end of the peer review process. Rather it is part of the process. Many studies that have made it through the peer review process to publication are demolished once exposed to hundreds of thousands of readers.

As part of an attempt to improve the *BMJ*'s system of peer review we drew a diagram of the process. The resulting flow chart was some five feet long and full of loops and swirls. What I have described above is a simplified version of the process. We imagined that some part of the process must be redundant, but—even with the help of outside consultants—we couldn't identify a piece that we could delete. Can it really be that this degree of elaboration is justified?

But does peer review 'work' at all? A systematic review of all the available evidence on peer review concluded that 'the practice of peer review is based on faith in its effects, rather than on facts'.[126] But the answer to the question on whether or not peer review works depends on the question, 'What is peer review for?'

One answer is that it's a method to select the best grant applications for funding and the best papers to publish in a journal. It's hard to test this aim because there is no agreed definition of what constitutes a good paper or a good research proposal. Plus what is peer review to be tested against? Chance, or a much simpler process? Stephen Lock when editor of the *BMJ* conducted a study in which he decided alone which of a consecutive series of papers submitted to the journal he would publish. He then let the papers go through the usual process. There was little difference between the papers he chose and those selected after the full process of peer review.[121] This small study suggests that perhaps you don't need an elaborate process. Maybe a lone editor, thoroughly familiar with what the journal wants and knowledgeable about research methods, would be enough. But it would be a bold journal that stepped aside from the sacred path of peer review.

Another answer to the question of what peer review is for is that it is to improve the quality of papers that are published or research proposals that are funded. The systematic review found little evidence to support this, but again such studies are hampered by the lack of an agreed definition of a good study or a good research proposal.

Peer review might also be useful for detecting errors or fraud. At the *BMJ* we did several studies where we inserted major errors into papers that we then sent to many reviewers.[127,128] Nobody ever spotted all of the errors. Some reviewers didn't spot any, and most reviewers spotted only about one-quarter. Peer review sometimes picks up fraud by chance, but generally it is not a reliable method for detecting fraud because it works on trust. A major question, which I will return to, is whether or not peer review and journals should cease to work on trust.

So we have little evidence on the effectiveness of peer review, but we have considerable evidence on its defects. In addition to being poor at detecting gross defects and almost useless for detecting fraud, it is slow, expensive, profligate of academic time, highly subjective, something of a lottery, prone to bias and easily abused.

The slowness of the *BMJ*'s system I've already described, and many journals and bodies conducting peer review processes are much slower. Many journals, even in the age of the internet, take more than a year to review and publish a paper. It's hard to get good data on the cost of peer review, particularly because reviewers are often not paid (the same, come to that, is true of many editors). Yet there is a substantial 'opportunity cost', as economists call it, in that the time spent reviewing could be spent doing something more productive—like original research. (Some high-quality researchers recognize this problem and refuse to review.) I estimate that the cost of peer review per paper for the *BMJ* (remembering that the journal rejected 60% without external review) was of the order of £100, whereas the cost of a paper that made it right through the system was closer to £1000.

The cost of peer review has become important because of the open access movement, which hopes to make research freely available to everybody. With the current publishing model peer review is usually 'free' to authors, and publishers make their money by charging institutions to access the material. One open access model is that authors will pay for peer review and the cost of posting their article on a website. So those offering or proposing this system have had to come up with a figure—which is currently between $500 and $2500 per article. Those promoting the open access system calculate that at the moment the academic community pays about $5000 for access to a peer reviewed paper. (The $5000 is obviously paying for much more than peer review: it includes other editorial costs, distribution costs [expensive with paper] and a big chunk of profit for the publisher.) So there may be substantial financial gains to be had by academics if the model for publishing science changes.

There is an obvious irony in people charging for a process that is not proved to be effective, but that's how much the scientific community values its faith in peer review.

People have a great many fantasies about peer review, and one of the most powerful is that it's a highly objective, reliable and consistent process. I regularly received letters from authors who were upset that the *BMJ* had rejected their paper and then published what they thought to be a much inferior paper on the same subject. Always they saw something underhand. They found it hard to accept that peer review is a subjective and therefore inconsistent process. But it is probably unreasonable to expect it to be objective and consistent. If I ask people to rank painters like Titian, Tintoretto, Bellini, Carpaccio and Veronese I would never expect them to come up with the same order. A scientific study submitted to a medical journal may not be as complex a work as a Tintoretto altarpiece, but it is complex. Inevitably people will take different views on its strengths, weaknesses and importance.

So the evidence is that if reviewers are asked to give an opinion on whether or not a paper should be published, they agree only slightly more than they would be expected to agree by chance. (I'm conscious that this evidence conflicts with the study of Stephen Lock showing that he alone and the whole *BMJ* peer review process tended to reach the same decision on which papers should be published. The explanation may be that by being the editor who had designed the *BMJ* process and appointed the editors and reviewers, it wasn't surprising that they were fashioned in his image and made similar decisions.)

Sometimes the inconsistency can be laughable. Here is an example of two reviewers commenting on the same papers.

Reviewer A: 'I found this paper an extremely muddled paper with a large number of deficits.'

Reviewer B: 'It is written in a clear style and would be understood by any reader.'

This—perhaps inevitable—inconsistency can make peer review something of a lottery. You submit a study to a journal. It enters a system that is effectively a black box, and then a more or less sensible answer comes out at the other end. The black box is like the roulette wheel, and the prizes and the losses can be big. For an academic, publication in a major journal like *Nature* or *Cell* is to win the jackpot.

The evidence on whether there is bias in peer review against certain sorts of authors is conflicting, but there is strong evidence of bias against women in the process of awarding grants. The most famous piece of evidence on bias against authors comes from a study by Peters and Ceci.[129] They took 12 studies that came from prestigious institutions and had already been published in psychology journals. They retyped the papers, made minor changes to the titles, abstracts and introductions, but changed the authors' names and institutions. They invented institutions with names like the Tri-Valley Center for Human Potential. The papers were then resubmitted to the journals that had first published them. In only three cases did the journals realize that they had already published the paper, and eight of the remaining nine were rejected—not because of lack of originality but because of poor quality. Peters and Ceci concluded that this was evidence of bias against authors from less prestigious institutions.

This is known as the Mathew effect: 'To those who have, shall be given; to those who have not shall be taken away even the little that they have.' I remember feeling the effect strongly when as a young editor I had to consider a paper submitted to the *BMJ* by Karl Popper.[130] I was unimpressed and thought we should reject the paper. But we couldn't. The power of the name was too strong. So we published, and time has shown we were right to do so. The paper argued that we should pay much more attention to error in medicine, about 20 years before many papers appeared arguing the same.

The editorial peer review process has been strongly biased against 'negative studies'—studies that find an intervention doesn't work. It's also clear that authors often don't even bother to write up such studies. This matters because it biases the information base of medicine. It's easy to see why journals would be biased against negative studies. Journalistic values come into play. Who wants to read that a new treatment doesn't work? That's boring.

We became very conscious of this bias at the *BMJ*, and we always tried to concentrate not on the results of a study we were considering but on the question it was asking. If the question is important and the answer valid, then it mustn't matter whether the answer is positive or negative. I fear, however, that bias is not so easily abolished and persists.

The *Lancet* has tried to get round the problem by agreeing to consider the protocols (plans) for studies yet to be done.[131] If it thinks the protocol sound and if the protocol is followed, then the *Lancet* will publish the final results regardless of whether they are positive or negative. Such a system also has the advantage of stopping resources being spent on poor studies. The main disadvantage is that it increases the sum of peer reviewing—because most protocols will need to be reviewed in order to get funding to perform the study.

There are several ways to abuse the process of peer review. You can steal ideas and present them as your own or produce an unjustly harsh review to block or at least slow down the publication of the ideas of a competitor. These have all happened. Drummond Rennie tells the story of a paper he sent, when deputy editor of the *New England Journal of Medicine*, for review to Vijay Soman.[132] Having produced a critical review of the paper, Soman copied some of the paragraphs and submitted it to another journal, the *American Journal of Medicine*. This journal, by coincidence, sent it for review to the boss of the author of the plagiarized paper. She realized that she had been plagiarized and objected strongly. She threatened to denounce Soman but was advised against it. Eventually, however, Soman was discovered to have invented data and patients and left the country. Rennie learnt a lesson that he never subsequently forgot but which medical authorities seem reluctant to accept: those who behave dishonestly in one way are likely to do so in other ways as well.

The most important question with peer review is not whether to abandon it but how to improve it. Many ideas have been advanced to do so, and an increasing number have been tested experimentally. The options include standardizing procedures, opening up the process, blinding reviewers to the identity of authors, reviewing protocols, training reviewers, being more rigorous in selecting and deselecting reviewers, using electronic review, rewarding reviewers, providing detailed feedback to reviewers, using more checklists or creating professional review agencies.

I hope that it won't seem too indulgent if I describe the far from finished journey of the *BMJ* to try and improve peer review. We tried as we went to conduct experiments rather than simply introduce changes.

The most important step on the journey was realizing that peer review could be studied just like anything else. This was the idea of Stephen Lock, together with Drummond Rennie and John Bailar. At the time it was a radical idea, and still seems radical to some—rather like conducting experiments with God or love.

The next important step was prompted by hearing the results of a randomized trial that showed that blinding reviewers to the identity of authors improved the quality of reviews (as measured by a validated instrument).[133] This trial, which was conducted by Bob McNutt, AT Evans, and Bob and Suzanne Fletcher, was important not only for its results but because it provided an experimental design for investigating peer review. Studies where you intervene and experiment allow more confident conclusions than studies you observe without intervening.

This trial was repeated on a larger scale by the *BMJ* and by a group in the United States who conducted the study in many different journals.[134,135] Neither study found that blinding reviewers improved the quality of reviews. These studies also showed that such blinding is difficult to achieve (because many studies include internal clues on authorship) and that reviewers could identify the authors in about one-quarter to one-third of cases. But even when the results were analysed by looking at only those cases where blinding was successful, there was no evidence of improved quality of the review.

At this point we at the *BMJ* thought that we would change direction dramatically and begin to open up the process. In the early 1990s the journal *Cardiovascular Research* published a paper arguing for open peer review and invited commentaries from several editors, including Stephen Lock, Drummond Rennie and me.[136,137]

Interestingly, we all concluded that the case for open review was strong. The main arguments for open review are justice, accountability and credit. Judgement by an invisible judge is ominous, and yet that is what happens with closed review. Reviewers should be fully accountable for what they say, but they should also receive credit. Both accountability and credit are severely limited when reviewers are known only to editors. Open reviewing should also reduce abuses of the system and make it more polite and constructive. Plus why should the burden of proof rest with those who want to open up the system rather than those who want to keep it closed? We live in a world where, whether we like it or not, what is not open is assumed to be biased, corrupt or incompetent until proved otherwise.

The main argument against open review is that it will make it difficult for junior researchers (often the best reviewers) to criticize the work of senior researchers. It might also lead to reviewers holding back their criticisms or create resentment and animosity when they let rip. Another argument is the classic 'if it ain't broke don't fix it', but I hope that most readers will agree that peer review is sufficiently broke for us to need to look for methods of improvement.

At the *BMJ* we began our pursuit of greater openness by conducting a randomized trial of open review (meaning that the authors but not the readers knew the identity of the reviewers) against traditional review.[138] It had no effect on the quality of reviewers' opinions. They were neither better nor worse. Because of the strong ethical arguments in favour of open review we thus went ahead and introduced a system of authors knowing the names of reviewers.

Other editors often asked about our experience, and my simple answer was, 'the earth hasn't moved'. Most reviewers were happy to put their names to reviews, and few problems have arisen—after three years of open review. Before we introduced the system we were challenged by Simon Wessely—a professor of psychiatry and a researcher who has conducted research into peer review—that we were irresponsible in that we were introducing a new 'drug' without any system of monitoring for adverse effects. We thus copied Britain's 'yellow card scheme' that asks every doctor to notify the authorities of possible adverse effects of drugs. All *BMJ* reviewers used to receive yellow forms asking them to notify us of any problems that they experienced through reviewing openly. We had a few yellow forms returned, but none told us of a serious problem. The most common occurrence (not really a problem) was that we discovered that reviewers had conflicts of interest that they haven't declared. Most journals have not, however, adopted open peer review.

Our next step was to conduct a trial of our current open system against a system whereby every document associated with peer review together with the names of everybody involved was posted on the *BMJ*'s website when the paper was published. Once again this intervention had no effect on the quality of the opinion. We thus planned to make posting peer review documents the next stage in opening up our peer review process, but that hasn't yet happened—partly because the results of the trial have not yet been published and partly because this step required various technical developments.

The final step was in my mind to open up the whole process and conduct it in realtime on the web in front of the eyes of anybody interested. Peer review would then be transformed from a black box into an open scientific discourse. Often I found the discourse around a study was a lot more interesting than the study itself. Now that I've left I'm not sure if this system will be introduced.

The *BMJ* also experimented with another possible way to improve peer review—by training reviewers.[128] It is perhaps extraordinary that there has been no formal training for such an important job. Reviewers learn either by trial and error (without, it has to be said, very good feedback) or by working with an experienced reviewer (who might unfortunately be experienced but not very good).

Our randomized trial of training reviewers had three arms: one group got nothing; one group had a day's face to face training plus a CD-ROM of the training; and the third group got just the CD-ROM. The face to face training comprised half a day from editors on what we wanted from reviewers and half a day on critically appraising randomized trials. Our trial dealt only with randomized trials and we admitted to the study only reviewers from Britain who had reviewed for the *BMJ* in the past year. All the reviewers were sent the same study to review before we did anything. The study had deliberate errors inserted. Everybody then received further papers with errors one month and six months after the training. We used our standardized instrument to measure the quality of the reviews and we counted the number of errors spotted.

The overall result was that training made little difference. The groups that had training did show some evidence of improvement relative to those who had no training, but we didn't think that the difference was big enough to be meaningful. We can't conclude from this that longer or better training would not be helpful. A problem with our study was that most of the reviewers had been reviewing for a long time. 'Old dogs cannot be taught new tricks', but the possibility remains that younger ones could. Most of those who had the face to face training both liked it and thought that it would improve their ability to review. The *BMJ* thus does offer such training, thinking of it more as a reward than something that will improve the quality of review.

One difficult question is whether or not peer review should continue to operate on trust. Some have made small steps beyond into the world of audit. The Food and Drug Administration in the United States reserves the right to go and look at the records and raw data of those who produce studies that are used in applications for new drugs to receive licences. Sometimes it does so. Some journals, including the *BMJ*, make it a condition of submission that the editors can ask for the raw data behind a study. We did so once or twice, only to discover that reviewing raw data is difficult, expensive and time consuming. I cannot see journals moving beyond trust in any major way unless the whole scientific enterprise were to move in that direction.

So peer review is a flawed process full of easily identified defects with little evidence that it works. Nevertheless, it is likely to remain central to science and journals because there is no obvious alternative and scientists and editors have a continuing belief in peer review. How odd that science should be rooted in belief.

Section 4: Problems in publishing medical research

►8

Research misconduct: the poisoning of the well

On Wednesday 11 January 2006 Seoul National University concluded that Hwang Woo-suk, a pioneer in stem cell research and a national hero in Korea, had fabricated much of his research. His claim in 2005 to have produced stem cells from adult cells had reverberated around the world because it opened up new ways to treat Parkinson's disease and other degenerative diseases. His disgrace was equally high profile, providing one of the most dramatic cases of scientific fraud ever.

Sadly history includes many egregious examples of fraudulent scientists, but they were until recently regarded as isolated oddballs who did little damage to science, a self-correcting enterprise. But in the past 20 years country after country has recognized increasing examples of fraud and come to think that it cannot be ignored but needs to be recognized and managed. It's a painful transition, which is why few countries have developed an effective, comprehensive, national process for responding to research fraud. The Nordic countries have done so, but none of the large countries of the European Union has yet succeeded.

Responses to fraud are driven by scandals. They accumulate to a point where the scientific community can no longer ignore them and 'something has to be done'. Usually this process is excruciatingly slow.

Stephen Lock in his 'imperfect history' of research misconduct in medicine dates the beginning of the modern story to 1974.[139] William Summerlin from the Sloan-Kettering Institute in New York, one of the world's leading biomedical research centres, claimed to have transplanted human corneas into rabbits. He also faked transplantation experiments in white mice by blackening patches of their skin with a pen, an extraordinarily crude form of forgery. Eventually Summerlin's misconduct could no longer be ignored, but his behaviour was attributed to a mental health problem. This is a response that is seen repeatedly. It's a form of scientific denial.

The cases that eventually led to action in the United States were those of Vijay Soman, John Darsee and Robert Slutsky. I mentioned Soman's case in chapter 7, but in summary he was a diabetologist and the author of 12 papers where data were either missing or fraudulent. One paper, which he co-authored with Philip Felig, was stolen from another author when Felig was sent a paper to review and passed it on to Soman. Felig had to resign. Senior figures putting their names on papers which eventually turn out to be fraudulent is a recurrent problem. Soman was exposed in 1980, and his 12 papers were retracted.

John Darsee worked in the department of cardiology at Harvard and was observed falsifying data. His boss, Eugene Braunwald, an eminent cardiologist, decided that this misconduct was an isolated incident and so did not fire him. A few months later, however, it became clear that results he had obtained in a study being conducted in several places were very different from those of the others. An investigation was started and went back to when he was an undergraduate. Many of his more than a hundred studies proved to be fraudulent and had to be retracted. Again many of the studies included distinguished authors—sparking a debate and a series of studies on 'gift authorship' ("authors", usually senior, being included as authors on a study but who have done little or nothing). This subject is discussed further in chapter 9.

Robert Slutsky, a cardiological radiologist from the University of California, published 137 papers between 1978 and 1985. At one point he was producing one every 10 days. A reviewer raised anxieties about some of Slutsky's work, illustrating how peer review sometimes can pick up on fraud. An investigation decided that 12 of Slutsky's studies were definitely fraudulent and 49 questionable. Many were retracted, although a disturbing number of journals either declined to retract the studies or did so in such a roundabout way that readers wouldn't necessarily understand that they had been retracted. Journals are too often unwilling to retract fraudulent research—either because the publishers' lawyers advise them against it on what I believe to be spurious legal grounds or because they see it as an admission of failure. Retractions are, I believe, like corrections. Good journals have more than poor journals, not because they make more mistakes and publish more fraudulent research, but simply because they are more willing to put the record straight. It's the same with newspapers: the *New York Times*, a world class newspaper, publishes several corrections every day, whereas British tabloid newspapers publish hardly any.

The Darsee case made the front pages of the newspapers in 1981, the year that saw the first of a series of congressional hearings into scientific misconduct. Drummond Rennie and Kristina Gunsalus have described how the first witness, the president of the National Academy of Sciences, 'asserted that problems were rare—the product of "psychopathic behaviour" originating in "temporarily deranged" minds'.[140] The chairman of the hearing, Al Gore, noted, however, at the end of the hearing that, 'one reason for the persistence of this type of problem is the reluctance of people high in the science field to take these matters very seriously'.[140] Huge sums of public money are spent on research in the United States, and the federal government has needed more reassurance that money is not being misspent than it has been able to get from the scientific community. The result after many bitter battles between scientists and politicians has been a federal Office of Research Integrity.

Many British scientists watched the American battles and scandals with smugness, believing that such things could not happen in the less cut throat and more gentlemanly scientific culture in Britain. Then came the case of Malcolm Pearce, which made it onto the front pages of the British newspapers.[141,142]

I first heard of this case when I had breakfast in 1994 with Geoffrey Chamberlain, editor of the *British Journal of Obstetrics and Gynaecology* and president of the Royal College of Obstetricians and Gynaecologists, the owners of the journal. Chamberlain, known to all as 'Bodger', was a kind of obstetric Falstaff, not only in his manner but also to look at. He was much liked, which is one reason why he was filling two prestigious positions in the college that many might have seen as providing a conflict of interest. The point of the breakfast, as I remember, was to discuss the best method of finding Chamberlain's successor as editor. One story was that Chamberlain had been brought into the editorship after his predecessor was run out for being 'too scientific'. By this time I had been involved in appointing several editors and had very much come round to the view that an open advertisement, perhaps supplemented by some direct invitations to apply, was the only acceptable method. I put this to Chamberlain, and he agreed and thought that the college would too.

Then he told me that there had been 'a bit of trouble'. Malcolm Pearce—an assistant editor on the journal and a senior lecturer in the department at St George's Hospital Medical School where Chamberlain was the professor—had published two papers in the August issue of the journal that were fraudulent. One was a case report of the embryo of an ectopic pregnancy being reimplanted and leading to a baby being born.[143] Obstetricians had been trying to do this for years, and the report when published received worldwide media attention. The second paper was a trial of treating recurrent miscarriage in nearly 200 women with polycystic ovary syndrome.[144] A whistleblower at the hospital had pointed out that the patient with the reimplanted pregnancy didn't exist and had also questioned whether Pearce could have found 200 patients with polycystic ovary syndrome. There had been an investigation at the medical school, and Pearce had been both fired and reported to the General Medical Council (GMC).

I knew that such a story would have to emerge in Britain, but I was still taken aback. I was impressed, however, with the way that the inquiry had been held quickly and how the medical school had not attempted the traditional cover up. I remember advising Chamberlain to think about how the story would be told to the media. 'You should tell the story as soon as possible in order to keep the initiative. If it leaks—as it surely will— it may work even more against you than it need do. You may have experienced fraud, but you've responded quickly and correctly.'

A day or two later there was a large picture of Chamberlain on the front of the *Daily Mail* together with the full story. (One anxiety I had was that Chamberlain would think that I'd leaked the story. I hadn't, and as far as I know he never thought I had.) Chamberlain, it emerged, had been an author on the fraudulent case report.[143] He was reported as not knowing until after publication that the case didn't exist and that it was normal for senior people to put their names on papers when they hadn't really done anything. He was, ironically, correct, but it was a strange idea to readers of the *Daily Mail* that you would put your name on a scientific paper when you had had little or nothing to do with it. That sounded to them like fraud.

I was subsequently a member of a working party set up by the college to consider the implications of the case for the college, the journal and the relationship between them.[141] Pearce had by this time been found guilty of serious professional misconduct by the GMC and struck off, and Chamberlain had resigned both as editor and president. Both were disgraced. The medical school investigated other studies by Pearce, and another four were retracted, including two that had been published in the *BMJ*. The working party, which was chaired by a senior lawyer, interviewed all the protagonists, including Pearce and Chamberlain, and offered a remarkable insight into what is still Britain's major case of research fraud.

The well written report we produced (which was not written by me) reads somewhat like a whodunnit. It made a great many recommendations which argued that the time had come to move from the long amateur tradition of editing specialist journals to something more professional.[141,142] The appointment, training, support, records and accountability of editors all needed to be modernized. These recommendations apply to all journals. What happened at the *British Journal of Obstetrics and Gynaecology* could easily have happened at other journals—and probably still could. Indeed, it probably will.

Alcohol played a prominent part in the Pearce story. It was at a dinner at the college that Pearce after drinking heavily told a colleague, Gedis Grudzinskas, that he had successfully reimplanted the embryo. Grudzinskas for his own reasons told the media, who then contacted Pearce regularly for news—putting him under extra pressure. It was during drinks to celebrate the editor's birthday that Pearce told the rest of the editorial team about his success. He told them he was thinking of submitting a case report to the *Lancet* or the *BMJ*. The editorial team wanted such a report for their journal. They told Pearce that if he wrote the paper immediately they could publish it in the August issue. He wrote the paper there and then, adding Chamberlain's name, and the study was rushed into the journal without any external review.

The paper on recurrent miscarriage had been reviewed, but the clinical reviewer saw the request to review the paper as a good opportunity to promote his own related paper. His review was cursory. The statistical reviewer, in contrast, saw many problems with the study and said that he assumed that it was performed better than it was reported. When the inquiry asked him directly, he said that it had not once crossed his mind that the paper might be fraudulent.

One of the most painful parts of the inquiry was interviewing a junior doctor who was a co-author on the fraudulent trial. She had had no training in research or the ethics of research, didn't really understand what was happening, and even felt guilty that Pearce had done so much of the work. She had been cruelly exploited by Pearce and badly let down by the medical school. Pearce himself had the most elaborate—and unbelievable—explanation of how records had been lost on both the single patient in the case report and the patients in the trial. Chamberlain's double tragedy was, first, to severely misjudge the character of Pearce, his protégé, and, second, to fail to notice that best practice had changed around him. When he was first an academic, a head of department might almost be expected to put his name on a paper even if he had done little—rather like countersigning a cheque. By the end of his career such behaviour was misconduct, although it persists as normal in many medical cultures.

The Pearce case sent a shock through the British academic medical community. It was soon followed by the case of John Anderton, an Edinburgh physician who had been an official of the Royal College of Physicians of Edinburgh. He had faked results in a drug trial. He was found guilty of serious professional misconduct by the GMC, as was Robert Davies, a professor of respiratory medicine in London. These were prominent figures in British medicine.

A more recent case involving Arup Banerjee brought up new issues.[145] He was found guilty of serious professional misconduct in 2001 for research fraud that dated back to the early 1990s. His fraudulent study was not retracted until more than 10 years after it was published. Later his supervisor, Professor Tim Peters, was also found guilty of serious professional misconduct for failing to take action over falsified research published by Banerjee. This fits with the line taken by the GMC on clinical practice: 'You are required to take action on a colleague who may be harming patients, and you may be found guilty of serious professional misconduct if you do not.'

But Peter Wilmshurst, a cardiologist who reported Banerjee to the GMC, has pointed out that people in a good many institutions knew about Banerjee's fraudulent work and yet failed to take action.[145] These included people at King's College School of Medicine and Dentistry of King's College London, the Royal College of Surgeons, the University of London and the British Society of Gastroenterology. Wilmshurst calls this 'institutional corruption', drawing a parallel with 'institutional racism', whereby an institution can behave in a racist manner even though none of the individuals within the organization is racist. He began his article by quoting Edmund Burke: 'For the triumph of evil it is only necessary for good men to do nothing.' Academic institutions in the United States, Britain and other countries have indeed been complacent about research misconduct.

Despite all these cases in Britain and despite a summit meeting of the relevant institutions agreeing in Edinburgh in 2000 that national action was needed, the biomedical establishment has not acted. (Two weeks before reading the final proofs of this book – in July 2006 – I attended the first meeting of the UK Panel for Research Integrity in Health and Biomedical Sciences.)

One of the many unanswered questions on scientific fraud or research misconduct is how commonly it occurs. (I've used the phrases scientific fraud and research misconduct interchangeably until now, but from now I'll use research misconduct. This term is now preferred to scientific fraud because it recognizes that misconduct takes many forms and is often minor. It also avoids confusion with financial fraud.) The question on the incidence of research misconduct obviously depends on how it is defined, another difficult question.[146]

The Americans have argued long and hard about the definition of research misconduct.[110] Researchers wanted a tight definition that would allow them to know clearly what was and what was not misconduct. They were also anxious that 'honest error' might be mixed up with misconduct and that a loose definition might allow academic disputes, which are distressingly common, to become accusations of misconduct. In 1995 the United States Commission on Research Integrity produced a definition some 400 words long.[147] Then at the end of 2000 the federal government produced a slightly shorter definition (only with long footnotes) together with requirements for a finding of misconduct.[148] The definition states:

'Research misconduct is defined as fabrication, falsification, or plagiarism in proposing, performing, or reviewing research, or in reporting research results. Fabrication is making up data or results and recording or reporting them. Falsification is manipulating research materials, equipment, or processes, or changing or omitting data or results such that the research is not accurately represented in the research record.

Plagiarism is the appropriation of another person's ideas, processes, results or words without giving appropriate credit.'

The definition continues by making clear that 'research misconduct does not include honest error or differences of opinion'.

A finding of research misconduct depends on three requirements. First, there must be 'a significant departure from accepted practices of the relevant research community'. Second, the misconduct must be 'committed intentionally or knowingly, or recklessly'. Third, the allegations must be proved 'by a preponderance of evidence'.

Drummond Rennie and Kristina Gunsalus, both members of the Commission on Research Integrity, believe that it's important to produce as precise a definition as possible but worry that the American definition may be too narrow, allowing behaviour that is damaging to science to escape from being called research misconduct.[140]

The Nordic countries and Britain have taken a different line from the Americans and opted for broad definitions. The Norwegian Committee on Scientific Dishonesty defines research misconduct as: 'All serious deviation from accepted ethical research practice in proposing, performing, and reporting research.'[149] The consensus conference held in Edinburgh went for something still broader: 'Behaviour by a researcher, intentional or not, that falls short of good ethical and scientific standards.'[150] This definition includes nothing about falling 'seriously' or 'significantly' short of good standards and does not depend on intention. Traditionally in law 'ignorance is no defence', and this definition places an onus on researchers to know what are 'good ethical and scientific standards'.

One question that has always fascinated me is the relation between serious and minor misconduct. We know that some forms of misconduct—publishing closely related material more than once without disclosure, declaring yourself to be an author of a paper when you have done very little, or failing to declare a conflict of interest—are extremely common. Indeed, it has been more common not to declare a conflict of interest than it has been to do so. Many like to think that serious and minor misconduct are different phenomena. Serious misconduct, they like to think, is very rare and nothing to do with minor misconduct. I have no good evidence one way or the other, but it seems unlikely to me that the two are wholly unrelated. I suspect that they exist on a spectrum with minor merging into serious misconduct, and that those who are prone to minor misconduct are more likely to progress to serious misconduct than those who are not.

I suspect too that misconduct may in some sense be contagious. There is a famous book by Harriet Zuckerman in which she analyses the behaviour of the 'tribe' of Nobel prize winners.[151] One conclusion she reaches is that one of the best ways to win a Nobel prize is to go and work with somebody who has already won one. Nobel prize winners beget other Nobel prize winners. I suspect that this may also be true of fraudsters. Working in an institution that allows, or even encourages, poor and sloppy behaviour may lead to misconduct. I can think of at least one family tree where fraudsters may have begotten fraudsters, remembering that research, clinical and financial fraud all tend to go together—and I would love to write the dark version of Zuckerman's book.

The relation between minor and serious misconduct matters when deciding how best to respond to the problem. Should those who want to respond concentrate simply on serious research misconduct or concern themselves as well with minor misconduct? This reminds me of the intense debate on how best to manage high blood pressure. Should doctors concentrate on treating those with very high pressure, or are resources better spent trying to reduce the blood pressure of the entire population by a little— 'shifting the curve [of the distribution of blood pressure in a population] to the left', as the jargon has it. The answer is that both are needed, but treating only those who have very high blood pressure will not be enough on its own because most of the problems caused by high blood pressure—strokes and heart attacks—occur in those with only slightly raised blood pressure—simply because there are more of them.

A similar argument arises over how best to improve the performance of doctors. Should you concentrate on removing the 'bad apples' or try to improve the performance of everybody? 'Bad apples' must of course be dealt with, but much more is to be gained overall by working to improve the performance of everybody. This is sometimes called 'a systems approach'. It recognizes that healthcare is a complex system and that little is gained by working only with individuals. You need to work with the whole system. Richard Horton, editor of the *Lancet*, shocked the consensus conference in Edinburgh by saying how many junior doctors he knew routinely invented data in audit projects they were required to do—because they were not given the time and resources to conduct the audit. The only way to get the job done was to invent the data. So that's what everybody did. The 'system' was pushing young doctors into misconduct.

'Cheating' seems to be endemic among medical students. A survey of 676 medical students in Dundee to which 461 responded (68% response rate) asked about various forms of dishonesty.[152] One in seven of the students didn't think that it was wrong, for example, to write in a patient's notes 'neurological system NAD [meaning "no abnormality detected"]' when the system had not been examined. Three-quarters did think it wrong, but one-third of the students had done it. (The somewhat anxious joke among doctors is that NAD really means 'not actually done'.) One in 10 thought that it was all right to copy text directly without quoting the source, and 14% had done it.

The debates on how best to define research misconduct continue, and so there can be no definitive answer on how commonly it occurs. As I've said, we do know that minor forms of misconduct are common, but we have less good information on the prevalence of serious misconduct. The United States, which has far more biomedical research than any other country and where the problem has been taken seriously for two decades, has seen hundreds of cases, many of them serious. It has also recently had a series of high profile cases in the physical sciences. The committees of scientific integrity in the Nordic countries have seen dozens of cases, few of them serious. Britain has had about two dozen general practitioners participating in trials conducted by pharmaceutical companies found guilty of serious professional misconduct for research fraud. There have also been about a dozen cases among medical academics. Germany has had a very high profile case in molecular biology, which sent shockwaves through the German academic system. The Dutch have also had a prominent professor found guilty of serious research misconduct, but many countries have had few cases.

Mike Farthing, the chairman of the Committee on Publication Ethics and who has been the dean of three medical schools, estimates that major institutions in Britain have roughly one serious case a year. That means about 50 cases a year.

Most cases are probably not publicized. They are simply not recognized, covered up altogether, or the guilty researcher is urged to retrain, move to another institution or retire from research. I have spoken perhaps a dozen times on research misconduct in several countries and often to audiences where people come from many countries. I usually ask the members of these audiences how many know of a case of misconduct. (I consciously don't offer a definition.) Usually one-half to two-thirds of the audience put up their hands. I then ask whether or not those cases were fully investigated, people punished if necessary, lessons learnt and the published record corrected. Hardly any hands go up. Stephen Lock got a similar result from a postal survey he did of friends who were professors of medicine.[153] These 'cover ups' explain why it is so hard to get good data on the prevalence of serious research misconduct, but some countries and disciplines have more cases not, I suspect, because misconduct is more common but because they have begun to face up to the problem.

It may also be that misconduct seems to be more common now not because it is happening more often but because cases are being detected and reported. I often draw an analogy with child abuse. It seems to be a recent phenomenon, but child abuse has gone on for centuries, it just wasn't recognized as such—partly because it was too horrible even to contemplate.

Why does research misconduct happen? The answer that researchers love is 'pressure to publish', but my preferred answer is, 'Why wouldn't it happen?' All human activity is associated with misconduct. Indeed, misconduct may be easier for scientists because the system operates on trust. Plus scientists may have been victims of their own rhetoric: they have fooled themselves that science is a wholly objective enterprise unsullied by the usual human subjectivity and imperfections. It isn't. It's a human activity.

A full response to the problem of research misconduct requires first, I believe, a national body to provide leadership. It needs to raise consciousness about the problem, provide guidelines on good practice, encourage research and teaching, offer help with investigations of misconduct, and probably provide a place for whistleblowers to report anxieties and for the hearing of major cases or appeals against local judgements. One problem with local bodies—universities or hospitals—dealing with cases is that they often lack competence and sometimes commitment. They also face a deep conflict of interest in that they fear that openly investigating and reporting a case will damage the institution.

The main emphasis in responding to the problem of misconduct should, as I've suggested, be on raising the overall level of scientific integrity rather than on investigating suspected cases—although there have to be good systems for investigating, judging and reporting cases. We need codes of good practice rather than simply lists of bad practices to be avoided, and we need to teach integrity rather than warn against dishonesty. Once their consciousness is raised, researchers will realize that they are constantly presented with ethically difficult questions around analysis of data, authorship, conflict of interest, informed consent and a dozen other issues. There are usually no 'right' answers that can be read from a rulebook. Rather researchers need to be able to think their way through the complexities to reach an ethically defensible answer. They may often need help and should not be afraid to ask for it.

Editors and journals have an important part to play in the response to research misconduct. Editors are often the first people to encounter the results of research, and journals are the conduit through which fraudulent research reaches the world. We editors have only comparatively recently recognized the important role we have to play. In my first 18 years as an editor I certainly encountered misconduct, but the cases seemed to be rare and I often did nothing. Problems usually arose with papers we planned to reject, and we didn't think that we had a duty to act. Indeed, the traditional 'confidentiality' of our relationship with authors almost made us think that we shouldn't act.

I do remember, however, some disturbing cases from 20 years ago. One concerned a general practitioner who had become convinced that electroconvulsive therapy was a good treatment for many more conditions than severe depression, the one condition for which it probably is effective. He had a portable machine and had given the treatment to hundreds of his patients, most with physical disease. We were appalled but did nothing. Perhaps the study was a spoof, but we didn't think so. In another case a doctor, who had worked in a psychiatric hospital, moved into general practice and conducted a study in which he took all the patients in the practice who were on antidepressants off them to try a particular test. The study was dangerous and wholly unscientific—and therefore meaningless—and he had neither consent from the patients to be in an experiment nor approval from an ethics committee (in those days there were no ethics committees for general practice). Again, we were astonished but did nothing.

Between 1997 and when I left the *BMJ* in 2004 I dealt with about 20 cases a year and I came to think that it would be misconduct on our part to turn a blind eye to misconduct in authors. This was the effect of the Committee on Publication Ethics (COPE), which was founded in 1997 primarily as a self-help group for editors of medical journals wondering what to do with cases of misconduct they encountered. Its biggest achievement may have been to sensitize editors to recognize misconduct and oblige them to take action.

Although a small group of editors—from *Gut, Lancet, BMJ, Journal of Bone and Joint Surgery* and other journals—began COPE to help each other, it was also prompted by the series of high profile cases of research misconduct in Britain that I've described. Around 200 journals now belong to COPE, most of them British.

The first aim of COPE was to advise editors on cases. The advice has had to be offered anonymously—for fear of libel and to avoid creating a kangaroo court—and the onus remains on the editor to take action. As well as helping editors, COPE wanted to begin to establish what forms misconduct took and how common they might be. So far COPE has dealt with around 250 cases, all of which are described anonymously in the committee's annual reports and are available in full text on the committee's website (www.publicationethics.org.uk).

An analysis of the first 137 cases suggested that there was evidence of misconduct in 106. This is a somewhat arbitrary judgement as COPE hears only one side of the case. The most common problem was publishing or submitting similar material more than once (43 cases), followed by problems with authorship (24 cases), falsification (17 cases), failure to get informed consent from patients (14 cases), 'unethical research' (for example, doing research that didn't need to be done or doing it so badly that no conclusion would be possible) (14 cases), failure to get ethics committee approval (13 cases), fabrication (nine cases) and plagiarism (six cases). We also saw cases of editorial and reviewer misconduct, undeclared conflicts of interest, breaches of confidentiality, clinical misconduct, attacks on whistleblowers, deception and failure to publish.

Many of these cases might be classified as serious, and most cases come from a handful of journals, including the founding journals. Most editors have not been sensitized to the problem of research misconduct. They fail to spot cases or do not feel an obligation to act even if they do. COPE is probably therefore dealing with only a small fraction of all the cases that may be passing through journals.

Experience gathered with these cases has been used by COPE to draft guidelines on good publication practice, so achieving its second aim. The guidelines are available in full on the COPE website. It has been keen to emphasize good practice, not just map poor practice. The guidelines cover study design and ethical approval, data analysis, authorship, conflicts of interest, peer review, redundant publication, plagiarism, duties of editors, media relations, advertising and how to deal with suspected misconduct. The guidelines are regularly revised in the light of new cases and experience.

The next two aims of COPE have been to offer teaching and encourage research. Members of COPE have lectured widely, and some simple descriptive research has been undertaken and presented. COPE has now formed committees for both education and research, but much more work is needed.

In its early days COPE was very much an experiment, and it seemed likely that it might fulfil its mission and disappear. In fact the opposite happened, and COPE formalized itself, adopted a constitution, prepared financial accounts, gathered members and elected officers. The work is simply not complete and the need remains.

One urgent need that continues is that of prompting the medical establishment in Britain to create a national body to lead on research misconduct. Members of COPE fear that otherwise public confidence in medical research may be undermined and that the government may be forced to regulate research in a way that could be counterproductive.

Another need that remains for COPE is to regulate editors. People are always keener on regulating others rather than themselves, and editors have been no exception. I will discuss editorial misconduct in chapter 12, but COPE has encountered eight cases of editorial misconduct. While COPE operated informally and primarily by advising editors it could not effectively regulate them. Now that it has a constitution and membership it can potentially do so. A code of practice has now been drafted, and COPE has developed a mechanism to regulate members.[154] It hasn't yet, however, heard a case, and a major challenge for COPE will be to demonstrate that it can respond to misconduct not only by authors but also by editors. If it can't, its credibility will plummet.

COPE is ultimately advisory. It remains for individual editors to act, and, although editors may be the first to encounter research misconduct, they are restricted in what they can do. They are in many ways simply privileged 'whistleblowers', privileged in that it is hard for researchers, universities or even national or international bodies to bully them. Conventional whistleblowers, who are usually junior researchers, are often the people who expose research misconduct. Unfortunately, they often encounter more problems than those on whom they blow the whistle—even when they are thoroughly vindicated.

Those accused of research misconduct have a right to due process—just like anybody against whom a serious accusation is made. Journals cannot provide due process. Furthermore, they do not usually have any legal legitimacy to hear a case and impose punishment. It's employers who do. Unfortunately, many editors do not understand their restricted powers and may take illegitimate actions. I sat on one of the subcommittees of the Danish Committee on Scientific Integrity where the editor of an international journal had been accused of misconduct by a Danish researcher for taking illegitimate action against him. We found fault with both the editor and the researcher, and the wise chairman told me that fault had been found on both sides in almost all the many cases he had dealt with. It's very hard—perhaps even impossible—to behave with complete integrity.

The role of editors is to pass on accusations to the relevant authority, usually an employer but sometimes a regulatory authority. A difficult question is to know how much evidence you need to have. There is an understandable tendency to think that you need a great deal of evidence to make such a dramatic allegation, but gathering it is often difficult, expensive and time consuming, and can create many problems. I made this mistake with one of the first cases I encountered.

We were about to publish a paper that suggested that cimetidine, a drug used to treat stomach and duodenal ulcers, might help people lose weight.[155] It was an unlikely and unexpected finding. We'd never heard or even thought of cimetidine being used in this way. Nevertheless, the paper had made it through our peer review process. But then we received a similar study that found no evidence that cimetidine helped with weight loss.[156] This made us re-examine the first paper. We noted that it came from a single author, a general practitioner from a rural area. A statistician with an interest in fraud looked at the paper and was worried. A clinical reviewer was also anxious now that the possibility of misconduct had been considered.

In retrospect this was enough evidence to ask the researcher's employer to investigate. At the time I thought I needed more evidence. I rang a friend from the country where the author lived. He made some inquiries, and the result was that many people in the country, including the researcher, knew about my anxieties. The researcher flew to London to see me, telling me stories of being abused by other academics. I was simultaneously accuser and comforter. The whole thing was a mess.

I did eventually ask her employers to investigate. They did and concluded that there was not a problem with the work. We published the study with a highly sceptical commentary.[155,157] This was years ago, and the idea that cimetidine might help with weight loss is dead. I'm not sure if the work was fraudulent, but I'm left with severe doubts.

That episode taught me not only that I don't have to assemble a watertight case before asking an employer to investigate but also that it may be risky to try and do so. When I contacted an employer or regulatory authority to say that I was worried about a paper I was not saying that the person was guilty of research misconduct. I was simply doing my duty in raising anxieties. The difference is crucial, and a lot less evidence is needed to raise anxieties than conclude that an author has been guilty of misconduct. This is not, however, to say that anxieties can be raised lightly.

I still remember how uncomfortable I felt the first time that I reported an author to the GMC. I did so because he had no employer. Eventually I posted my letter, feeling awful. The next day somebody rang from the council to say, 'You do know that this doctor has already been found guilty of serious professional misconduct.' I didn't.

Sometimes editors should 'blow the whistle' to encourage organizations to clarify what is good practice. When Sir Richard Peto, one of Britain's leading researchers, rang me once to say that I had broken every one of COPE's principles, I suggested that he make a complaint about me to COPE. This was not masochism but an attempt to achieve greater clarity on the principles and what they mean. He didn't make the complaint.

I once complained about a *BMJ* author to the GMC because the author, who was a private practitioner (and so had no employer), told me that he couldn't get approval from a research ethics committee because there was no committee covering private practice. I also accused him of doing research on patients without informed consent, but he told me that what he had done was routine clinical practice rather than research. I thought he had done wrong. He disagreed. But we agreed that it would be good for everybody to know what private practitioners should do about ethics committee approval and also to be given guidance on where clinical practice ends and research begins.

Although editors cannot undertake investigations, they do have a duty, I believe, to persist in making sure that justice is done. As I've said repeatedly, institutions are inclined to let accusations fade away. Every time I wrote making an accusation I made a note in my diary to follow it up a month later. Often I had to write again a month later after hearing nothing. Another major advantage that editors have over lone whistleblowers is that the institutions know that journals can publish their concerns. They have a means to expose laggard institutions.

Despite the power of journals many institutions still do nothing when anxieties are raised. It is difficult for institutions in Britain not to respond to the *BMJ* because it knows how to oblige institutions to respond—resorting to the GMC, the Department of Health or a similar national body if all else fails. (Despite this, the medical director of one district general hospital responded to an accusation by saying to me that the hospital would investigate 'if the *BMJ* was willing to pay'. The hospital didn't want to pay because it was strapped for cash and had already suspended the doctor I was complaining about because of problems in his clinical practice. I was flabbergasted and responded by saying, perhaps melodramatically, that if I rang the police to say that I thought the man next door had murdered his wife I didn't expect to be asked to pay for the investigation. The hospital did eventually comply.)

Over the years I made complaints to employers and authorities in Australia, Canada, Egypt, Germany, Greece, India, Jordan, Russia, Britain and the United States, and often I received no response. I usually wrote again at least once, but often I then gave up, thinking that I had discharged my duty in alerting the authorities.

But sometimes the case was so serious that I persisted. I pursued for over 10 years one case of an Indian researcher, RB Singh, who had published dozens of what I thought to be fraudulent studies. The case started in the days when I thought that I needed to assemble a convincing case before I approached an authority to investigate. Assembling the case took years. Then I spent years trying to find an institution to investigate the case. The researcher owned his own institution. Nobody would investigate, so I decided that we ought to publish the whole story in the *BMJ*. The *BMJ* Ethics Committee agreed, and a year after I left the story was published.[158]

At the same time that this story was published, the *BMJ* published further information on a case of a Canadian researcher, RK Chandra, whom the journal had also been pursuing for years.[159] We had severe doubts about the authenticity of a trial submitted to us. We thought that the data had been fabricated or falsified. Three reviewers, each from different disciplines, agreed with us. I wrote to the Memorial University, Newfoundland, asking it to investigate. One immediate response was a letter from the author's lawyers demanding to know the name of the reviewers. (The *BMJ* has a peer review system whereby the authors know the names of reviewers [see p 93], but suspected fraud is the one set of circumstances where we kept the names of reviewers back—to protect them.) I declined.

The university investigated and found no problem. We were unconvinced by the thoroughness of the investigation, and asked it to look again and provide answers to specific questions. The next letter from the university said that it wouldn't be able to investigate because Chandra had left its employment and the country, leaving only a poste restante address in Switzerland. We took this as an admission of guilt.

We then discovered that the author had published the paper we were querying in the journal *Nutrition*.[160] The study that concerned us was closely related to a study published by Chandra in the *Lancet* more than 10 years previously.[161] Our ethics committee agreed that we had a responsibility to notify these other journals about our doubts. We discovered as well that the researcher had published a great many randomized trials on his own in major journals over the past 10 years. There are always doubts about such studies because a randomized trial is a major undertaking and difficult—if not impossible—to do on your own.

Nutrition eventually retracted the study,[162] and the *Lancet* published a letter raising severe doubts about the study.[163] In 2006 Canadian television broadcast programmes showing that Chandra had a long history of misconduct and that the university had investigated him for fraud in the mid-1990s and found severe problems. Chandra had, however, gone on working and publishing.

Both Singh and Chandra have published dozens of studies in major journals, and I and others have severe doubts about all of them. Hardly any of the studies have, however, been retracted. There is simply nobody willing to take on the responsibility of investigating all those past studies. Surely, however, they should be marked in some way as suspect in Medline and other databases.

The Chandra and Singh cases have led to an article on the front page of the *Wall Street Journal* and the Canadian television programmes but very little reaction from the scientific community. It could be that the *BMJ* is utterly unique in coming across two such cases of repeated fraud, but it seems more likely to me that such fraud is happening equally commonly in the other 30,000 or so scientific journals. Why should the *BMJ* be unique?

These cases illustrate, I hope, why journals need to persist in asking employers to investigate. But it can be a long drawn out and risky business, and it's easy to understand why smaller journals without the resources of the *BMJ* might think it beyond them. Journals cannot, I believe, simply publish their doubts without attempting to get an institution to investigate. That could amount to 'trial by media' without due process. Journals may, however, have a duty to publish their doubts when they run out of other options—when they cannot get any institution to take responsibility to investigate properly. So far there are very few examples of journals taking such a course, illustrating, I fear, how many researchers may get away with misconduct. Institutions won't investigate properly and journals don't see it as their duty to act.

This is a global problem, which is to be expected as the conducting and publishing of research is a global enterprise. Many countries do not seem to have adequate means for responding to research misconduct. Plus an increasing number of trials are conducted in several countries simultaneously. There is clearly a case for an international body to respond to the problem of research misconduct.

▶9

The death of the author and the birth of the contributor?

When Anthony Trollope sat down at 5.30 in the morning day after day to write his 47 novels he wrote every word. Editors and publishers no doubt proposed ideas and suggested changes. But the work was his. He was a true author. Mostly it doesn't work like that in research. Many people with different skills are essential. Writing the paper may be one of the easiest parts of the process, and sometimes may be undertaken by a professional writer who has had nothing to do with the research. Authorship is thus, I will argue, the wrong concept for research studies, but it's a concept with great tenacity. It is the coinage of academia, and academics have proved reluctant to move away from it to something call contributorship.

Authorship is about credit and accountability. Authors are most interested in the credit, whereas editors are most concerned about accountability. Publishing papers in important journals is the main way to progress in the academic world. Those who publish the most will be promoted the fastest, win the most grants, get paid the most, and find their way to the best universities and departments. Increasingly departments and institutions are themselves judged on the amount they publish and where they publish. The cliché 'publish or perish' is known beyond the academic world—and is largely true. It's often also more a matter of quantity than quality. So there are huge incentives to publish as much as possible.

The number of authors on papers has increased steadily in recent years. Some studies in molecular biology have over a hundred authors. Some of this increase is no doubt legitimate in that it reflects the increasing complexity of science and the need for teams of people with different skills. But some of this increase is probably illegitimate, driven by the need of individuals and institutions for publications: authors are included who have done little or nothing, a practice that has been called 'gift authorship'.[164–166]

Putting your name to a paper should be like signing a cheque, a major undertaking, but often it isn't.[167] Gift authorship is a form of deception. It's particularly troublesome to editors when there turn out to be serious problems with the paper and yet the gift authors will not accept any responsibility. I described several florid cases in chapter 8.

So who should be an author? Some academic institutions have attempted definitions, but the best known definition is that produced by the International Committee of Medical Journal Editors (which is widely known as the Vancouver group because it first met in that city in 1979).[168]

What is the legitimacy of this group to define something so important for academic life? One answer might be 'none'. The group, of which I've been a member, is self-appointed and comprises the editors of the major general medical journals from the

United States and Britain. There are some editors from other countries but very few, and only one or two editors are from journals not published in English. International is a misnomer. It has no constitution, no clear mission, no secretariat, no funds and no leaders. It was started by Stephen Lock, my predecessor as the editor of the *BMJ*, and Ed Huth, the editor of the *Annals of Internal Medicine*. And its great achievement was to get these major journals (and subsequently many others) to agree to use one system of referencing. This meant—in the days before word processing—that authors (or in reality their secretaries) did not have to keep retyping manuscripts as they worked their way down the food chain of journals. The group has continued to meet every one or two years and has now produced guidance on many aspects of publishing medical research. Some of this guidance has been used in institutions like the Supreme Court in the United States.

The legitimacy of the group to produce a definition of authorship (and other statements) stems partly from the fact that nobody else was doing so and partly from its potential ability to enforce the definition. Its initial definition of authorship was produced by the editors without any consultation. This meant, I judge, that it produced a definition that didn't work in the real world. It has now, however, moved substantially towards supporting a policy of contributorship, but it continues to offer guidance on when a contributor might qualify as an author.

This is its current position:[168]

'An "author" is generally considered to be someone who has made substantive intellectual contributions to a published study, and biomedical authorship continues to have important academic, social, and financial implications. In the past, readers were rarely provided with information about contributions to studies from those listed as authors and in acknowledgments. Some journals now request and publish information about the contributions of each person named as having participated in a submitted study, at least for original research. Editors are strongly encouraged to develop and implement a contributorship policy, as well as a policy on identifying who is responsible for the integrity of the work as a whole.'

While contributorship and guarantorship policies obviously remove much of the ambiguity surrounding contributions, it leaves unresolved the question of the quantity and quality of contribution that qualify for authorship. The International Committee of Medical Journal Editors has recommended the following criteria for authorship; these criteria are still appropriate for those journals that distinguish authors from other contributors.

- Authorship credit should be based on 1) substantial contributions to conception and design, or acquisition of data, or analysis and interpretation of data; 2) drafting the article or revising it critically for important intellectual content; and 3) final approval of the version to be published. Authors should meet conditions 1, 2 and 3.
- Acquisition of funding, collection of data, or general supervision of the research group, alone, does not justify authorship.

- All persons designated as authors should qualify for authorship, and all those who qualify should be listed.
- Each author should have participated sufficiently in the work to take public responsibility for appropriate portions of the content.

One important change introduced by these criteria is that authors are now publicly accountable for 'appropriate portions of the content'. It used to be that authors were expected to be publicly accountable for the whole document. Indeed, the way that I remembered the definition and explained it to others was by the story of the lead author who was about to fly to Acapulco to present the results of the study and then was suddenly taken ill. If you could get on the plane to Acapulco that day, present the paper and answer all questions you were an author. If you couldn't, you weren't.

Raj Bhopal, at that time a professor at Newcastle Medical School, and others conducted a study in 1996 of what academics from every part and every level of the medical school thought about the Vancouver group's earlier definition of authorship.[169] They approached 70 academics and achieved a 94% response rate. Three-quarters of those they interviewed thought that there should be criteria for authorship, but few knew of any criteria. Only 16 knew of the Vancouver group, and only five knew the three criteria, which survive in the definition quoted above. One academic of the 76 knew that you had to satisfy all the criteria in order to qualify for authorship.

Most of the academics agreed with the individual criteria of the Vancouver group, but most thought it unreasonable to expect all three to be fulfilled. The need to fulfil all three criteria was viewed as inflexible and restrictive—and prejudicial to junior researchers. Many thought that the (then) requirement to be publicly accountable for the whole study failed to recognize the real world of multidisciplinary research.

More than half of those interviewed thought that the criteria were not usually adhered to, which fits with what is now a large body of evidence that shows that only a minority of authors of studies meet all three criteria.[164-166] Indeed, something like one-fifth don't meet any of them. The Vancouver group criteria just don't fly in the real world. Many of those interviewed in Newcastle thought it inevitable that the criteria would be breached—often for reasons of 'power, status, and "nepotism"'. Some didn't recognize the authority of the Vancouver group to produce a definition of authorship.

Many of those from Newcastle—and particularly the junior researchers—thought that the Vancouver definition gave too much emphasis to intellectual input and too little to practical work. Indeed, the Vancouver definition has been called 'a senior author's charter'. I know about this because, although I hesitate to describe myself as a researcher, I have conducted research on aspects of medical publishing with colleagues and medical students. Often the idea is mine, and I have a rough proposal for an experimental design. But it is the others who do all the hard work, sticking stamps on envelopes, chasing those who don't respond, and compiling and analysing the data. Without them there would be no research.

One of those interviewed in Newcastle put it this way: 'There needs to be a difference between intellectual contribution and the execution of work. You need to have made a contribution to one or the other but it may not be realistic to have both. The criteria seem to overlook the practical, doing the experiments. They seem to say if you have ideas you become an author, if you work in the laboratory 12 hours a day you don't get on. It should be teamwork.'

Gift authorship was seen by those in Newcastle as 'unethical, dishonest and unacceptable', and yet it was thought to happen commonly. The reasons given for gift authorship were (in order of importance) pressure to publish, enhancing the chances of publication (by including a 'big name'), to repay favours, to motivate a team and encourage collaboration, and to maintain good relationships. The 'solution' that was most favoured was to require researchers to sign a statement justifying authorship and to specify the actual contribution of each author. Limiting the number of publications listed in a curriculum vitae or a system of fixed credits per publication found less favour.

An important aspect of the Newcastle study was to show that problems with authorship are common. Two-thirds of the academics had experienced problems, most commonly being excluded from authorship when they felt that they deserved it. Many had vivid and bitter memories of disputes over authorship. At Harvard disputes about authorship accounted for 2.3% of 355 complaints brought to the Ombuds Office in 1991–2 and 10.7% of 551 complaints in 1996–7.[170] One-third of 51 German students who had published papers reported honorary authorship of the department head, and 16 among 201 students who had done research reported that they had been omitted as author from a publication despite having contributed.[171] Disputes over authorship are often the origin of the long running feuds for which the academic world is notorious. Despite most respondents in Newcastle disapproving of gift authorship, one-third of the academics had included as authors people who had done little. Gifting authorship is one of the currencies of academic life.

The overall conclusion of the Newcastle study was that: 'The strategy for communicating and implementing the criteria of the International Committee of Medical Journal Editors has largely failed. New initiatives should engage researchers and meet their legitimate needs. Future guidelines should be developed collaboratively and not be imposed on researchers by editors.'

So the academic community and medical journals have a problem. Authorship is of fundamental importance in the academic world and yet it is corrupted. Many people appear as authors when they have done very little, but at the same time people who have done a great deal of work, usually the practical work, are excluded. How can journals respond?

One response—tried by the American journal, *Obstetrics and Gynecology*—was to limit the number of authors. If your paper had more than six authors you were asked to justify why. One result was that a great many papers had six authors but another was that authors submitted studies that had more than six authors elsewhere. This may have damaged the journal because major studies—like randomized controlled trials—often have more than six authors. It was a crude response to a complex problem.

Another solution suggested by the Newcastle researchers and tried by us at the *BMJ* was to ask everybody to sign to say that they met the Vancouver group criteria. We also tried to respond to the problem of people being excluded from authorship by asking the authors to sign to say that there wasn't somebody who met the criteria but hadn't been included. This solution hasn't worked. The number of authors has not changed, and later research has shown that many people who appear as authors do not meet the criteria. Editors can go only so far in 'enforcing' a solution, and it doesn't feel comfortable to be operating like a policeman.

Something much more radical was suggested in *JAMA* in 1997 by Drummond Rennie, Veronica Yank and Linda Emmanuel.[172] They suggested abandoning the concept of authorship and moving instead to contributorship. Instead of making an inevitably arbitrary decision on who was and was not an author people would simply describe their contribution. It should be possible for people to agree on who did what. It's simply a descriptive not a judgemental exercise. The sorting of people into the sheep of authors and the goats of the merely acknowledged seems to be based, unsurprisingly, on power. The powerful even if they have done little become sheep, while hardworking goats are excluded.

The great benefit of the contributorship system in my mind is that it can be informative, precise and honest. Contributors describe exactly what they did, and readers make up their mind on the value of the contribution. By making people either authors or not lots of information is lost, and there is a pressure to be dishonest. You want to include as an author somebody who has done a great deal of work but who doesn't feel comfortable with being publicly accountable for even part of the work. So currently they are included as an author, but readers are deceived.

One immediate problem with such a system is the need to ascertain who will take overall responsibility. Otherwise, we may be left with the problem of a dishonest paper and only 'honest' authors. Rennie and others suggested that all papers should have guarantors, people who accept responsibility for the full paper.[172] 'Guarantors,' they wrote, 'are those people who have contributed substantially, but who have also made added efforts to ensure the integrity of the entire project. They organize, oversee and double check, and must be prepared to be accountable for all parts of the completed manuscript, before and after publication.'

At the *BMJ* we were convinced that we needed guarantors, but we were not convinced that they had to have double checked every aspect of the research. Would this be possible if the study includes molecular biology, statistics and economics? More controversially, did the guarantor necessarily have to have contributed substantially? Mightn't the guarantor sometimes be the person who hired all the researchers even if he or she hasn't contributed much to the particular study? In other words, guarantorship might be akin to the responsibility of a government minister. While sat in Venice writing this book I was the guarantor of the *BMJ*. The buck stopped with me. I fulfilled this role not through double checking every word in the *BMJ* and every decision taken, but by hiring good people and creating good systems. The *BMJ* thus adopted the 'ministerial' version of the guarantor, and, interestingly, it potentially revived in some way the tradition of heads of department putting their names on papers just as people countersign cheques.

The idea of Rennie and others was radical—and so naturally there were objections. People have described the contributorship system as being like 'film credits', and one anxiety was that studies would accumulate enormous lists of contributors—down to the 'principal lady's baggage carrier'. This has not happened. In fact the opposite has happened in that the sum of the contributions turns out to be less than the work that clearly had to be done. For example, papers have been published that nobody has written. Those journals—like the *Lancet* and the *BMJ*—that have adopted the system have so far allowed contributors to produce their own statement in straight text. The *BMJ* did plan to experiment with a matrix system, where the journal would list the activities that we knew had to be undertaken to complete and publish a study (conception, design, data collection and analysis, writing and correcting the paper) and then ask for an indication of which author did what. We didn't want to be restrictive and would have allowed authors to add tasks that were not in our routine list.

Another objection is that the contributorship devalues authorship. All sorts of ragamuffins are now included. But the beauty of the system in my mind is that there should be no pretence, no deceit. If the ragamuffins simply made the tea then the contributorship statement will say so. Disclosure is once again a panacea.

One problem that is potentially solved by the system of contributorship is the problem of the 'ghost author', somebody who simply writes the paper. Such people are often employed by pharmaceutical companies, which has prompted great anxiety. Clearly nobody can be happy with a distinguished doctor receiving a ready written review article that is to be submitted to a major journal and being asked to append his name in exchange for $10,000. A bold doctor might be willing to declare that his contribution was to sign his name and bank the cheque, but this is a degree of deception that cannot be tolerated. Unfortunately, it happens, although I know of no data that say how often.

I did, however, recently meet a professor who told me that he sat next to a woman on a plane—in business class—who boasted that she had published more papers in major medical journals, including the *BMJ*, than any other living author. Yet her name, she said, never appeared. She was a champion ghostwriter and employed by pharmaceutical companies.

What is known to happen commonly is that a professional writer writes the paper. The other contributors will read the paper and make changes, but the professional writer does the donkey work of getting the first draft written. To my mind, this is no different from using a statistician, somebody with special skills, and is perfectly acceptable so long as it's declared. Others differ. They think that the process of writing creates ideas and allows bias to suffuse through the paper. Professional writers should thus be banned. If a scientific paper were a novel or a poem I would agree, but it's not. It should be as clear a statement as possible of what was done and found. Those parts of a scientific paper that are closest to a novel—the introduction and discussion— should be cut back ruthlessly. Furthermore, the other contributors—and particularly the guarantor—must approve every word of the final study. They are, I keep repeating, signing a cheque.

A more important objection to the system of contributorship is that the academic system of credit depends on authorship, and some journals moving away from authorship messes up the academic system. People who have contributed small amounts to a study will be seen as authors by a system that simply counts the names attached to a study. I can see the problem, but for me it is an argument not for editors abandoning contributorship but for academics adopting a more sophisticated system.

The information included in contributorship statements should be very useful to those awarding credits or making appointments. Do you want to appoint an 'ideas' person or somebody who is better at implementation? Contributorship statements will give you this information in a way that lists of authors will not.

Despite my enthusiasm for the concept of contributorship it has not been widely adopted. This is, I think, mainly a matter of time and conservatism—and there has been steady movement in the direction of contributorship by the International Committee of Medical Journal Editors. It can't, however, take the logical step of abandoning authorship and moving wholesale to contributorship. Nor, I have to say, did the *BMJ* while I was editor. Academic medicine is stultifyingly conservative. It's something to do with fear. Those academics who have fought their way to the top of the pile have done so through the present system. Any change in the system might expose the fragility they feel in their hearts.

A subject that I must discuss despite its unimportance is the order of contributors— because, although unimportant, it causes great distress. When correcting the first draft of this chapter I was in correspondence with a contributor ready to take extreme steps in a dispute over order of contributorship. I argued that she was fighting a battle without meaning, but she didn't agree. I argued that the battle was meaningless because order of contributorship is uninterpretable. The traditions over order vary among disciplines, specialties, institutions and departments. Sometimes the 'senior' contributor (in itself a phrase with little meaning) is first, sometimes last, sometimes in the middle. Unless readers have the traditions explained to them they can't infer anything from the order.

The Vancouver group has this to say:[168]

'The order of authorship on the byline should be a joint decision of the co-authors. Authors should be prepared to explain the order in which authors are listed.'

The adoption of contributorship statements would make the debate over the order of contributorship irrelevant. The information a reader might need is in the statement. But Rennie and others suggest that contributors meet together and agree on the relative sizes of their contributions and then list themselves in order of size of contribution. This is of course a matter of comparing apples and oranges (how does having the idea while in the bath compare with six weeks of data collection in the street?), and with such processes the powerful are likely to come out on top.

I want to end this chapter by commenting on an interesting paper by Richard Horton, the editor of the *Lancet*, that suggests that the idea that all the contributors to a study agree with its conclusions is often false. He builds on the insight of the French philosopher Simone Weill that, 'All sentences that begin with "we" are lies.' We can never know exactly what each other thinks. I use the quote whenever I talk about the media, a plural noun. The same might be said of sentences that begin 'Doctors...' or 'Medical journals...' There are probably many such sentences in this book. They are inescapable.

Horton began with the observation that there have been some high profile studies— for example, an Italian trial on the treatment of acute stroke where contributors have disagreed openly, and sometimes bitterly, about the meaning of their study.[173–175] He selected 10 papers published in the *Lancet* in 2000 and wrote to the 54 contributors asking about the studies' results, strengths and weaknesses, interpretation, implications, and meaning for further research. Overall he found substantial disagreement among contributors, but this diversity of views was not reflected in the published papers. Weaknesses of the study were played down, and the discussion section of papers was poorly organized and didn't address many scientific questions that they should have addressed.

Perhaps we shouldn't be surprised by this. Simone Weill has pointed out the problem, and we know that many people describing a comparatively simple event will give very different descriptions. As the film maker Robert Evans said, 'There are three sides to every story: yours, mine, and the truth.' This might be extended upwards to any number of people, and the only version that I would disbelieve completely would be that labelled 'the truth'. Who would produce it?

One response to the problem Horton has identified might be to require structured discussions, a suggestion that I made together with Mike Doherty, who was at the time the editor of the *Annals of Rheumatic Diseases*.[176] But a more interesting response might be to make discussions exactly what the word implies. Instead of presenting one discussion contributors might display their different views.

Moves away from authorship towards contributorship, and possible future moves to reflect the diversity of views of contributors, all help to move us beyond the illusion of a scientific paper as an objective artefact to a living, human and therefore imperfect document.

▶10

Publishing too much and nothing: serious problems not just nuisances

'Redundant publication' means republishing material that is closely related to material already published. There are many circumstances in which this is perfectly acceptable if the connections between the papers are made explicit. Often, however, researchers repeatedly publish closely related papers without making clear the connections. This might seem to be simply impolite and not a serious problem. Indeed, that's how most academics view redundant publication, but I want to try and convince you that it's an important problem—because it introduces a bias into medical evidence. The result may be that treatments seem more effective than they are, misleading doctors and patients. Bias also arises from failing to publish studies altogether, another common problem.

Academics, as I keep repeating, gain credit from publishing. The credit comes as much—and possibly more—from the quantity than from the quality of publication. There is thus a strong incentive to slice up studies into the smallest possible unit in order to maximize the number of publications that might result from any piece of research. This is known as 'salami' publication. You may also benefit from publishing the same material repeatedly.

You publish a case report of a patient with a new condition. Then you publish a series of three patients followed by another paper describing 20 patients. Next you might make a comparison with another group of patients or give an account of how the condition affects the kidneys, then the heart. Perhaps you participate in an international study of the patients. The Australian results are published in an Australian journal, the Brazilian results in a Brazilian journal, and so on for 15 countries. You, as a world authority and discoverer of the condition, are an author on all of the papers. You review all your studies, sometimes on your own initiative, sometimes at the invitation of editors. Very soon you can have dozens of publications, a professorship, an international reputation and invitations to international conferences in exotic places. ('A successful scientist,' a longstanding joke goes, 'is one who converts data into airmiles.') At each conference you give closely related papers that are published in supplements to journals.

When somebody attempts a systematic review of your work he or she will become very confused. Are the same patients being described repeatedly? What is new material and what is old material being recycled? The confusion is particularly profound if the author has obscured the links. The reviewer finds what he or she thinks is a new study but takes time to realize that it's the same as a study reported in another journal. Worse, the studies are often not by one person but by several. Authors are trading authorship. Sometimes the same studies have the same authors, but often the authors appear in different combinations and different orders.

Medical evidence is in this way polluted. As I hope I've made clear in chapter 6, medical studies are hard to do and to interpret. Making sense of medical evidence—or as it's pretentiously called, the medical literature—is hard if everything is optimal, but this pollution makes the job much harder.

I am perhaps being too cynical. A minority of researchers are wickedly and consciously inflating their publications through deception, but it requires both concentration and integrity to minimize rather than maximize the number of papers you publish from a given body of work. There is the ever present pressure—from your head of department, the university, your own insecurity—to publish more, and there are what sound like good reasons for publishing more rather than fewer papers. Too much material in one paper will make it indigestible for readers. You need to reach different audiences with papers with different emphases in different journals. It would be impolite to your charming host at that conference in Rome to refuse to write a paper. Your lecture in Beijing had enough new material to merit a paper, and the new material would not make sense if you didn't include a considerable amount of the material you had already published.

Another group with an interest in material being republished is the pharmaceutical industry. Research and marketing have become intertwined, as I will discuss further in chapter 16, and the publication of a trial favourable to a company's product in a major journal is worth hundreds of thousands of dollars spent on advertising. Furthermore, big trials cost millions of dollars to perform. Companies would thus like to see as many publications as possible coming out of trials. Many trials are conducted in several countries at once. As well as publishing the overall results in an international journal it might seem reasonable to publish the German results in a German journal, the French in a French journal, and so on. The German results will have an author who is an acknowledged leader in Germany, prompting German doctors to pay close attention to and trust the work. Sometimes the German and French results will be combined. Sometimes there will be yet another combination. It might so happen that emphasis will be given to the more favourable results. Favourable comments by leading doctors and researchers are invaluable, and they thus receive many invitations to speak at conferences, some of them huge, which are mostly funded by the industry. The industry also funds supplements to journals to report material presented at the conferences. These reports commonly include recycled material.

Editors and journals tend to see themselves on the side of the angels in this vexed issue of redundant publication, but that is to oversimplify. Although some journals are overwhelmed with material, many are not—and are by no means unwilling to publish material closely related to material already published. Many journals are keen to have the 'top experts' write for them and don't worry too much if the 'top expert's' paper is not much different from 50 he has already published. Supplements can be an important source of revenue and profit to journals and commonly contain recycled studies. The *BMJ* when I was editor was involved in republishing material. We had local editions of the *BMJ* in many countries and regions, including the United States, China and South Asia, and these reproduced material published in the weekly *BMJ*. We always, however, provided a reference to the original publication, and only the original publication is referenced in databases like Medline.

Editors and authors often tussle over whether papers are redundant or not. Editors see redundancy where authors see effective communication. Arguing over the degree of overlap and how much it matters can be fruitless, but what is important is transparency. Ideally, when submitting a study authors should send editors at the same time copies of any related material, published and unpublished. In addition, the manuscript should make clear any links to other material, particularly published material. And this should be done not with a reference half way through the discussion of a paper but with a clear statement at the beginning.

With such openness editors cannot accuse authors of misconduct. They may, however, decline to publish the paper submitted.

Often, however, authors are not open, and various studies have suggested that something like one-fifth of medical studies are redundant.[177-180] In other words, redundant publication is common. It is the form of misconduct most commonly seen by the Committee on Publication Ethics. But does it matter? The world has tended to see it as sloppiness, a minor misdemeanour, but might it be more?

A group from Oxford have provided the most compelling evidence on how redundant publication can be misleading and potentially dangerous. They conducted a systematic review of the effectiveness of a drug called odanstetron in reducing the sickness that patients commonly experience after an operation.[178] The group found 84 trials that included information on 11,980 patients. But when they looked closely they found that there were in reality only 70 trials and 8645 patients. In other words, 17% of the studies had been published more than once and the number of patients had been inflated by 28%. The Oxford group confirmed this duplication of results by going back to the original authors. The published papers did not make clear that trials had been published more than once. The duplication was covert.

The reviewers had to work hard to spot the duplication. One trial had been conducted in several centres, which is very common for trials of drugs. The results from the overall trial had been published, but then researchers from four centres had published their part of the trial. These papers all had different authors, adding to the difficulty of spotting that they were the same trial. It's easy to understand the temptation of both the authors and the pharmaceutical company to publish in this way. The authors get a publication to themselves, and the companies have the benefits of their drug publicized four times—in different journals and probably different countries.

In addition, four pairs of identical trials, the Oxford group found, were published by completely different authors without any common authorship. This has to be misconduct. I discussed in chapter 9 how authorship carries both credit and accountability. Readers and editors need to know who did the work. Clearly in these reports important information is missing. The work reported is the same but the authorship is completely different. This is deception.

Equally worrying was the Oxford group's finding that duplicate reports used different numbers of patients or patient characteristics from the original. In another trial the sex distribution was different in the two reports. We will all be inclined to think that this is sloppiness not misconduct, but such discrepancies are always worrying.

Thus far this study from Oxford had confirmed what we already knew—that redundant publication is common, that the redundant studies often don't refer to each other, and that often the authorship is different. The group then went on to look at which studies were most likely to be duplicated, and—perhaps you've guessed already—it was the ones with the most positive results. The group presented the results as 'number needed to treat'—which means the number of patients you needed to treat in order to stop one patient from vomiting. (Clearly the lower the number the more effective the treatment. This is a measure that seems to be useful for both doctors and patients. Often dozens of patients need to be treated in order to prevent one death, heart attack, or whatever.) The number needed to treat for the trials that were not duplicated trials was 9.5, while it was 3.9 for the duplicated trials. In other words, the duplicated trials suggested that the drug was more than twice as effective. If all the trials were combined without duplication the number needed to treat was 6.4, whereas if reviewers had combined all the trials without spotting the duplication the apparent number needed to treat improved to 4.9. The effectiveness of the treatment was overestimated by one-quarter.

Authors of systematic reviews—which, as I've discussed, are widely regarded as the best evidence on which to base decisions about treating patients—do not usually go to the lengths of the Oxford group to exclude results that are published more than once. It was a major undertaking to do so, made much more complicated by the lack of cross references and the change in authorship. Systematic reviews may thus be routinely misleading patients and doctors because of redundant publication, which is why redundant publication is serious.

Perversely, I believe, some people see this as a problem not of redundant publication but of systematic reviews. It's important to recognize, however, that systematic reviews simply do systematically what reviewers and doctors do more haphazardly— synthesize evidence. The problem lies not with the systematic review but with the underlying evidence. The Oxford group illustrated this in its review by showing how various experts and a textbook had cited duplicate publications without recognizing that they were duplicates.

How can we respond to the problem of redundant publication? Perhaps the first response should be to cease regarding it as simply impoliteness. It is more—and may be very much more. Prevention must be next, producing and promoting codes of good practice—as, for example, the Committee on Publication Ethics (COPE) has done. Authors should be actively encouraged to send editors any other papers related to their submissions. This can be done through guidance to authors (which are famously unread) and through specific reminders at the time of submission. Reviewers may sometimes spot duplicate publication, and the best reviewers will do a search for related papers. The electronic world may make it easier to spot redundant publication, although it may also make it easier to publish redundantly—as outlets proliferate and it becomes ever easier to copy and transmit words and data.

What about punishment? Editors like other groups divide into hawks and doves. Some see redundant publication as a dreadful sin (more sometimes because it wastes their resources rather than distorts and pollutes medical evidence) and want redundant publishers punished by their employers, publicly shamed, and perhaps banned from receiving further submissions to their journal for some period. Certainly if redundant publication is detected after publication then 'notices of redundant publication' should appear in both journals—to alert readers of both journals to the redundancy. The figures suggest, however, that such a notice appears for perhaps one in a thousand cases. Redundant publication seems to be like speeding, so common a 'crime' as to be normal. Nevertheless, when I was at the *BMJ* if we identified a case we tended to bring it to the attention of heads of departments, deans or employers—largely to raise consciousness of the problem and its consequences.

I doubt, however, that we will make much progress while redundant publication is seen as a trivial issue. We will probably make even slower progress with a common sin of omission—simply not writing up and publishing studies. Iain Chalmers, one of the founders of the Oxford Cochrane Collaboration, has argued this is a form of misconduct, and slowly but surely he is being taken seriously.[181] Again the problem is that medical evidence is biased, because 'negative studies' (studies that find that an intervention doesn't work) usually are not published and the evidence is consistently biased towards making treatments seem more effective than they actually are.[182,183]

It is well established that negative studies are less likely to be published, and it's becoming steadily clearer that this is not so much because journals reject them (as has been commonly supposed) but because authors don't write them up and submit them. People have looked at research protocols approved by ethics committees, doctoral dissertations and abstracts presented at scientific meetings, and followed them up to see if they resulted in publications. Consistently, negative studies are less likely to be published.[182–184]

These studies also show that authors are more likely to write up and submit positive studies. Now a large study from *JAMA* has shown that it is just as likely to publish negative as positive studies.[185] This was a study in just one journal and only on particular sorts of trials, but it fits with other evidence suggesting that the problem lies more with authors than editors.

Perplexingly, academics want nothing more than to be published. So paradoxically they may not be writing up and submitting studies because they don't think that they will be able to get them published, even though that seems not to be the case.

Pharmaceutical companies, in contrast, might prefer not to have negative studies published, and some three-quarters of trials published in four of the major general journals (*Annals of Internal Medicine, JAMA, Lancet* and *New England Journal of Medicine*) are funded by the industry.[186] (Interestingly it's only one-third of those published in the *BMJ*.) The industry thus has a chance to be highly influential. I think it unlikely that big companies are actively suppressing negative studies, but they may well be less energetic in encouraging their writing up and submission. Many studies have shown that published papers sponsored by pharmaceutical studies are more likely to be positive than studies they have not been sponsored.[187,188] This could be because editors are preferentially selecting positive papers by pharmaceutical companies, but this seems highly unlikely.

As many as one-half of trials reported in summary form are never published in full, and the bias introduced into medical evidence may be huge. Nobody can know the extent of this bias, but there are stories. Iain Chalmers quotes the work of RJ Simes, who found that published trials showed that a combination of drugs was better than a single drug for treating patients with advanced ovarian cancer. If unpublished trials were included then the combination was no longer better.[181]

Chalmers also tells how failure to publish a study on how best to look after women about to give birth to twins led to an unnecessary delay in moving to the best management.[181] Obstetricians were split 50:50 on whether these mothers should be routinely admitted to rest in bed before delivery. A study conducted in Zimbabwe in 1977 showed that the practice actually led to a worse outcome for mothers and babies. But the study wasn't published until visitors to Zambia learnt about the study years later. Once published in the *Lancet* the study helped to lead to a change in policy across the world.[189]

One response to this problem of people failing to publish is to raise awareness of the problem, and this has happened to some extent. I used to think of publication bias as a small, almost technical problem, but I've increasingly come to think of it as a serious problem—although I'm not sure exactly how serious.

In the late 1990s around 100 journals joined together to publicize an amnesty for unpublished trials.[190] We urged people who had conducted trials and never published them to register that the trial had been conducted. Anybody doing a systematic review on the subject could then contact the authors for data. Many dozens of trials were registered, but they must constitute only a tiny fraction of all unpublished trials. This was more a publicity stunt to raise awareness of the problem rather than a solution to the problem.

A much more serious response is the creation of registers of trials underway. The hope is that eventually every trial that begins anywhere will be registered. There are now many registers and a register of registers. American law requires the registration of trials, and the International Committee of Medical Journal Editors now requires trials submitted to journals that follow its guidance to include a registration number.[191]

These registers should allow the identification of trials that had been started but never published—and so counteract publication bias. They will also make it easier for doctors to encourage patients with problems where the best treatment is not clear to enter trials.

Those who conduct systematic reviews are well aware of the problem of publication bias, and various statistical techniques have been developed to try and identify missing studies. To identify what is not there is clearly a difficult problem, and no technique can be foolproof. It is even more difficult to try and adjust results to compensate for the missing evidence. Many would say it can't really be done at all.

I hope that I have convinced readers that publishing studies more than once and failing to publish are both potentially serious problems, not simply minor misdemeanours. The combination of the two—with positive results being published more than once and negative studies not being published at all—may be particularly dangerous. The result can be patients being given toxic and expensive treatments that are thought to work but which in reality don't.

►11
Conflicts of interest: how money clouds objectivity

I want to begin this chapter with a fantasy, one that has a powerful hold in the minds of many. Doctors treat patients using simply the best evidence and their experience. They are not influenced by money or self-interest. Similarly, researchers try to answer the important questions in medicine, specialist societies are concerned only with what is best for a population of patients, and editors of journals publish only what is true and important for medicine. Unlike people who work in the venal worlds of commerce, politics or journalism we in healthcare are untainted by money and 'the pursuit', in the words of Sigmund Freud, 'of fame and the love of beautiful women (or perhaps men)'.

This is of course nonsense. Those who work in healthcare are human beings and just as prone as any other humans to acting in their own interest, responding to economic incentives, and stumbling into frank fraud and corruption. Anybody who has knocked around in the world and read Dante, Juvenal, Balzac and Dickens knows that this is how human beings behave. Yet somehow in medicine we have fallen prey to the fantasy that we are superhuman. We are not. We are exposed to conflicts of interest, like everybody else. Our response should not be to pretend that they don't exist but rather to acknowledge and disclose them always, and sometimes to accept that they are so extreme that the doctor should not treat a particular patient or an author write an editorial in a medical journal.

Academia and industry are becoming increasingly entangled. In the United States industry support of biomedical research grew from one-third in 1980 to almost two-thirds in 2000.[192] In 1986 just under one-half of life science companies in the United States funded research in academic institutions. This had increased to 92% of them by 1996. About two-thirds of universities in the United States invest in businesses that sponsor research in the same institutions. Meanwhile, pharmaceutical companies spend billions on the influencing, education and entertainment of doctors around the world. The scope for conflicts of interest is vast.

Conflict of interest has been defined as: 'A set of conditions in which professional judgement concerning a primary interest (such as patients' welfare or the validity of research) tends to be unduly influenced by a secondary interest (such as financial gain).'[193] It is important to understand that it is a *condition* not a *behaviour*. Many doctors fail to declare a conflict of interest because they are confident that the conflict has not caused them to behave in a different way. This is to misunderstand conflict of interest. It is hard—perhaps impossible—for us to know whether the conflict of interest has caused us to behave in a different way. We do not understand our own motivations. Double blind randomized trials are so important not because researchers are consciously dishonest but because bias is pervasive and unconscious. It is the same, I suggest, with conflicts of interest.

There is a tendency to concentrate on financial conflicts of interest, but the conflicts might be personal, academic, political or religious. Many things may cause conflicts of interest. Once when writing an editorial on animal research in the *BMJ*, I declared as a conflict of interest that my pet rabbit had been killed by a fox just a few days earlier.[194] This might seem absurd, but I strongly suspect that the rabbit's death influenced what I wrote. It may be that some non-financial conflicts of interest may have more powerful effects than financial conflicts, but they are hard to pin down and define. What's more, much of the research on conflict of interest has concentrated on financial conflicts, which means that our actions on financial conflicts can be more firmly based on evidence. Policies on conflict of interest thus tend to concentrate on financial conflicts.

At the *BMJ* when I was the editor we *required* authors, reviewers and editors to declare financial conflicts of interest but simply *encouraged* them to declare non-financial conflicts. We had required people to declare all conflicts, including non-financial conflicts, but the policy proved unworkable.

Conflicts of interest may be almost universal. Doctors in many countries are paid at least in part according to what they do. If doctors are paid to perform investigations, to admit patients to particular hospitals or to carry out treatments or investigations, then they have financial conflicts of interest. Similarly if they have lunch bought for them by pharmaceutical companies, are paid as consultants by those companies, or have shares in those companies, then they have conflicts of interest. There are very few doctors who have not been given something by a pharmaceutical company.

A major review in *JAMA* systematically collected all the evidence on financial conflict of interest in biomedical research and concluded that about one-quarter of researchers have received research funding from the pharmaceutical industry.[192] Whether or not people are deemed to have conflicts of interest obviously depends on the definition used, and a survey in 1998 found that nearly one-half of researchers had received 'research-related gifts'—materials or money.[195] An analysis of 789 articles from major medical journals found that one-third of the lead authors had financial interests in their research—patents, shares or payments for being on advisory boards or working as a director. These conflicts were mostly not disclosed to readers.[196]

A study in the *New England Journal of Medicine* looked at the financial conflicts of interest of authors of 75 pieces in prominent medical journals on calcium channel antagonists.[197] They asked the 89 authors of the articles whether they had received from pharmaceutical companies reimbursement for attending a symposium, fees for speaking, fees for organizing education, funds for research, funds for a member of staff or fees for consulting. They also asked about the ownership of stocks and shares in companies. (The questionnaire used in the study and adapted for use by the *BMJ* can be viewed at http://bmj.com/cgi/content/full/317/7154/291/DC1.) Sixty-nine (80%) of the authors responded, and 45 (63%) had financial conflicts of interest. Yet only two of the 75 pieces disclosed the conflicts of interest. This is despite the fact that the uniform requirements for authors submitting articles to medical journals have required them to declare conflicts of interest since 1993.[198]

A study that I undertook with a medical student looked at 3642 articles in the five leading general medical journals (*Annals of Internal Medicine, BMJ, Lancet, JAMA* and the *New England Journal of Medicine*) and found that only 52 (1.4%) declared authors' conflicts of interest.[199] One positive sign was that there was a trend towards more declarations over time.

The journals now have a policy of requiring authors of randomized trials funded by industry (about three-quarters of trials published in the journals[186]) to declare the role of the sponsor in the study and who controlled the decision on publication.[200] A study of trials in the same five journals in 2001 showed that only the *Annals of Internal Medicine* had ever published such a statement.[201] Frank Davidoff, former editor of the *Annals*, explained that he had been sensitized to this issue after one set of authors repeatedly failed to tone down their conclusions despite editorial requests. When Davidoff phoned to ask why, they explained that the unidentified sponsors didn't want them to do so. An extension of the study looking at whether or not the major journals describe the role of the sponsor found that in only eight of 100 studies funded by industry was the role of the sponsor spelt out—and even when spelt out it often wasn't clear.[202]

Anxiety on this issue has risen steadily, and *JAMA* now requires not only that the role of the sponsor is declared but also that the data are analysed by an independent statistician not employed by the sponsor.[203] This policy has been described as both discriminatory and unworkable ('independent' statisticians are not easily found),[204] but the editors of *JAMA* have hit back with an impressive list of cases where studies with commercial sponsors have included serious examples of bias.[205]

The picture that emerges is that financial conflicts of interest are very common among authors of studies in medical journals and yet these conflicts have been rarely declared—despite editors saying that they require such declarations. Editors themselves, I must note, hardly ever declare their own conflicts of interest. The *BMJ* posted competing interest statements for the members of the editorial team, the editorial board and the management team in 2003, but this was several years after it required authors and reviewers to declare their competing interests. A study of 37 general medical journals found that only nine had an explicit policy to deal with the editors' conflicts of interest and that the *BMJ* was the only journal that publicly declared the conflicts of interests of its editors and editorial board.[206]

Several studies have shown that financial benefit will make doctors more likely to refer patients for tests, operations or hospital admission,[207–209] or to ask that drugs be stocked by a hospital pharmacy.[210] Caesarean section rates vary dramatically across the world and are higher when women are cared for by private practitioners who are paid for the operation.[211,212] Doctors in Britain performed screening examinations on older people when paid to do so—even though most argued that there was no evidence to support such screening. Dentists in Britain have carried out many unnecessary fillings because they are paid much more to fill teeth than to simply clean them. Doctors, in other words, do respond to financial incentives, and it would be surprising if they didn't.

The *JAMA* review found 11 studies that compared the outcome of studies sponsored by industry and those not so sponsored.[192] In every study those that were sponsored were more likely to have a finding favourable to industry. When the results were pooled the sponsored studies were almost four times more likely to find results favourable to industry. When we remember that industry sponsors about three-quarters of the randomized trials in the major weekly journals, then we can see that there is substantial room for bias.

One study included in the *JAMA* review looked at 69 randomized trials of non-steroidal anti-inflammatory drugs, which are prescribed on a huge scale for arthritis.[213] All of these trials were sponsored by industry, and the drug being investigated (the sponsor's drug) was as good as the comparative treatment in three-quarters of the studies and better in one-quarter. In not a single case was the drug being investigated worse than the comparative treatment. This suggests something is wrong. Supposedly researchers conduct trials when they are in a charmed state called 'equipoise', which means that they are genuinely uncertain which is the best treatment. If they think that one treatment is better than another then they shouldn't be conducting the trial. The implication is that the results should half the time favour one treatment and half the time the other. The fact that none of these 69 trials found that the comparison treatment was better suggests that the trials might have been done more for marketing than medical or scientific reasons. Or it could have been that the trials that found against the sponsor's interest were somehow 'lost'.

(Richard Lilford, a researcher from Birmingham, has recently made the interesting point that although traditionally it is the researcher who is required to be in equipoise, it is the patients who are receiving the treatments with the possibility of both benefit and harm.[214] In a genuinely 'patient-centred' world it would the equipoise of patients not doctors that mattered.)

The study I have already quoted on calcium channel antagonists classified 70 articles from major journals as critical of the drugs (23 articles), supportive (30) or neutral (17). Almost all the supportive authors (96%) had financial relationships with manufacturers, compared with 60% of the neutral authors and 37% of the critical authors.[197]

An important study from *JAMA* looked at what characteristics determined the conclusions of review articles on passive smoking.[215] The authors identified 106 reviews, with 37% concluding that passive smoking was not harmful and the rest that it was. They then considered all the factors that might mean that authors of reviews reached different conclusions. One was the quality of the review. Perhaps better done reviews reached one conclusion and poorly done ones another. Another factor they considered was whether or not a journal was peer reviewed. It might be that journals that had a peer review system would publish better reviews that reached the same conclusion. Or could it be the year of publication? Perhaps recent studies had changed the direction of the evidence. The authors of the *JAMA* study expected to find that the quality of the review would be the most important determinant of whether or not authors of reviews found that passive smoking was harmful.

In fact the only factor associated with the review's conclusion was whether or not the authors were affiliated with the tobacco industry.[215] Three-quarters of the articles concluding that passive smoking was not harmful were written by tobacco industry affiliates. The study authors suggest that 'the tobacco industry may be attempting to influence scientific opinion by flooding the scientific literature with large numbers of review articles supporting its position that passive smoking is not harmful to health'. Again, only a minority of the articles (23%) disclosed the sources of funding for research. The review's authors had to use their own database of researchers linked with the tobacco industry to determine whether authors had such links.[216]

This is a disturbing finding. It suggests that far from conflict of interest being unimportant in the objective and pure world of science where method and the quality of data are everything, it is the main factor determining the result of studies. But the *JAMA* study was of reviews and concerned the tobacco industry, which is notorious for trying to corrupt science. Could the same thing apply with other sorts of studies and with industries less louche than the tobacco industry?

The systematic review of all studies suggests that the answer to the question is yes,[192] and a powerful example comes from studies of whether or not third generation contraceptive pills carry an increased risk of thromboembolic disease. This is a question that matters greatly to women and their doctors. Women who take the contraceptive pill are young and healthy. All medicines have some risks, and those people who have life threatening illnesses are often willing to accept serious and common side-effects. But small risks of side-effects are much more of a problem when millions of healthy people are going to use a drug. Third generation pills were heavily promoted by manufacturers as being an improvement on second generation pills. Many women were switched to the new pills.

New drugs are also important to the companies who make them. It costs hundreds of millions of dollars to bring new drugs to market, and for a new drug to be banned or lose favour in the market can cause companies serious financial damage. Furthermore, some companies have just one or two successful drugs. If just one of those drugs comes under suspicion and loses market share then the whole company may fail, with hundreds or thousands losing their jobs. The incentive is thus enormously strong for companies to conduct studies and interpret their findings in ways that will be favourable to their drugs. There's also a strong incentive to find ways to undermine any studies that are unfavourable to your products. Researchers who work on studies funded by industry may be handsomely rewarded in many different ways. It seems not unlikely that the motivations of the companies may be transmitted to the researchers—albeit in ways that stop short of conscious dishonesty.

Drug authorities in Britain issued a warning on the dangers of third generation contraceptive pills increasing the risks of clots before the studies that raised this possibility were published. There was wide media coverage of the warning, and many women stopped taking the new pills immediately.[217] Other studies soon appeared—and disturbingly for those who believe in the objectivity of science—studies funded by the pharmaceutical industry found no increased risk, whereas studies funded by public money mostly did.[218]

Jan Vandenbroucke, a Dutch epidemiologist and a leading researcher in this area, observed in 2000 that the eight studies that had not been funded by the industry found (when combined) that there was just over twice the chance of developing a clot on the new contraceptive pills compared with the old.[218] One study that had not been funded by the industry found no increased risk.[219] Three of four studies that had been funded by the industry found no increased risk, but one did. This study has been repeatedly re-analysed by statisticians funded by the industry—until the extra risk disappeared. Another study funded by the industry that found an increased risk was never published—but discovered later by Dutch journalists.[219] (I explained in chapter 10 why some argue that failure to publish completed trials is research misconduct.)

If the possible extra risk of third generation contraceptive pills had been high then perhaps all the trials would have found the same result, but the difference was 'small'. The publicly funded trials found that women on third generation pills had about twice the chance of developing clots when compared with those on older pills. A systematic review of all available trials, including those funded by industry, found the risk to be increased by about 70%.[220] Another way to present the results is to say that the chance of a young woman developing a clot in any one year is increased from five per 100,000 person-years [one person taking the drug for one year would be one person year as would two patients taking the drug for six months each] if she is not taking any pill to 15 if she uses the second generation pill and to 25 if she uses the third generation pill. About 1–2% of people who develop a deep venous thrombosis die, which means that the chance of a woman on the third generation pill dying of clots in her lungs is about 2 per million users. In other words the chance of a woman dying from a clot is very low, so an increase in the risk of developing one of 70% seems trivial from the point of view of any individual woman. But when we remember that hundreds of millions of women around the world take these pills, many of them for 10 years or more, then the increased risk if true means a good many dead mothers and motherless children. The risk doesn't seem trivial to relatives of patients who die and to patients who are affected.

Women who developed clots and relatives of patients who died took legal action against the manufacturers of third generation contraceptive pills. Seven women, one of them aged 16, had died. Of those who survived one had lost part of her leg, one had had a stroke, one had been in a coma for weeks, and one had had much of her bowel removed. Both sides in the case agreed that it would be necessary for the plaintiffs to make a case that the risk of developing clots was doubled by taking the pills. They failed, and the case was dismissed. David Skegg, an epidemiologist from New Zealand and one of the leading researchers on the subject, called the judgement bizarre in an editorial in the *BMJ*.[221]

This case was very interesting to us at the *BMJ* because the judge was strongly influenced by Ken MacCrae, a first class statistician who had been an adviser to the *BMJ*. There might be better statisticians than Ken, I don't know, but I've never met one with a better sense of humour and with such an ability to explain complex statistics to people with little or no knowledge of statistics. This ability was obviously invaluable in court cases and made Ken highly desirable as an expert witness. Another characteristic of Ken was a delight in being as politically incorrect as he could and still be amusing. He belonged to the Savage club, a club of heavy drinking wits. Anybody could join who wasn't a bore or a woman.

The *BMJ* had reluctantly had to part company with Ken when he agreed to give evidence on behalf of tobacco companies. He would be giving evidence against Sir Richard Doll, Britain's leading epidemiologists and one of the first scientists to identify smoking as the main cause of lung cancer. Ken's argument was that he was no different from a barrister. Britain has an adversarial legal system, and each side makes the best case it can. Justice required that the tobacco companies had good statistical advice. Most statisticians wouldn't dream of advising tobacco companies, but Ken's delight in political incorrectness meant he would. He would also be very handsomely rewarded, earning in a few weeks what he might earn in a year as an academic.

The same thinking meant that he had always been willing to give evidence on behalf of pharmaceutical companies, and in the case of the third generation contraceptive pills he won the case for the companies. The judge relied primarily on his evidence—despite it being a complex and controversial re-analysis of a study that as published (in the *BMJ*) showed that the third generation pills did carry a higher risk.[222,223] Hours after giving his evidence Ken, who was around 60, collapsed and died.[224]

Discussion of conflict of interest and journals rarely extends beyond authors and reviewers, and the fact that all of us are much more interested in the conflicts of interest of others than our own conflicts means that we have little evidence on the prevalence, extent and effects of editorial conflicts of interest. But the 'black box' of peer review leaves huge scope for conflicts of interest to have powerful effects. I will discuss, for example, the problem of editors publishing their own research in their own journals in chapter 12.

But I want to describe here some of the other conflicts than arise. The one that seems to me most stark arises in relation to reprints of articles. Pharmaceutical companies will often spend thousands (and occasionally millions) of dollars buying reprints of single articles from journals. As I described in chapter 2, the company Merck reportedly bought a million reprints of the highly controversial VIGOR trial that suggested that its drug, rofecoxib, had fewer gastrointestinal side-effects than naproxen.[46] The companies usually buy reprints of studies that they have funded themselves. Unsurprisingly, they buy them only when the results are positive for their drugs, and they use these reprints as a form of marketing. They are given to doctors, and the prestige of the journal adds to the marketing message.

Editors know which sorts of articles are likely to be purchased as reprints by pharmaceutical companies. If they accept such an article then their journal may receive hundreds of thousands of dollars in income—and these reprints are very profitable. If they reject the article then the money is gone. Some editors are directly responsible for the budgets of their journals, and all editors are concerned about their budgets. A healthy budget means job security, praise from the owners, and often the freedom to expand and innovate. A failing budget means the opposite, and for many journals reprint income is an important source of revenue—sometimes the most important. Editors may be faced with a choice as stark as accepting a study that will bring a substantial income or making some editorial colleagues redundant in order to stay within budget. A million dollar order may mean $600,000 profit, which is the equivalent of several editorial salaries for a year.

Sometimes companies will ring when an article is submitted and make clear that they will purchase reprints if the article is accepted. This is effectively a bribe, and 'everybody has their price'. A woman from a public relations company once rang me at the *BMJ* to say that if we accepted a paper then she would 'take me to the restaurant of my choice'. She was very effusive and stopped just short of saying she would go to bed with me if we took the paper. This was actually the most brazen bribe I was offered in 25 years as an editor. Readers will be relieved to know that the *BMJ* did not accept the paper.

I don't know how other editors handle this conflict of interest, but I think that the answer is that they reassure themselves that their judgement is not affected. The evidence that I've quoted on conflicts of interest in other contexts suggests that they are wrong. I was somewhat relieved of any conflict in that I rarely attended the meetings where the final decision was taken on which papers to publish. The *BMJ* was highly unusual (some would say irresponsible) in that the decisions on which original research papers to publish were taken largely by outside advisers. They had no responsibility for the budget, and most (at least until reading this book) were unaware of the money attached to reprints.

Another conflict of interest for editors relates to advertising, a major source of income for many journals. Most of the advertising comes from pharmaceutical companies. Advertisers would always prefer an editorial plug to an advertisement— because they know that readers discount advertising. They want to tie advertising and editorial material as closely together as possible and have various ways to do this, as I discuss in chapter 16. Advertisers may also object to particular studies and withdraw— or threaten to withdraw—their advertising. This may mean death for some journals, and editors may be faced with the stark choice of agreeing not to publish a particular piece or seeing their journal die.

The *BMJ* faced something close to this with one of its local editions (selections from the weekly *BMJ* published in around a dozen different countries). The local edition was heavily dependent on advertising and just breaking even. One company which bought advertising threatened to withdraw it if the local edition republished an article that had been published in the weekly *BMJ* and was critical of the company and one of its products. For the staff, including the business staff, in London this was an easy decision—what the Americans call a 'no brainer'. If the *BMJ* succumbed to such pressure there would be no point in publishing the local edition and—worse still—the independence of the weekly edition, perhaps its greatest attribute, would be undermined. It wasn't so easy for the local publishers, who stood to lose their investment and damage their relationship with an important customer who bought advertising space in their other publications. But the *BMJ* stood firm and published the article. (The local edition did not die at that point but did later through lack of income from advertising.)

In 2004 the *BMJ* devoted the whole issue to the relationship between doctors, including their journals, and the pharmaceutical industry.[225] The cover of the journal— which summed up the whole issue for many showed doctors as pigs gorging at a banquet and playing golf with the drug company representatives as lizards; a patient— depicted as a guineapig—sat amazed at the whole escapade. The *BMJ*'s target was more doctors than drug companies, but the companies were very upset and threatened to withdraw £750,000 of advertising. As far as I can tell, they didn't: it's impossible to know for sure because you can't know exactly what they were intending to spend.

For many editors, however, it isn't so easy to resist the threats and blandishments of the advertisers. If they resist the journal may die, and the owners of the journal—perhaps a specialist society—may be far from pleased. Indeed, the society may be financially dependent on profits from the journal. The *Annals of Internal Medicine* suffered a severe drop in advertising income after the journal published a study that showed that pharmaceutical advertising was often misleading.[226] The episode contributed to the premature departure of the editors, Bob and Suzanne Fletcher, two outstanding editors.

A financial conflict of a different form for editors and journals arises in relation to allowing their studies to be posted on electronic databases—like PubMed Central—that allow everybody free access. If the journals and their owners are primarily interested in advancing science and medicine, as most medical organizations claim to be, then surely the material should be made available for free—particularly as most of the cost of generating it, the research costs, have been met with public money. But making material available for free may cause a loss of subscriptions to the journal—and so reduce profits and perhaps ultimately kill the journal.

Most editors and journals have dealt with this conflict by not recognizing it. Most have stayed with the status quo and declined to make their studies available on PubMed Central. I will discuss this issue further in chapter 17, but this issue illustrates how there is constant conflict between what might be best editorially and financially. This is analogous to the conflict between what doctors and patients might want to do given unlimited resources and what can be afforded. Some argue that the best way to resolve the conflict is for editors (and by analogy doctors) to have no responsibility whatsoever for money. This responsibility should lie with somebody else—owners, publishers or managers.

The trouble with this 'solution' is that it leads to constant—and often increasingly bitter—battles. The conflict between editorial (or medical) and financial needs is real. It cannot be avoided. It has to be resolved, and if the conflict is institutionalized in different individuals or parts of the organization it isn't resolved efficiently and effectively. Rather, much grief is generated. I think it better that one individual (the editor) or one team has responsibility for both editorial quality (or medical excellence) and finance. The conflicts can then be resolved within the individual or team. We are all used to doing this in our daily lives. If I want to make a journey I trade off comfort, speed and cost—and perhaps travel standard class on a train. But if I didn't have to think at all about cost I might charter a plane or at least travel first class.

So we have expanding evidence that conflicts of interest do affect how doctors treat patients and what conclusions researchers reach in studies, but we have little evidence on the conflicts of interest of editors and journals. This could be a rich area for study.

There has also been little evidence on how statements on conflicts of interest affect readers, but together with others (whom I should confess did most of the work) I have conducted two studies to investigate this.[227,228] We took a letter posted on the *BMJ* website that reported that the impact of pain from shingles on patients' daily functioning may be substantial. It came from authors associated with a drug company, and they kindly gave us permission to use a version of the letter in our study.

We sent a random sample of 150 readers the letter with no competing interest declared and another random sample of 150 the letter with a statement that the authors were employees of a fictional company and held stock in the company.[227] We asked the readers to score the letters for interest, importance, relevance, validity and believability. We thought that readers might rate as less believable the version that had a conflict of interest statement. In fact the 170 responders (a 52% response rate) rated the version with a competing interest statement lower on every criterion—of interest, importance, relevance, validity and believability.

This study suggested that doctors, although not inclined to declare their own conflicts of interest, do believe that such conflicts are important. They discount in every way studies where authors have substantial conflicts of interest.

We then repeated the study, but this time the competing statement declared that one of the authors was a recipient of funding for studentships and research grants from the fictional company.[228] This statement did not lead readers to judge the study any differently from the version that had no competing interest statement.

In the second study we also investigated whether different statements would affect readers' judgement of a non-clinical study—one on the use of problem lists in letters between hospital doctors and general practitioners.[228] The statements were analogous to those in our first study: no statement; a statement that one of the authors was an employee of the company making the software and held stock options within the company; and a statement that one of the authors was a recipient of funding for studentships and research grants from the company making medical management software. Each statement was sent to a random sample of 150 readers. This time—with a 66% response rate—there was no difference in how readers rated the interest, importance, relevance, validity and believability of the three versions.

We are at the beginning of understanding how competing interest statements alter the readers' judgement of papers, but it looks as if they do discount studies where there is a 'strong' conflict of interest. A 'strong' conflict is when the authors are employed by an organization that might benefit from the results of the study, although this didn't seem to be true in the second case where the software company might have benefited from the positive results associated with its software. Perhaps doctors are more sensitized to conflicts of interest associated with pharmaceutical companies.

The greatest difficulty with conflict of interest is to know how to respond. It is impossible to eradicate conflicts of interest. They are part of life. The *New England Journal of Medicine* did try to have its editorials written only by doctors without any conflicts of interest. One result was that the editors had great difficulty finding authors to write on some subjects. Within some medical specialties—rheumatology and dermatology, for example—it is impossible to find anybody who doesn't have a conflict of interest. The *BMJ* once snootily dismissed a television programme by saying that it was full of people with vested interests. The producer wrote and, rightly, pointed out that the only people who don't have vested interests are those who don't know anything about a subject—and what would be the point of having them on the programme. (This always reminds me of another correct aphorism that 'the only people who don't have personality disorders are people who don't have personalities'.)

Another result of the policy of the *New England Journal of Medicine* was that sometimes editorials were written by people with conflicts of interest but readers—and editors—didn't know. The editors were embarrassed when the *Los Angeles Times* published a piece entitled, 'Medical journal may have flouted own ethics 8 times.'[229] The journalist had identified eight cases where editorials had been written by authors with undeclared conflicts of interest. The journal has now changed its policy and allows editorials from authors who have a financial conflict below \$10,000.[230] The policy states:

'The key provision of the definition sets an upper limit on the annual sum that a person may receive before a relationship is automatically considered significant (the limit, currently \$10,000, is referred to as the *de minimis* level). We also regard as a significant interest any holding in which the potential for profits is not limited, such as stock, stock options and patent positions.'

This too, I fear, will be hard to enforce. Measuring the size of a financial conflict is hard. But to its credit the journal has tried to grasp the nettle of defining when a conflict is so large that the person must be excluded. The *BMJ* had not done that in my time as editor.

A more common policy is to ask people to declare conflicts of interest. Those sitting on government committees must declare conflicts. In some circumstances doctors treating patients are required to declare conflicts—for example, telling patients that they are receiving a payment for entering them into a post-marketing trial of a drug, or that they have a financial interest in the hospital to which they are referring them. Mostly, however, doctors do not declare conflicts of interest to patients. Increasingly, I suspect, they will be required to. The Declaration of Helsinki, which is written by the World Medical Association, now requires researchers to tell participants about their conflicts of interest.[231] Why should the same not apply in everyday medical practice?

Most journals are moving towards asking authors and reviewers to declare conflicts of interest. The *BMJ* asks all authors and reviewers to complete a questionnaire on conflicts of interest, and authors' statements are published.[232] As mentioned above, the journal *requires* people to declare financial conflicts of interest and *encourages* them to declare non-financial conflicts. This is not because the journal thinks non-financial conflicts of interest unimportant. Indeed, many would say that non-financial conflicts—personal, academic or religious—may be more powerful than financial conflicts.

The *BMJ* concentrated on financial conflicts of interest for three main reasons. First, they are easier to define. Second, most of the research on conflicts of interest has looked at financial conflicts. Third, the journal editors thought it more likely to be able to persuade people to declare conflicts of interest if it began by concentrating on financial conflicts of interest.

The journal did used to require authors and reviewers to declare both financial and non-financial conflicts of interest but had little success.[233] The editors sent everybody a form describing what they meant by conflicts of interest and asking authors to let them know if they had any. Few people declared conflicts of interest, as the research showed. But research also showed that most people had them. Why were they not being declared?

One reason is that the culture was not to declare them. It wasn't an issue that doctors thought important. That is now changing. People also didn't declare conflicts of interest because they were confident that they were not influenced by them—in the same way that most of us, and certainly most doctors, are confident that we are not influenced by advertising. 'Other people must be—otherwise advertisers wouldn't bother—but I'm not.' I suspect too that authors and reviewers thought that it was in some way 'naughty' to have a conflict of interest. By declaring a conflict you suggested that you had been 'bought'. I believe that it is by no means naughty to have a conflict of interest but it is not to declare one.

The *BMJ* changed its policies in order to try and get more authors and reviewers to declare conflicts of interest. First, it changed the phrase from 'conflicts of interest' to 'competing interests'. This, the editors hoped, would reduce the feeling of 'naughtiness'. Second, the journal abandoned requiring people to declare non-financial conflicts. Third, authors and reviewers were sent a specific questionnaire that authors have to complete. The form was derived from that used in the study on calcium channel blockers,[197] and it asks specifically about shares, employment, reimbursement for attending a meeting, fees for speaking, and funds for a member of staff, research, consulting or organizing education.

Whatever the reason, many more authors and reviewers do now declare a competing interest.[234] The culture seems to have changed, and it has become acceptable and normal—at least within the *BMJ*—to declare competing interests. The journal started with original papers but slowly extended the practice to every part of the journal. Letters to the editor—for the *BMJ* and other journals—have been a hotbed of conflict of interest. Many authors who described themselves simply as doctors had close links with pharmaceutical companies and were often prompted by the companies to write. Almost all letters to the editor to the *BMJ* now arrive electronically, and the software will only allow submission of the letter if authors either declare a competing interest or click to say they don't have one.

The *BMJ*'s policy is 'if in doubt, declare'. Problems rarely flow from declaring conflicts of interest, but problems do arise when they are discovered to exist when not declared. We live in a world, whether we like it or not, where what is not transparent is assumed to be biased, corrupt or incompetent until proved otherwise.

Disclosure alone cannot solve the problem of conflict of interest. Clearly some conflicts are so extreme that they preclude a person from writing or reviewing. Thus a journal would not commission an editorial on a drug from somebody employed by the manufacturer of the drug. Nor would a journal ask an author to review his sister's book. But where is the cut-off point? Most journals have not been explicit about where it is—but they surely should be.

And what about the problem that not a single study on non-steroidal anti inflammatory drugs has findings unfavourable to the manufacturers or that almost every study funded by manufacturers finds no increase in clots in women taking third generation contraceptive pills? Disclosure won't solve what seems to be a deep bias. Something more is needed, and that something seems to be beyond the power of editors and journals. The answer might be that there need to be many more large, publicly funded trials where drugs are compared directly with each other.

It might even be that we need a completely different way of publishing trials, as I have argued elsewhere with Ian Roberts, a triallist and professor at the London School of Hygiene and Tropical Medicine.[235] We argue that trials should not be published in journals, where they are 'spun'. Instead, the whole process should be conducted openly on the World Wide Web. First, there should be a systematic review showing which questions need answering—because so many trials don't need doing scientifically but are done for marketing. Second, the protocol should be placed on the web for scrutiny and the trial registered. This would allow the wider world to agree that the trial needed doing and that the methods would allow a confident conclusion. It would also mean that authors could not drift from the protocol without adequate justification and prevent the suppression of results that proved unfavourable to the sponsor. Third, the full data would be posted on the web, preventing selective publication of results and allowing detailed critique of the results. There would be no discussion of the results—because often this proves to be simply spin.

This radical proposal is unlikely to happen anytime soon because it would work against the interests of both sponsors, who would have less room for marketing, and journals, whose income and scientific credibility depend on publishing such trials.

Problems remain even with the policy of disclosure.[234] Reviewers' conflicts are not published because reviewers are not named in most journals. The *BMJ* was planning to do so when I left and then it would have disclosed reviewers' competing interest. But the *BMJ* remains highly unusual with its policy of open review, and it would seem odd to disclose the reviewers' conflicts of interest if their names were not disclosed. Next, journals usually give no information on the scale of the financial competing interest. It might be that an author was bought a cheese sandwich by a company or that he has a sizeable vineyard funded from consulting fees. I think it likely that the scale of the competing interest is important, but it would be a bold step to require it— especially in Britain where people find it even more difficult to talk about their financial affairs than their sex lives. Then, journals should surely at some time try again with *requiring* people to declare non-financial competing interests.

Conflicts of interest are common in healthcare, and yet until recently they have rarely been declared. We have increasing evidence that conflicts of interest affect behaviours like the referral of patients and the interpretation of the results of studies. Editorial conflicts of interest may be particularly stark, and yet they are largely unstudied. Readers seem to discount studies where conflicts of interest are declared, but much more research is needed to understand this more fully. The best response to conflicts of interest seems to be disclosure rather than attempted eradication, but sometimes conflicts of interest will be so strong that they will rule people out from actions like referring patients or writing editorials. The bigger problem of profound bias within trials conducted by pharmaceutical companies cannot be solved by journals.

►12

Editorial misconduct, freedom and accountability: amateurs at work

If editorial freedom is thought to mean that editors should be free to do whatever they want, then it is a myth. Editors must balance the demands of many different groups, from readers to owners, and must be accountable. Perhaps because of the power of the myth of editorial freedom editors are often much less accountable than other professionals, and there are many examples of editors abusing their positions without any retribution. But at the same time, if editors are slaves to the political commands of their owners then the journals they edit will never be respected. How can the right balance be achieved? This is a question that some very grand medical organizations have failed to answer.

Sir Cyril Burt stars in the classic case of editorial misconduct.[132] His important—and much disputed—work on intelligence was important in designing education systems. He founded a journal called the *British Journal of Statistical Psychology* and was its editor. He published 63 of his own articles and often altered the work of others without permission, sometimes adding favourable references to his own work. Once he published a letter he wrote himself under a pseudonym and a response he also wrote himself under another pseudonym in order to attack a colleague.

Another psychologist, Hans Eysenck, used the journal he edited to publish his extraordinary work that must have been fraudulent. He started a journal called *Personality and Individual Differences* and published in the journal studies that suggested that personality was a much bigger risk factor for cancer and vascular diseases than smoking, diet or any other known risk factor. He also proposed that psychological therapies could reduce deaths from cancer and vascular diseases. Anthony Pelosi and Louis Appleby exposed the severe deficiencies in this work, and nobody else has found similar results.[236]

These cases illustrate the dangers of editors publishing in their own journals, and I described in chapter 8 the case of the editors of the *British Journal of Obstetrics and Gynaecology* publishing fraudulent research in the journal. Many thus argue that editors should not publish in their own journals. Even if they are not involved in peer reviewing the research (as they surely shouldn't be), then it will be impossibly hard for other editors, particularly junior ones, to turn down the research. The result might be that inferior work will be published and the reputation of the journal damaged.

It is not so hard for editors of general journals to adopt this position as they are mostly not active researchers, but it's much harder for editors of specialist journals. They are often appointed to be editors of journals because they are leading researchers.

If the journals cannot publish their research then the journals may suffer from the appointment.

I must confess that I have submitted research to the *BMJ* and had it published. (The covering letter says: 'We must declare a competing interest in that one of us is the editor of this journal.') I've also had it rejected, as did my predecessor, who had his still often quoted research on peer review rejected. My reason for submitting our research to the *BMJ* was that it was usually research on the processes of the *BMJ*—for example, open peer review—performed on *BMJ* authors, readers and editors. Plus the research provided the evidence on which we changed our policies. It would seem strange to publish such research in another journal that would be read by only a small fraction of *BMJ* readers.

Disclosure—yet again—is a large part of the answer. Readers should know exactly what process the study has gone through before publication. The *BMJ*, which began an active research programme and had in-house researchers, developed a system whereby papers produced by the staff were peer reviewed only by external editors and not by editors employed by the *BMJ*. This was possible for the *BMJ* because external editors were central to the peer review process. This system was described on the *BMJ*'s website, and editors indicated at the end of the study that this is how it had been peer reviewed.

This system is of course acceptable to the *BMJ* team, but critics would prefer an absolute ban on editors publishing in their own journals. What does seem to me unacceptable is for editors to publish original research in their own journals without any indication of what peer review process they have been through. This is, however, the norm.

The Burt and Eysenck cases of editorial misconduct are well known, but—just as with conflict of interest—editors have been much more interested in the misconduct of others than in their own misconduct. Editorial misconduct is thus less well described, but we begin to have a collection of cases.

Doug Altman, Iain Chalmers and Andrew Herxheimer described three cases at the Second International Congress on Peer Review in Chicago in 1993 and subsequently in *JAMA*.[237] They argued that all three cases showed editorial misconduct and the great difficulties in making editors accountable. They called for an international scientific press council. In their first paper they were unable for legal reasons to name names, but in 2003 the same authors made a second presentation—at the annual meeting of the Committee on Publication Ethics.[238] They were able to give more detail of one of the cases and add two further cases. They observed that very little progress had been made in a decade to develop ways to respond to editorial misconduct.

In the first case Richard Mattingly, the editor of *Obstetrics and Gynecology*, republished in 1983 a paper that had appeared in the *Journal of Pediatrics* without the permission of the authors—although Mattingly stated that permission had been obtained. This paper by Jon Tyson and others reviewed 86 'therapeutic studies' in perinatal medicine published in various journals, including *Obstetrics and Gynecology*, and concluded that in less than one-fifth of the studies were the conclusions supported by the data. Mattingly accompanied the paper with an editorial that described the republished paper as 'a poor study'. Tyson and colleagues sent a response as did two others, one of whom was Iain Chalmers. Mattingly did not acknowledge the letters. Tyson then sent letters to all the members of the editorial board, and eventually an editorial assistant rang him and said his letter would be published. The letter was published a year after the article was published, but the sentence that said that the paper had been republished without the authors' permission was deleted. Again there was a hostile editorial. A letter in response by Doug Altman was not published.

Chalmers and Altman considered this poor editorial conduct and decided that the story needed to be told. They had their paper rejected by six journals, including *Obstetrics and Gynecology*, although brief, anonymized reports of the story appeared—including in the JAMA paper.[237] *Obstetrics and Gynecology* said that it wasn't interested in the misconduct of its former editor. Two journals said their readers would not be interested in misconduct at another journal. Two further journals didn't think that they had any obligation to publish the material when they had not been involved, and one journal simply never responded (itself poor conduct). At least two of the journals were concerned about the risk of a libel action from publishing such material.

Mattingly died in 1985, and Chalmers pursued the new editor asking for an apology to the authors. The new editor declined, but Chalmers, ever persistent, asked the next editor for an apology—and finally one was forthcoming in 2003.

In a second case a scientist was invited to write a review for a journal. It was accepted, and the scientist corrected proofs. But the article never appeared. Subsequently the journal published an article with the same title but by different authors. When the scientist read the article he discovered that much of the text was identical to that in his own article. He could get no response or explanation from the editor.

A third case concerned a randomized trial of two active drugs against a placebo. The study reported serious side-effects with one of the drugs. The authors did not know this, but the editor of the journal was a paid consultant to the company that made the drug with the serious side-effects. The editor sent the paper to several reviewers, including an employee of the company. Altman, Chalmers and Herxheimer did not think it wrong that the editor used a reviewer from the company, but they argue that the combined conflicts of interest of the editor and one of the reviewers must have counted against the study. It was rejected and published in a less prominent journal two years later.

In a fourth case Dr K had a letter accepted that drew attention to possible misconduct. Despite being accepted the letter was later rejected. Dr K tried several other journals but none would publish. One journal editor said that the allegations were serious but that they were none of his business. The letter should be published in the journal that published the papers, but that journal was the problem.

These cases inevitably look like editors closing ranks, and they come from a time— before the late 1990s—when unfortunately it was normal in academia and clinical practice to turn a blind eye to research and clinical misconduct. I'm not trying to excuse editors, but it's another example of a complacent culture. Considering these cases now, the first two seem to provide strong *prima facie* evidence of editorial misconduct. The correct response, to my mind, was not simply to publish the case but to persist in obliging the owners of the journals to investigate the behaviour of their editors. It is the owners who have the legal legitimacy to do so and the ability to ensure due process. The culture that meant that authorities turned a blind eye also meant that the complainants didn't persist. As I've discovered after years of turning a blind eye myself, it's exhausting to persist and often leads to disputes, threats and legal fees.

There are few fully described accounts of editorial misconduct—perhaps because there is no regulatory body anywhere—but another incomplete, although colourful, story emerged in 2003.[239] Antonio Arnaiz-Villena, head of the immunology department at a large public hospital in Madrid and professor of immunology and cell biology at Madrid's Complutense University, was invited to be the guest editor of a theme issue of the journal *Human Immunology*. The theme issue was on anthropology and genetic markers. Nicole Suciu-Foca, the editor-in-chief of the journal and a professor in New York, invited Arnaiz-Villena to edit the issue because he was an expert in 'historic genomics'. The guest editor was given little or no guidance on what was expected. Nor was it clear whether or not the language would be (or actually was) copy edited—despite English not being the first language of most of the contributors, including the guest editor.

Controversy erupted when the issue was published. Arnaiz-Villena's keynote paper concluded that Jews and Palestinians are genetically very close and that their 'rivalry is based on cultural and religious, but not genetic, differences'.[240] It wasn't the science that caused the problem but words and phrases in the article that seemed political—particularly in the highly emotional climate that followed the attacks on New York and Washington on 11 September 2001 (the issue was published in November 2001). Karen Shashok—an American who lives in Spain and works as a translator and editor—argues that most of the problems arose from lapses in translation and editing rather than political intent.[239] Whatever the cause the response was dramatic. The editor fired the guest editor from the editorial board and had the article retracted from Medline and deleted from the online edition of the journal. Subscribers were even invited 'to physically remove the pages' from their copies of the journal.

Was this an over-reaction? Was the editor making the guest editor the scapegoat for her own failures? The editor, the owners (the American Society of Histocompatibility and Immunogenetics) and the publishers (Elsevier Science) have not answered these questions, and this might be an ideal case to refer to an international medical scientific press council. As it stands, we have no trustworthy ruling on the degree of transgression (some might argue it was close to nothing), why it happened, whose fault it was, whether or not it was right to retract the article and whether or not the editor over-reacted. Everybody is smeared; nobody is cleared.

The Committee on Publication Ethics (COPE) concerned itself initially with advising editors about author and reviewer misconduct and only recently concerned itself with editorial misconduct.[241] Nevertheless, it has had cases of editorial misconduct reported to it—and so provides further case studies.

The first COPE case is reported in the annual report for 2000 and is headed, 'Who ensures the integrity of the editor?'[242] The discussion of the case asks: 'What can be done to stop/prevent corruption within the editorial office of a scientific publication?'

and notes that this is 'an issue that has virtually escaped discussion and consideration within the scientific community'. The case was reported to COPE by an editor who was sacked for raising questions about the behaviour of the editor-in-chief. It's obviously unsatisfactory that the case is anonymous (as it has to be to avoid libel) and that COPE has only one side of the story. One recommendation that came from the case was that it be published in full in a major journal. But that hasn't happened.

The story is complex and begins with the editor who was eventually sacked (whom I'll call 'the editor') discovering that the editor-in-chief had written a letter saying that he, the editor, had accepted a paper when he'd rejected it. The paper was a guideline on a common medical condition and recommended a new expensive drug as the best treatment. Reviews had been mixed, but the meeting of scientific editors had decided to reject the paper. The editor-in-chief spoke to the principal author of the paper at length and asked for a third review. Despite this being unfavourable the editor-in-chief had accepted the paper.

Editors-in-chief are 'free' to make idiosyncratic decisions, but the worrying feature of the first part of the story is the editor-in-chief lying, writing that the editor had accepted the paper when he'd rejected it.

The next event in this story was that the association that owned the journal stipulated that any editorial material published in the journal must have an elected official as an author even if written by somebody else. This not only seemed to compromise editorial independence but also to undermine good standards of authorship. Next, the chief executive of the association announced that the journal could not publish any letters critical of the association. The editor-in-chief said that he would protest, but the journal never did publish any more critical letters.

The editor then had further battles with the editor-in-chief over him publishing papers that were poorly supported by evidence and strongly criticized by reviewers. The editor-in-chief was also cavalier, the editor alleges, in rejecting a paper by the editor. Relationships broke down completely, and the editor was sacked. His view was that the chief executive of the organization and the editor-in-chief had made a Faustian bargain whereby the editor-in-chief compromised the independence of the journal in exchange for being able to publish what he wanted without being constrained by usual editorial standards.

The editor-in-chief would no doubt have a different story to tell, but this case illustrates how it could be difficult or impossible to do anything about an editor-in-chief who might make a bargain like the one the editor alleges. The owners would see no problem, but the journal would be debased. There is no professional accountability but only accountability to the owners.

A second COPE case is minor and concerns a journal publishing an editorial that had already been published elsewhere without disclosing the fact—despite the editors discovering the previous publication during the peer review process.[243] Nor had the editors sought copyright permission. When it was later pointed out that the two articles were essentially the same the editors agreed that they had been at fault and published a notice of duplicate publication.

In the third case an editor was accused of publication bias because he had invited the same trainee in radiology to write 14 commentaries in five years. The most recent commentary covered the same ground as previous commentaries and cited mostly the trainee and the accused editor. The editor was failing to let other authors and viewpoints come through. This case was referred to the journal's ombudsman (see discussion below) who judged it unfounded.[244]

As I described in chapter 2, a similar complaint was made against me. A group of readers and authors complained that the *BMJ* presented a one-sided view of the condition known as chronic fatigue syndrome or myalgic encephalomyelitis. The *BMJ*, they alleged, published only material that supported the idea that the condition is psychological, used the same reviewers (most of whom are psychiatrists), and refused to publish studies that show that the condition is a physical condition. The complainants conducted an analysis of what the *BMJ* had published on the subject, and their anger was increased when we declined to publish the analysis. (One objection to the analysis was that it included information only on papers we published and not those submitted to us—so how could it show bias?)

My response was that the *BMJ* did not have a position on the nature of chronic fatigue syndrome or myalgic encephalomyelitis. We selected the best research studies submitted to the journal and published them. Often studies contradicted previous studies that we had published. Bias seemed to arise because we were more likely to accept randomized trials of treatments (including a psychological treatment called 'cognitive behavioural therapy') than we were studies reporting a small series of patients who had evidence of a previous infection. We thought of this as a bias towards rigorous science, a bias that it was right for us to have.

In addition, we would ask a variety of people to write commentaries for us, selecting those who know about the condition, argued well using evidence and wrote clearly. It did so happen that most of the experts thought that the condition does have a substantial psychological component and that it is highly unlikely to be entirely a physical condition. Indeed, most of them believe that most conditions have a physical and psychological component. They are also distressed by the implication of the complainants that a physical condition is somehow more 'real' than a psychological condition. This seems to perpetuate the stigma against those with mental health problems.

When it comes to letters anybody can comment, and the *BMJ* carries many letters from people who disagree with most of what the *BMJ* publishes. When I left the *BMJ* received well over one hundred rapid responses (electronic letters to the editor) each week and we were able to publish fewer than 10% in the paper journal. This arrangement provided a rich test bed for studying editorial bias: what were the characteristics of the fewer than 10% that we selected? We'd like to think that they were more interesting, sound and readable, but no doubt other forms of bias were at work.

This is a question of where editorial judgement ends and misconduct begins. Editors are expected to discriminate, but they should discriminate on grounds of evidence, importance, relevance, quality and clarity rather than on personal foibles. But it is also widely believed to be the job of the editor to give a publication a 'personality'—and that's likely to be related to his or her personality. So some personal selection seems desirable.

The complaints against me alleging misconduct in relation to selecting material on chronic fatigue syndrome—to the British Medical Association (BMA), the owners of the *BMJ*, and the Press Complaints Commission—were dismissed, but the complainants saw this as an establishment cover up. Perhaps it was.

A more substantial—and justified—complaint was made against me through the website of the World Association of Medical Editors (WAME). We at the *BMJ* had made the mistake of selecting too many papers for our education and debate section (a section of the journal where we published not original research but essays, 'think pieces'). We discussed what to do and decided that we would 'cull' the papers—weed out and reject the poorer ones. In the past we'd done this with letters to the editor and personal views (short, subjective essays).

Some editors thought that we shouldn't do it for these longer papers, but I argued that this was a trade off between the needs of present authors and readers and future authors. If we published all these papers then we would have to reject most of the papers we received in the next few months, which would be unfair both to future authors (some of whom would undoubtedly submit papers better than those we were about to publish) and to readers (because we would be giving them a collection of less good papers). I carried the day (probably because of my position rather than the strength of my argument), and we culled the papers.

'Culled' authors were furious, and one wrote to WAME asking for advice. WAME decided that an anonymized version of the case should be put on the list serve. A flood of comments followed. Virtually every commentator thought that 'unknown editor' (me) had behaved unethically and many were strongly abusive—as is often the case with list serves. I was on the list serve, and I recognized the case. There was a delicious irony in the debate in that I had been one of three people on the stage at the only meeting that WAME had ever held on ethics. Having been displayed as some sort of 'ethical expert' I was now being accused of the most unethical behaviour yet shown by a WAME editor.

I weighed in with a signed contribution, starting it, 'I am that wicked editor…' I advanced my argument and was perhaps too cocky and unapologetic—but I did agree that I had done the wrong thing and would publish the papers. A torrent of criticism and abuse followed, and the chairman of the ethics committee of WAME was obliged to ask for calm.

Firing editors can be hard—because the editor may well invoke editorial freedom—but it's my misfortune to have fired four editors. In one case the processes of the journal had collapsed. Authors had waited years for a response, papers had been lost, and the journal was close to disintegration. In two cases the editors had simply run out of steam, and their journals were sliding down. In both cases the editors walked out during our conversations, and I've never seen them since. In the fourth case we had taken over a moribund journal and decided that we needed new blood if we were to have any chance of making the journal a success.

We have no good data, only stories, but I suspect that cases of editors performing poorly far outnumber cases of frank misconduct. But most editors like being editors. It gives them a platform and status. People are inclined to flatter editors—because they want them to publish their papers and advance their views. Grandiosity and self-importance are thus occupational hazards of editors, and getting rid of them may prove difficult. Many associations go on with poorly performing editors for fear of the fuss that might result from firing him or her. One way to avoid this predicament is to give the editor a fixed-term contract, usually for five years, and that is what we did with the editors of the *BMJ* journals.

Although it may be hard to fire editors, the world of medical editors has seen a spectacular case that made the lead story on CNN. As I first described in chapter 2, it was in 1999 when E Ratcliffe Anderson, the executive vice president of the American Medical Association (AMA), fired George Lundberg, the editor of *JAMA*. In characteristic style Anderson rang Lundberg, who was at home with a wrist in plaster, and told him not to come back. He was fired not for publishing but for speeding up the publication of a small paper that suggested that many American students did not think of oral sex as sex.[29] This was important because of the impeachment of President Clinton which featured a discussion of whether or not he had had sex with Monica Lewinsky and lied about it. As one of the newspaper commentators observed, it was strange to fire an editor for publishing something highly topical.

Perhaps what was remarkable was that Lundberg hadn't been fired sooner. Many, perhaps even most, editors of *JAMA* had been fired, and Lundberg had come close a few times—not least when, as an ex-pathologist, he said on television that doctors were 'burying their mistakes'. The AMA has a firing culture—Anderson was himself fired not long after—and there is, I believe, a structural problem in the relationship between the AMA and *JAMA*.

The AMA now has less than 30% of doctors in membership—and compared with non-members they tend to be older, less likely to work in managed care and Republican. They are, in short, highly conservative. But the editors of *JAMA* are trying to produce a journal that will appeal to all the doctors in America and to doctors beyond the United States (in a world where the gap in attitude between Americans and the rest of the world seems to be growing). This, it seems to me, is bound to produce tensions. The *BMJ* has tensions with the BMA, but the BMA is a much broader church than the AMA. About 80% of doctors belong—as do 60% of students. There is not a major mismatch between the beliefs and attitudes of the owners of the journal and the target audience.

Anderson, when he fired Lundberg, argued that he was—paradoxically—respecting editorial freedom. It would have been wrong, he said, for the AMA to interfere with individual decisions of the editors but it had to have the 'nuclear option' to fire the editor when he went too far.

Lundberg didn't do badly from the firing. A lover of publicity, his firing received massive media coverage worldwide—almost all of it sympathetic (partly because many journalists hate the AMA). Although many editors around the world found Lundberg's egocentricity unattractive, they all rallied round—supporting him and condemning the AMA. Some researchers called for a boycott on submitting papers to *JAMA*. Full of dirt on the AMA, Lundberg was paid a substantial sum for signing a confidentiality agreement. And he got another highly paid job, only this time with equity. Fired in the upswing of the dot.com boom, he was appointed as editor of Medscape and reappeared on the editorial scene dressed in black with gold rim glasses.

The firing of Lundberg was the most dramatic firing of a journal editor of recent years, but the firing of the editors of the *Canadian Medical Association Journal* (*CMAJ*) came close. John Hoey, the editor, and Anne Marie Todkill, the deputy editor, were fired at a moment's notice on 20 February 2006. The Canadian Medical Association (CMA) insisted that the firings were nothing to do with editorial independence but simply that a fresh approach was needed. Most of the world, including the *CMAJ* editorial board, found this unbelievable. The journal had improved dramatically in the 10 years that Hoey had been the editor, and even if the CMA did want a fresh approach why would it put the whole journal at risk by such precipitous action?

Plus there had been lots of disputes over editorial independence. Indeed, the CMA, like the AMA, has a firing culture—and many editors have been fired. Hoey's predecessor almost came unstuck by publishing a picture of a person holding a mug saying, 'My GP is a nurse practitioner.' The general practitioners in the CMA were not amused.

The issue that caused the final rupture was an article about how pharmacists were collecting too much information from women seeking over-the-counter emergency contraception. The *CMAJ* journalists working on the story had asked 13 women to go to a pharmacy, ask for the drug, and describe how they were treated. The Canadian Pharmacists Association found out about the article and contacted the CMA to ask if the research was being conducted in an ethical manner. The chief executive officer of the CMA asked Graham Morris, the publisher of the *CMAJ*, and he told Hoey not to run the story because it had not had ethical approval. The editors argued that the 'research' was simply investigative journalism and didn't need ethical approval. The editors and Morris agreed that the story should be run without the quotes from the women.

Hoey set up a committee to investigate the episode. The committee included Jerry Kassirer, former editor of the *New England Journal of Medicine*, who had himself had plenty of battles with the Massachusetts Medical Society, the owners of the *New England Journal of Medicine*. The committee ruled that Hoey had transgressed in giving in to the CMA but also judged that the CMA was guilty of 'blatant interference with the publication of a legitimate report'.

Another battle that came just before the end was caused by an online news report that was critical of the new Canadian health minister, referring to him as 'two tier Tony'. The CMA was upset, and the version that appeared in the paper version of the journal was toned down and included positive quotes about the new minister from the CMA president.

After Hoey and Todkill were fired one of the other editors, Stephen Choi, took over—but he couldn't reach agreement with the CMA and so left together with another editor. The editorial board was very critical of the CMA but attempted to reach agreement. The board wanted the editors reinstated and a written guarantee of editorial independence from the CMA. Neither happened, and so the editorial board resigned. Prominent Canadian researchers have also said that they will not submit studies to the journal, and the *CMAJ* faces extinction. As I write, attempts are being made to rescue the journal with a temporary editor and a former chief justice of the Supreme Court of Canada preparing a report on future governance.

Two other major general medical journals in North America—the *New England Journal of Medicine* and the *Annals of Internal Medicine*—also lost editors in inauspicious circumstances. The Massachusetts Medical Society, did not fire Jerry Kassirer, editor of the *New England Journal of Medicine*, but they did not renew his contract—which is effectively a firing. Relationships between the editors and the society had long been fraught, mostly over commercial matters. The society, which is financially heavily dependent on the journal, wanted to exploit its asset through activities like launching a *New England Journal of Primary Care*. The editors were anxious about the quality of such publications and worried—in marketing speak—that the brand would be devalued.

Having declined to renew Kassirer's contract, the society appointed Marcia Angell, a longstanding deputy editor (and, many thought, the power behind Kassirer's throne) for a year. The hostility between the journal and the society was there for all to see, and then the society appointed Jeffrey Drazen to a blaze of publicity about his extensive contacts with the pharmaceutical industry. Ironically, the journal's strict rules on conflict of interest would stop him writing editorials in his own journal.

Business problems were also the main cause of the American College of Physicians losing Bob and Suzanne Fletcher, the editors of the *Annals of Internal Medicine*. There were probably several factors that led the Fletchers to decide that they would rather be professors at Harvard than editors of the *Annals*, but one factor was them publishing a study that showed that many drug advertisements in medical journals made unwarranted claims.[226] The advertising revenue of the journal fell, heightening tension with the business side. The Fletchers were keen to have more involvement with the business side. What was the point in them producing a great journal if the marketing was lousy? The chief executive of the college, however, didn't want them bothering 'their pretty heads' about that kind of thing. There was tension. Somebody had to go. It was the Fletchers, not least because the college was heavily involved at the time in political lobbying that was led by the chief executive.

The British mostly do these things more quietly. Richard Horton just after he was appointed editor of the *Lancet* showed a graph of the average tenure of a *Lancet* editor. At the time it was almost a straight line down from the more than 30 years of Thomas Wakley, the founder and first editor. Horton joked that his editorial life expectancy was months, but he has now been editor for approaching 10 years.

In contrast, I was only the sixth editor of the *BMJ* since 1898. The journal has, however, had a famous bust up between the editor and the association—in 1956. Hugh Clegg, the editor, was a fierce fellow who loved a fight. Very interested in medicopolitics, he might well have preferred to be secretary of the association rather than editor. His relationships with the secretaries were difficult, and when I met him once towards the end of his life he told me that one of the secretaries, Charlie Hill (later Lord Hill), was 'evil incarnate'. I can report it now because both are dead.[245]

The battle with the association arose after he wrote and published an editorial entitled 'The gold-headed cane'.[9,246] The title was a reference to the cane that belongs to the president of the Royal College of Physicians, and the editorial was an attack on the college—arguing that it was archaic, degenerate, confused, rudderless and out of touch with its members and fellows. Clegg also criticized the college for electing Lord

Brain to a seventh year as president. In the first draft of his editorial—which as always he wrote standing up while drinking a bottle of claret, his invective becoming stronger as his blood alcohol rose—he compared this election to Caligula electing his horse to the Senate. This image, much treasured by subsequent editors, disappeared from the final version.

The college was furious about the editorial (perhaps because it contained much truth), and the BMA wasn't pleased because it was trying to get closer to the college. The council of the association tried to persuade Clegg to get approval for all political editorials from BMA officers. He refused, and the council passed a motion disassociating itself from the editorial. At its annual representative meeting (the supreme body of the association) a motion was debated that said that *BMJ* editorials should reflect association policy. The motion was heavily defeated, with some speakers emphasizing that editorial freedom was essential if the journal was to remain at 'the top in world approbation'.

BMJ editors remember this vote as if it happened yesterday and think it crucial in securing editorial freedom for the *BMJ*, but Peter Bartrip, the journal's historian thinks that the editorial 'changed nothing'. He quotes Clegg some years after the episode as saying that he didn't feel he had a right to advocate a policy contrary to that of the association.

The *BMJ* has, however, many times in recent years—almost routinely—published editorials that depart from BMA policy. Indeed, we would ask somebody to write us an editorial on a political issue in just the way that we asked somebody to write an editorial on liver pathology. We identified authors who know about the subjects and let them say whatever they want. We also wrote editorials ourselves that contradicted BMA policy. Leaders of the association would write us letters for publication disagreeing with the editorials, and there might be mutterings about 'foolish editorials'. But there were no serious attempt to have me sacked or to pass motions saying that *BMJ* editorials must comply with BMA policy. There was a debate of a motion regretting me cutting coverage of BMA political affairs from 10 pages to one—but it wasn't passed.

Somehow editorial independence has got deep into the BMA culture. This is partly because there is another publication—*BMA News*—that is the association's creature. There is no pretence of editorial independence. It was increasingly accepted that the *BMJ* was an international journal and not expected to record the activities or views of the BMA. We did have news stories on the BMA, but we covered the BMA as we covered other organizations. The news stories and editorials being signed probably helped (editorials were not signed in Clegg's day), but perhaps the biggest factor securing independence for the *BMJ* is its financial independence. The journal has been highly profitable, and money flows from the journal to the association. Most BMA members imagine that a big chunk of their subscription goes to the journal—but in fact none of it does. If money flowed from the association to the journal then independence would, I suspect, be severely compromised.

Another factor that may have accounted for the editorial stability of the *BMJ* was that the editor of the *BMJ* was also the chief executive of the BMJ Publishing Group and on the same level as the secretary of the association. It was the secretary of the

AMA who fired Lundberg and the publisher of the *CMAJ* who fired Hoey and Todkill. This couldn't have happened at the *BMJ*, and as the two main pressures on editors come from politics (the central activity of the associations) and from business (the main concern of the publisher) the position of the editor of the *BMJ* may have protected him. After I left, however, the relationships changed so that the editor now reports to the chief executive of the BMJ Publishing Group who in turn reports to the chief executive of the association. It remains to be seen if this will cause problems as it has for the editors of other association journals.

Editorial freedom cannot mean that editors are free to do what they want and are wholly unaccountable. The difficult question is how to make them accountable—because editors have to balance the interests of many groups: owners, readers, authors, reviewers, staff, advertisers, the broader medical community, patients and the media. And editors must obviously ensure that their journals comply with the law and pay attention to financial constraints.

The relationship with owners is the one that seems to cause the most difficulty. Often owners are not very clear what they want from their journals. Nobody from the BMA ever told me what they want from the *BMJ*. Stephen Lock, my predecessor, said that all I needed to do was to make sure that the journal came out regularly and be sure not to introduce American spelling. It was for me to try and divine what the BMA wanted. The BMA cannot really know what it wants because there is no BMA: instead, there are over 100,000 members, all probably with different ideas on what they want from the *BMJ*, and many different factions. The leaders of the BMA understandably spend little time thinking about the journal. They have a hundred more immediate problems.

Rarely, I suspect, are the owners of medical journals clear about what they want. The most precise they can be is that they want more of the same, only better. They appoint the best editors they can find and let them get on with it. The owners hope for improvement, but they accept the status quo and resort to firing the editor only if something goes horribly wrong.

This lack of clarity of what owners want from their journals and editors is the starting point of a cascade that has been appallingly amateur. There was no job description for the editor. Selection of the editor was more opaque than the selection of a pope. There was no training for the editor and no adequate system of accountability. I exaggerate—but only just.

I've now been involved in appointing around 40 editors—mostly of *BMJ* journals—but also of some other journals. My first experience was having to appoint an editor for the *British Journal of Ophthalmology*. There seemed to be no system. When I asked the retiring editor how he had been appointed he said that the previous editor had put his hand on his shoulder and said 'You're it.' Without direction, training or much support he'd muddled through for many years.

We clearly needed a better system for appointing a new editor, but in 1991 it seemed far too dramatic a step to advertise (which is what now happens routinely). I decided that I would identify three possible candidates and then make a selection. I rang various ophthalmologists to get suggestions and was astonished by their willingness to make poisonous comments about colleagues to somebody they didn't know.

Eventually I identified three candidates—from Aberdeen, Belfast and Manchester. The candidate from Aberdeen began to emerge (probably the best verb to describe the process) as the likely editor. At this point I was visited by a senior consultant in a very expensive suit who told me that nobody outside London knew anything about ophthalmology and that the candidate was 'a boy'. (He was actually in his 40s and older than me.) I ignored him, and appointed the professor from Aberdeen. He did an excellent job, and now the journal is edited by a professor from San Francisco who was appointed—against stiff opposition—by a panel after open advertisement.

Most editors of the world's 10,000 or so biomedical journals have received no training. One day you're a professor of cardiology; the next you're editing a journal with a turnover of £5m a year. For an editor with no training in cardiology to become a cardiologist overnight would be unthinkable, but it's routine the other way round. I wouldn't argue that being an editor is as complex as being a cardiologist or that the consequences of working without training will be so dire, but editing—like most other occupations—is becoming steadily more complex. Journals are the main route for the research that underpins medicine to reach doctors and patients. If the process is poor—as I'm arguing in this book it often is—then something is rotten at the root of medicine.

The lack of training is compounded by many editors working largely alone. The World Association of Medical Editors was founded with the idea of providing training, support and guidance to editors, particularly in the developing world. But ironically the position of many editors in the developed world is similar to that of editors in the developing world in that they are untrained and work alone: the difference might be that the journal, although often not the editor, has a substantial budget.

There does now begin to be training for editors, but the courses available are few and short—and most editors still learn on the job. The major general medical journals are different in that they are edited mostly by professional editors, people who might have been doctors once but who have become full-time editors. Most of the journals provide training positions, although the training is unstructured and mostly through apprenticeship. There is no college of editors, no formal qualification, no obligation to stay up to date and competent. Perhaps these things will come if medical editing becomes more professional, but many of us, including me, revelled in the amateurishness.

There is a major difference between the big American and the big British journals in that the American journals appoint distinguished academics as editors, whereas the British journals appoint professional editors who have come up through the ranks. This difference probably relates to the differences in the journals: the British journals are much more journalistic. My bias is that the American journals will need to move to having professional editors. The American system works now only because the academic editors have teams of professional editors under them. The *Lancet* experimented with the American model, appointing an academic, but the owners quickly reverted to the traditional British model.

The lack of training of editors has been matched by the lack of a research base for what editors do. I've often been struck by how, for example, neurologists on editorial boards who would expect to base their treatments of patients on evidence will make dogmatic statements about editorial processes without any evidence whatsoever. Until recently professional editors behaved in the same way. We spent a great deal of time scrutinizing the evidence in the studies submitted to us but didn't think to examine systematically and experimentally what we did ourselves. Now we do, but there are still many editors who don't agree with studying journal processes. They see it as unproductive navel gazing. Drummond Rennie, the force behind the congresses on peer review, lambasted editors at the end of the last congress for neglecting their craft. Only a small fraction of all the editors in the world attended the conference, and yet it is the only editorial conference that presents evidence and data rather than opinion.

Perhaps standards would rise if editors were more accountable and organizations expected more of their editors. Similarly editors might expect more of their organizations. In the case of the major general medical journals both the owners and the editors are stewards of the journals. The editors take responsibility for the journal for a limited period, and ideally they will hand on an improved journal. But owners are also stewards in the sense that these major journals are important for the international medical community. The AMA, I would argue, abused its stewardship of *JAMA* when it fired George Lundberg to suit its short-term aims. John Hoey and colleagues argued the same when they were editors of the *CMAJ*: 'Any medical journal belongs, intellectually and morally, to its contributors, editors, editorial boards and readers…The American Medical Association doesn't own the *Journal of the American Medical Association*, it is the custodian of it.'[247] Seven years after writing that Hoey was fired by the CMA in conflict with the journal's contributors, editorial board and readers.

As I learnt at business school, all problems are opportunities, and the firing of Lundberg led to some deep thinking—by Huw Davies, a scholar, and Drummond Rennie, the deputy editor of *JAMA*—on what is needed for a trusting and productive relationship between owners and editors.[248]

First, the two need to recognize their mutual accountability. Second, there should be 'a clearly defined and shared vision for the enterprise'. For most journals, I suspect, this is missing, but logically the owners should know what sort of journal they want before they appoint an editor. If they appoint an editor who wants to produce a very different sort of journal from them then there is sure to be trouble. Editors and their teams will want to develop and enhance the vision, but it's primarily for the owners to define the vision. Increasingly we did this at the BMJ Publishing Group before appointing a new editor.

Third, editors should be responsible for delivering measurable objectives—perhaps an increase in the impact factor of the journal or the time to process manuscripts—from a defined and agreed strategy. [The impact factor of a journal is the number of times articles in the journal are cited divided by the number of articles that could be cited. It's a rough and ready measure of quality that is easily abused and manipulated.] Again this is, I think, unusual. Fourth, the editors should be free to decide the tactics to deliver the strategy. Regular interference with short-term objectives is ruinous for a journal. Fifth, there should be a regular flow of information for communication rather than for judgement. This should help build trust. Sixth, owners and editors should always try to resolve disputes informally, but there needs to be a formal system as a back-up.

Most journals don't have these things. They muddle through, and there are many who think that mutual trust and respect between owners and editors are enough. If they are present, the journal will flourish. If they are lacking, then elaborate governance cannot compensate.

Editors need other forms of accountability. They must be accountable to readers, authors, reviewers and the broader medical community. Most of this accountability is far from explicit, and there are no institutions to enforce it—but we perhaps need some. I will discuss the *Lancet*'s ombudsman and the *BMJ* ethics committee in chapter 19, but I want to consider now whether or not editors might develop institutions to make themselves professionally accountable—in the way, for example, that doctors are accountable to professional bodies. Such accountability may be important not only for raising standards but also for counterbalancing the accountability to owners.

The Committee on Publication Ethics (COPE) has made a start by publishing a code of conduct for editors, and readers, authors, peer reviewers, other editors or publishers can make complaints to COPE—so long as the complainants have first been through the complaints procedures of the journals.[241,249] There are, however, no sanctions apart from expulsion from COPE.

Altman, Chalmers and Herxheimer in their paper on editorial misconduct proposed an International Medical Scientific Press Council.[236] They imagined that the council might produce a code of good conduct and a taxonomy of misconduct. Journals would sign up to abide by the code and agree to abide by a specified investigation procedure. Readers and authors would know which journals agreed to follow the code, and any failure to follow the code would be publicized. If a complaint against a journal or editor was upheld then the judgement would be published, and the owners of the journal might decide to take some action.

A model for the International Scientific Press Council is Britain's Press Complaints Commission, a successor to the Press Council.[250] The commission is funded by the press that it regulates and has a code that editors must follow. The first chairman, Lord Wakeham, describes how the commission was 'established in break neck speed …[because] a Damoclean sword—in the shape of the Calcutt Report, a privacy law and statutory controls—dangled menacingly over our free press'.[251] The commission includes editors but has a majority of independent outsiders.

There is no cost to those who complain, and in 2002 the commission received 2630 complaints that editors had breached the code. Most are settled by conciliation, and in 2002 only 36 went to the commission for adjudication. There is no hearing. The commission makes its decision based on the offending article and correspondence between the complainant and the editor.

Although 92% of those who complain to the commission are satisfied with the response they receive, there are many anxieties about the commission. Complainants feel that the commission favours the editors. The commission has very little capacity for investigation, and the only punishment if editors are found in breach of the code is that they have to publish an account of the adjudication. They are inclined to bury this at the back of the publication and will sometimes publish a more prominent piece explaining why they disagree with the adjudication. A House of Commons select committee was critical of the commission, and some day there may be legislation to make the press more accountable.

The problem is that freedom of the press is undoubtedly a major asset, enshrined, for example, in the American constitution. The press acts for the governed not the governors and can act powerfully against despotism, corruption and misconduct. In what I always think of as the strongest argument for press freedom, the Nobel prize winner, Amartya Sen, has shown that famine does not occur in countries with a free press.[252] Famine arises not because of total lack of food but because of maldistribution: a free press will expose those eating three-course dinners while others starve. So how do you strike a balance between allowing the press the freedom that is ultimately good for all and making it accountable? It isn't easy, and the wise thing is probably to err on the side of freedom, accepting that some will be abused.

Complaints about the *BMJ* have been made several times to the Press Complaints Commission, but only once has a complaint got as far as an adjudication. As I described in chapter 2, we published an obituary of a doctor, David Horrobin, in which we made clear that he was unusually clever, charming, and creative but also suspect.[50] The obituary suggested that his ethics were 'dubious' and that he 'may prove to be the greatest snake oil salesman of his age'.

His family unsurprisingly were distressed, and his many friends were furious. We received over one hundred rapid responses to our website, almost all of them protesting strongly against the obituary. We published three alternative obituaries,[253–255] all positive, in the paper edition of the journal together with a summary of the responses.[95] The obituary also contained some errors that we corrected. We did, however, stand by the obituary as we believed it to be essentially 'true'. Initially I declined to apologize because it seemed hypocritical to do so: we knew that publishing such an obituary would cause distress. But then I was persuaded that I was sorry about the distress to the family—which I was—and that therefore it wouldn't be hypocrisy to apologize. So we did.

The complainants said that we had breached article one of the code by publishing 'inaccurate, misleading or distorted material' and article five by intruding into grief by handling the obituary 'insensitively'. The commission noted that we had published corrections and said it was not set up to decide whether the obituary was 'true' or not. It also decided that we had not breached article five. In short, we 'got off', but I can easily understand that the complainant would feel let down in that he strongly believed that the obituary was 'untrue'.

This account of the Press Complaints Commission and one experience of its workings illustrates why creating a body to regulate international scientific journals and making it work would be formidably hard. This is one reason—in addition to lack of will and the absence of a sword of Damocles—that it hasn't happened. The body would experience the greatest difficulty when there was a dispute between the organization and the journal. The journal might simply walk away, or lawyers might become involved generating large bills and finding large defects in the constitution of the organization. Nevertheless, COPE has made a beginning. The creation of a forum to hear cases against editors could be useful not only for making editors more accountable but also for setting standards. The vision of an International Medical Scientific Press Council, which is already 12 years old, is probably at least another 12 years away.

Section 5: Important relationships of medical journals

▶13
Patients and medical journals: from objects to partners

The relationship between doctors and patients is undergoing a profound change, which is reflected in medical journals. Until recently patients expected to do as the doctor told them. The doctor was an authority. Now patients and doctors are becoming partners—sharing uncertainty and decision-making. This change can be uncomfortable for both parties, but the evidence shows that with such a partnership patients do better and costs are lower. Medical journals have reflected this change by moving from a world where patients' involvement with journals was to be described within them, usually without consent, to a world where patients are partners in creating journals. I mustn't pretend that the changes within medicine and journals are complete. They are not. The changes are messy, patchy, often backwards rather than forwards, and still have a long way to go.

When I was training in medicine in the early 1970s we usually did not tell patients that they had cancer. We'd mutter something to them about 'a small growth' and tell the relatives that the patient had cancer. I never stopped to think at the time that this conflicted fundamentally with the ethic that the doctor's relationship with the patient was confidential.

I remember too watching a television programme where a professor of surgery worked with actors who acted out a real case. The professor had operated on a man and discovered that he had inoperable cancer. He asked to see the man's wife and daughter. They were naturally anxious. 'Is everything all right? Did the operation go well?'

'Everything is fine', answered the role playing professor. 'The operation went very well. I'm afraid, however, that Mr Jones has cancer and that we won't be able to cure it.'

'This is the technique of the Spanish inquisition', said a commentator on the television after the role play was over. 'You tell the victim that everything is fine and follow it up with the bad news.'

This was also a world where it was routine for students as part of their training to perform vaginal examinations on anaesthetized women without their consent. A study of medical students in Bristol published at the beginning of 2003 shows that unfortunately this world still exists.[256]

In 1974 I went to Africa as a medical student. A friend and I planned to do a study on gastritis in Africans. We wanted to put tubes into patients' stomachs and take samples. We didn't think about consent from patients either for the procedure or for participation in an 'experiment'—an experiment which in retrospect was scientifically hopeless and therefore, I would say now, unethical.

I don't think that either my friend (now a consultant cardiologist) or I were bad people. Indeed, we thought of ourselves as highly principled. We were very concerned about injustice in the world. I tell these stories to illustrate how unconsciously we adopted practices that now seem almost barbaric.

Most doctors practising today trained in a world where patients were expected to follow the commands of doctors, not to ask too many questions, and to be grateful for the attention they received. In fact, of course, patients often ignored the commands of doctors, but they pretended to comply. About one-half of patients, for example, do not take the drugs they are prescribed in the way that doctors advise.[111] It isn't easy—for either doctors or patients—to change from the old world to the new world of partnership. The tendency is always to slip back.

I can remember when as an editor I was expelled—hardly too strong a word—from the old world. It was the early 1990s, and we had published a picture that looked like six stones. In fact they were pieces of fetal skull that had leaked out from the uterus of a woman who had had a termination of pregnancy some months previously that had gone wrong. The gynaecologist had failed to remove all of the fetus. I'm not sure all these years afterwards why we wanted to publish such a picture—but it was probably because it was a dramatic story and had some lesson, albeit an unoriginal one. There was probably, if I'm honest, some 'freak show' element to the decision.

Some weeks after the publication I was rung by the woman. Her sister was a nurse and had seen the picture and recognized the story. We hadn't, of course, published the woman's name, but we had published the names and addresses of the doctors who had sent us the report. It was easy for the woman and her sister to be sure that this was the woman's story. And what to us was a picture of six stones was to the woman a picture of her dead baby—a lost baby for whom she was still grieving. Plus she was suing the doctors who had performed the termination. She was both furious and very upset that we had published the picture. 'I feel like killing myself', she told me.

We simply hadn't thought through our actions. We did what we had always done and what other journals did. We never published the names of patients, but we didn't think it necessary to get consent. We might 'anonymize' the story as much as we could by cutting out detail, and some journals would even change a few facts in order to make it more difficult to identify the case. But the journal was intended for doctors, and the vast majority of readers wouldn't be able to identify the patient. We somehow overlooked the fact that we tended to publish only case reports that we thought were remarkable in some way. They would thus always be identifiable to some people, particularly to the patient. Plus a journal like the *BMJ* is seen by hundreds of thousands of people, many of them not doctors. Indeed, now that the journal is available in full text and for free on the World Wide Web almost anybody can access the journal.

The *Lancet* had a similar experience. It published a hugely important paper that gave details on the first patients to develop new variant Creutzfeldt–Jakob disease—the 'human form' of bovine spongiform encephalopathy ('mad cow disease').[257] This paper was important for science, public health, politics and business. It was the first clinical evidence that an animal disease caused by prions (infectious agents made only of protein) could cross to humans. It might presage (and still could) an epidemic that could kill hundreds of thousands. The British government was greatly embarrassed because it had repeatedly said that there was no risk of the disease crossing from cows to man. The effect on business was a dramatic drop in the consumption of beef and a worldwide ban on British beef exports.

The *Lancet* study, which must have been carefully scrutinized by hundreds of thousands of people, gave fairly limited information on 10 patients. But it wasn't difficult to identify patients because deaths from new variant Creutzfedlt–Jakob disease were of course very rare. One patient happened to be from a religious group who were not supposed to eat meat, and the paper made it clear that she had done. The published paper thus included information that seemed innocuous to most readers (and to the editors) but which was highly damaging to the girl's memory and her family.

Doctors generally, or at least in Britain, became more aware of this problem of disclosing information about patients without consent when in 1995 three doctors were accused of serious professional misconduct for doing so. They had published a study in the *British Journal of Psychiatry* that described three patients with bulimia nervosa who had bled themselves.[258] The journal included the information that one of these patients was 'a 26-year-old preregistration doctor'. Perhaps nobody should have been surprised when a story appeared in the *Aberdeen Press and Journal* giving the medical history of the junior doctor. She was not named but a friend identified her.

The doctor made a complaint to the General Medical Council about the three authors. She had given consent for her case to be used in research but not to be published. 'I would absolutely not have given the go ahead to the article which appeared. I was very shocked, very angry, very upset. Several things stated in the article were untrue. They were really hurtful and judgemental because they blocked out everything I had based my healing and therapy on because it was based on trust.'[259]

The council held a public hearing but did not find the doctors guilty of serious professional misconduct. This case—and the changing climate—did, however, lead the council to issue guidance on the subject. If any doctors were today to publish a paper like that in the *British Journal of Psychiatry* then they probably would be found guilty of serious professional misconduct.

The council, the International Committee of Medical Journal Editors and various journals, including the *BMJ*, shifted in the mid 1990s from a policy of anonymizing reports to requiring written consent from patients.[81,260,261] Patients should see what was written about them before publication. The argument behind this policy is that patients rightly assume that information disclosed in their relationship with doctors is confidential. Such information needs to be confidential so that patients are willing to tell doctors everything. Only then can doctors be fully helpful to patients, understand their problem, make the correct diagnosis and advise the best treatment. The confidentiality of that information extends to every use of it, including publication in a medical journal. Breaching confidentiality requires the consent of the patient.

Some thought this policy extreme. It would stand in the way of science. Sigmund Freud, some said, would never have been able to publish his classic case reports with such a policy. Public health doctors were worried that it might be impossible to report cases that could be of great importance for public health. The needs of individuals were being put before those of the broader community. Forensic psychiatrists were worried because their discipline is based very much on detailed case reports of the activities of highly disturbed people who had committed serious and often gory offences. Would it ever be possible to get informed consent from such patients? And what about confidential inquiries, where doctors examined in detail cases where things had gone badly wrong—perhaps mothers had died in childbirth or patients had died on the operating table? Such inquiries are very important for the progress of medicine.

Perhaps most difficult of all—and this problem is far from solved—what about consent for the publication of family trees, an essential part of genetics? They may give very important (and possibly damaging) information on large numbers of people. Clearly it could be extremely distressing for people to learn from a medical journal that they might have serious genetic traits that they didn't know about. (I do not know of a case of this happening, but it surely could.) But could it ever be possible to get consent from everybody included in a family tree, including perhaps people who had no idea that they were at risk? An option might be to leave out some members of the family tree, but this could mean publishing untrue and scientifically misleading information. Readers will understand why the problem is not solved.

I know of a case where doctors had tested the fetus of pregnant women for Huntington's disease without the consent or even knowledge of their partners. Huntington's disease is a condition that leads to early dementia and severe neurological problems. It is genetically dominant, meaning that if one of your parents has the condition you have a one in two chance of developing the disease. The doctors, with ethical guidance, had decided that they would test the women, and they— rightly—thought that a paper should be published so that the dilemma could be widely discussed. The journal decided that it could not publish the case reports without the consent of the partners, and such consent could clearly not be obtained. Part of the argument was that it was possible to discuss the general problem without disclosing information on specific cases.

One response that I as an editor make to critics who think the policy of obtaining consent extreme is that patients almost always will give consent. People want to be helpful. My next response is that there could be circumstances where the public benefit from publishing is so great that it would be right to override the objections of a patient to publication. This is analogous to the circumstances where a doctor might judge it right to break confidentiality. I've already referred to the hypothetical case of a jumbo jet pilot who refuses to report his epilepsy. But it is hard to think of an analogy for such an urgent need for publication, and I don't know of an example. One example might have arisen if one of the patients who first had AIDS had denied consent to publication. But there was a series of patients, and was it necessary to report all of them?

Because this is such a complex subject on which to have simple rules editors have both toughened and weakened their policies. The *BMJ* toughened—or at least clarified—its policy after a high profile court case. We had published a very dramatic radiograph of a patient's skull with a long knife embedded in the skull. The patient had made a remarkable recovery and given written consent for the publication of the picture in the *BMJ*. Problems arose when the radiograph was presented in the trial of the man who had stabbed the patient. The media, unsurprisingly, were keen to reproduce the picture, and somebody made a connection between the trial and our picture. Despite the patient not wanting the radiograph reproduced in the mass media, they simply took (perhaps I should say stole) it from our website. Some asked permission. We denied it, but they still took the picture.

We threatened to sue the media for breach of copyright and to make complaints to the various regulatory authorities—like the Press Complaints Commission. We thought that the media should have the same standards as us and use the pictures only with written consent. The case was, however, complicated by the pictures having been presented in court. This perhaps meant that they could be reproduced. We didn't pursue the case, but we did introduce a consent form that made clear to patients who gave us consent just how widely the pictures would be distributed and what the risks are. So now authors must get patients to sign the *BMJ*'s consent form rather than produce one themselves.

The *BMJ*'s policies were also made less stringent. We had problems with brief anecdotes that we publish in the journal. These anecdotes are often about patients. They tell a story, usually with some sort of lesson. But they are slight, sometimes amusing, often strange, and very much about the art rather than the science of medicine. Readers like them a lot, and we had many submitted. Many are stories from years ago or from brief encounters in distant places. Did we need to get written consent for these as we did for contemporary case reports? We thought that sometimes we probably didn't need to, and we introduced a set of conditions for when consent wasn't needed.[82]

We could not, we concluded, produce completely specific guidelines on when we might be able to publish a patient's story without consent. The decision depends on balancing the importance and interest of the information against the likelihood that a patient might be damaged. Publication without consent may be acceptable in the following cases:

- The patient is long dead and has no living relatives.
- The interaction with the patient was long ago—perhaps more than 15 years.
- Because the interaction was long ago and the patient was elderly or terminally ill, the patient is likely to be dead.
- The piece is to be published without the authors' names attached, making it unlikely that anybody could identify the patient.
- All extraneous information that might help identification is excluded.
- Even if the patient were to identify himself or herself, the events described are unlikely to cause offence. We must remember, however, that it is difficult to know what will cause offence: some patients will be offended simply by the fact that the information they gave to their doctors was published without consent.

Various authors and editors still thought that these guidelines were still too restrictive and insufficiently clear. We thus took the issue to our ethics committee, and it agreed with the critics. There were two particular cases that prompted a debate. One was a story of a doctor briefly encountering a patient in a very poor country in South America. The story was poignant and illustrated the extreme difference between what patients in the rich and poor world might expect—an issue of the greatest importance. Another case told the story of a doctor in a patriarchal society failing to convince a father that his daughter ought to be allowed to attend school.

The committee drafted the following policy:

1. Publication of any personal information about a patient will normally require the consent of the patient. This will be so even if identifying details are removed.
2. Personal information about a patient will not be published over the patient's refusal, except in the most exceptional circumstance of overriding importance to public health.
3. Publication without the consent of the patient will be permitted if *all* of the following conditions are met:
   a) The patient who is the focus of the article is untraceable without an unduly burdensome effort and it is also impossible or unreasonable to expect consent to be obtained from the patient or the patient's next of kin.
   b) The article contains a worthwhile clinical lesson or public health point which could not be as effectively made in any other way. ('Worthwhile' is intended to sit on a spectrum between 'interesting', which is the publication threshold with patient consent, and 'overriding public health importance', which is the publication threshold over patient refusal.
   c) A reasonable person in the patient's position would not be expected to object to the publication of the case. (This requires an assessment of the intrusiveness of the disclosure and the potential that it has for causing the patient, or the patient's family, embarrassment or distress. Particular attention must be paid here to differences of cultural and social attitudes. It must not be assumed that what is a matter of indifference in one society will have the same status in another.)
   d) The risk of identification of the patient is minimized by measures designed to prevent the identity of the patient being revealed either to others or to the patient himself or herself. (These measures will include anonymization of the case and/or the author. The publication without consent of photographs will require particular scrupulous attention to anonymization.)

The *BMJ* is auditing these guidelines, and it might well be that they will prove to be more restrictive than those they replaced. Requirement 3b may well disallow pieces that could have been published under the previous policy. The committee applied these criteria to the two particular cases that had prompted a review of the policy. It recommended publication of the case from South America but recommended against publication of the case of the patriarchal family on the grounds the patient might well be embarrassed and so a reasonable person would object to publication.

One issue that arises repeatedly is the *BMJ*'s apparent 'double standard' when it comes to the news section of the *BMJ*. The *BMJ* has a policy of publishing a picture on every page of the news section—to make the pages look 'newsy' and to distinguish them from other parts of the journal. (This in itself gives rise to objections: 'If you didn't publish all those silly pictures you might have had space to publish my important paper.') Sometimes the *BMJ* publishes pictures of patients on the news pages, and we did so without signed consent. These pictures, we argued, did not arise from the doctor–patient relationship, and so there was not the same logic of breaking confidentiality without consent. News photographers do sometimes get some form of consent, but it is not the same quality of consent as we expect for information about patients coming from doctors. Next, nothing would be gained by the *BMJ* declining to publish photographs that are in the public domain. So we do have a 'double standard', but it is thought through and intentional. We debated the 'double standard' with the ethics committee, and it supported the policy.

Another issue that flows from the policy is whether or not doctors are entitled to the same kind of confidentiality as patients. So if a patient wants to tell stories about their interactions with doctors, does the *BMJ* need consent from the doctors? The answer is 'no'. The duty of confidentiality runs one way.

Patients sometimes want to tell stories about doctors because they are highly critical of doctors. Journals are interested in improving medical care and so should be interested in stories of things that have gone wrong. In the credo of continuous quality improvement 'every defect is a treasure'—because it shows a route for improvement. Journals must be careful, however, of 'trial by media'. If serious accusations are made against people—as I've argued in chapter 8 with research misconduct—they have a right to due process being used in any hearing. Journals cannot apply due process.

The *BMJ*'s policy did, however, allow us to publish stories of poor practice where the point of publication is not to accuse the doctors involved but to allow learning. We anonymized the stories, but we knew that anonymization is not 100% effective. That's why we needed consent from patients, but we did not from doctors in these circumstances. This upset some doctors who argued that 'there are two sides to every story' and that we were telling only one side. A particularly sore point was that if doctors wanted to respond to criticisms of themselves that they had identified then they might be restricted from doing so because they were bound by confidentiality when the patient was not. We debated this issue with our ethics committee and agreed that if we were going to publish stories by patients that were critical of doctors then we should ask the patients to agree—in writing—that if the doctors should choose to respond they were not bound by confidentiality.

The publication of material about individual patients is a very direct concern of journals, but they are also concerned with the quality of informed consent in studies that they publish. This is primarily a concern for ethics committees or institutional review boards (as they are called in the United States), but, as I argue in chapter 18, journals also have a role. We did not accept that a study was automatically 'ethical' because it was approved by an ethics committee.

The Committee on Publication Ethics (COPE) dealt with a case where it thought that an ethics committee—or at least its chairman—had behaved unethically.[262] A journal was considering for publication a study that involved an allergic challenge to a group of children known to be allergic. A reviewer thought the study unethical because he could not believe that parents would consent to a study where their children might experience a severe allergic reaction and even die. The editor agreed and investigated.

He discovered that the ethics committee had recognized the problem and asked for further expert advice. But instead the author talked to the chairman of the ethics committee and convinced him that the study was part of normal clinical practice and so did not require ethics committee approval. The study went ahead, and the information leaflet given to parents did mention the possibility of an allergic reaction but did not mention the possibility of death. The editor's judgement was that the test was not part of normal practice and that parents had not been adequately informed. He asked the authorities to investigate.

In 1997 the *BMJ* became embroiled in what proved to be a rich and productive debate over studies where patients have not given informed consent.[263] We published two such studies in one issue together with a collection of articles arguing that we were very wrong to do so and another collection arguing the opposite.[264–272] The journal received some 50 letters in response, most of them remarkably well argued, and they split 50–50 into those who thought us wrong and those who thought us right.[273] Subsequently we held a conference that extended the debate beyond research into clinical practice and education, and in 2001 we published a major book on informed consent in medical research.[274]

The issue of informed consent leads back inevitably to the Nuremberg trials that followed the Second World War. Nazi doctors had conducted wholly unacceptable experiments on people, many of them Jews. The Nuremberg Code, which emerged in the final judgement of the trials, determined that consent for research was essential and should be voluntary, informed and prospective.

Later the World Medical Association built on the Nuremberg Code and produced the Declaration of Helsinki. It distinguished between 'non-therapeutic' and 'therapeutic' research and was less than absolute in the requirement for informed consent in therapeutic research. The version that was current when the *BMJ* published the two studies that did not include informed consent allowed doctors sometimes to do without informed consent in the context of 'medical research combined with professional care (clinical research)'.[275] There is a general requirement for informed consent, but a 'let out' paragraph said: 'If the physician considers it essential not to obtain informed consent, the specific reasons for this proposal should be stated in the experimental protocol for transmission to the independent committee.'

Both the studies that the *BMJ* published complied with the Declaration of Helsinki and both were approved by ethics committees. One of the studies, from Edinburgh, investigated whether 'stroke family care workers' made life better for patients with stroke and their families.[265] The authors decided against seeking consent for the experiment because they thought that a full understanding of what was being investigated would bias the result of the experiment, making it impossible to conclude anything with confidence. In addition, the authors couldn't see how being looked after by the 'stroke family care worker' could be harmful and the patients and their families could always decline to see the worker.

Sheila McLean, a professor of law and ethics in medicine, argued that their reasons were insufficient to justify deviation from the general rule that good research must at all times respect the subject.[266] 'Any failure,' she writes, 'to offer this respect is in itself a harm, even if its consequences are not physical.' People are being treated as objects not people.

The second study, from South Africa, looked at whether patients infected with the human immunodeficiency virus (HIV) did worse when admitted to an intensive care unit than patients not infected.[267] This was an important question because many intensive care units would not admit patients infected with HIV—partly because they thought that they would inevitably do badly. The scarce resource of intensive care should be kept for those who could most benefit. Patients did not give consent to be in the study or to have their blood tested for HIV. The authors argued that consent could not be obtained from most cases because they were too sick and that the research was of such importance that the patients' right to informed consent could be waived.[268]

The chairman of the ethics committee explained in an accompanying commentary why the committee supported the research after its immediate reaction that it would not be possible to give ethical approval.[269] The explanations included the facts that the study entailed no interventions of any sort different from those that are necessary and arc carried out in standard intensive care, and that the injury done to the patients would be small.

Rajendra Kale, an Indian neurologist at the time but now an editor at the *BMJ*, argued that the ethics committee was wrong to approve the research and that the *BMJ* was wrong to publish it.[270] He thought that such research would not have been allowed in a fully developed country and worried that it may be too easy to flout fundamental human rights in the developing world.

Editors at the *BMJ* were divided on whether we should publish these papers. In the end we decided that, rather than restrict the debate to ourselves, we would do better to invite our readers to join in. (This is something we did regularly and might be described as a 'value' of the journal.) We accompanied the papers together with an argument from Len Doyal, a professor of medical ethics, that the *BMJ* should not in future publish papers like these.[271] He proposed a policy that all medical journals might follow.

'Our abilities to deliberate, to choose, and to plan for the future are,' he wrote, 'the focus of dignity and respect which we associate with being an autonomous person capable of participation in civic life.' To deny patients participating in research full information on that research was, he argued, a clear breach of their moral rights. He then examined the arguments against fully informed consent: patients may be distressed by detailed information; it may not be necessary when the risks of the research are negligible; and the interests of the public in medical progress will be undermined by too much emphasis on the rights of individual patients. He found all these arguments unconvincing.

But he then identified three sets of circumstances in which informed consent may not be necessary. First, so long as a set of conditions are met then research might be allowed without consent on patients not competent to give consent—including children, patients with learning difficulties, and unconscious or semiconscious patients. Otherwise, such patients might be denied the benefits of research. Second, epidemiological research on medical records might be acceptable in certain strict circumstances when, for practical reasons, consent could not be obtained. Third, research without informed consent might sometimes be acceptable on stored tissue from anonymous donors.

Jeffrey Tobias, a radiotherapist and researcher, argued that the *BMJ* was right sometimes to publish studies where patients had not given informed consent.[272] His argument revolved around the facts that patients trust their doctors and that what is clear in 'fine and lofty places' like the letters pages of medical journals was much less clear in the 'real world', where 'the doctor must somehow juggle the multiple responsibilities of expert, humane, and above all respectful support for the patient...with the wider healthcare concerns and requirements of society as a whole'.

The patient's voice was provided with an anonymous patient who was included in 1987 in a British trial of a new radiotherapy protocol for cervical cancer without being asked for fully informed consent.[276] She suffered severe consequences from the treatment and later discovered that she was one of many patients who had been included in trials without consent. She felt abused and quoted another patient who wrote, 'Somewhere, somehow, I have to expose this abuse of power. The doctors never got my informed consent. This is abuse of society's most vulnerable people. Where is there a platform for my voice to be heard, to make the public aware and the establishment accountable?'

One point that was raised repeatedly by researchers in the correspondence was the hypocrisy of demanding elaborate consent for research while accepting that consent within clinical practice is rudimentary. (At our conference a professor of surgery put up a slide of a signed consent form that said, 'Removal of right leg.' It was supposed to say, 'Removal of varicose veins from right leg.') Much of the time doctors are working with inadequate evidence. The best treatment is not clear. If—in an ethically responsible way—a doctor decided that she ought to conduct a trial then she would need to get ethics committee approval and fully informed consent for not only the different treatment options, perhaps including a placebo, but also for randomization—and randomization often doesn't feel comfortable to patients. If, however, the doctor chose to follow her hunch she would probably simply get consent for the treatment she recommended. (She should really explain all options plus her uncertainty, but doctors rarely do this.) Those who want the easy life—and most do—will not opt for research.

When the furious debate that followed the *BMJ* issue that included the trials without consent began to abate we asked Len Doyal and Jeff Tobias whether they wished to change their position.[277] Neither did. We also sought the help of others, including Mary Warnock, one of Britain's leading philosophers who chaired Britain's Committee of Inquiry into Human Fertilization. She argued that 'the principle of non-exploitation has come to seem to many to be by far the most important moral principle that should govern research using human subjects.'[277] She thought it a 'misuse of words' to suggest that not obtaining informed consent in itself constituted a harm, 'sometimes it amounts to exploitation, sometimes it does not'. She encouraged editors to continue to live in a morally hazardous world, to shun dogma and to follow a prayer from Hertford College Chapel, 'to distinguish things that differ'.

This encouragement was impossible to resist because morally hazardous worlds are, I believe, right and proper for journals. Dogma is not only dangerous but also boring. Reflecting the world from which we are slowly emerging, we largely forgot about the voices of patients themselves first time round. This time we commissioned several to comment. Heather Goodare, who had been a participant in the notorious Bristol Cancer Help Centre study (see chapter 2), argued that we should take a strong line and reject all studies that do not include informed consent.[277] Lisa Power, health advocacy manager for the Terrence Higgins Trust (an AIDS charity), asked us to consider the broader issue of patients in planning research and thought that 'any hard and fast rule that the *BMJ* made about publication would probably have to be broken at some point'.[277] Hazel Thornton, chairwoman of the Consumer's Advisory Group of Clinical Trails, took a similar line: 'Collaboration is the name of the game. Research is for the benefit of us all: all should be involved in debates about its improvement and promotion.'[278]

Patients, in other words, should cease to be 'subjects'—'human guineapigs', as Maurice Pappworth called them in his book on how patients had been abused by researchers (see p 226)—and become 'participants'. They should be part of the planning, designing, carrying out and interpreting of research. This does, of course, depend on learning new skills and jargon, and there is an anxiety that by the time that the patients have learnt what is necessary they are no longer patients. I have, however, watched many 'patients' make important contributions to research that could not have been made by researchers who didn't have that patient perspective. Such people will, I hope, be one of the major audiences for this book.

We decided at the *BMJ* to continue not having an absolute policy on informed consent in studies but rather to make up our minds on the merits of particular cases.

The Declaration of Helsinki was substantially revised in 2000, and it doesn't now have the 'let out' clause that allows doctors to forego informed consent when they think it right in the context of therapeutic research.[279] It does touch on the very difficult question of where research and clinical practice merge, requiring the doctor to make clear what is research.

The declaration is now much more specific on what is meant by 'informed consent':

'In any research on human beings, each potential subject must be adequately informed of the aims, methods, sources of funding, any possible conflicts of interest, institutional affiliations of the researcher, the anticipated benefits and potential risks of the study and the discomfort it may entail. The subject should be informed of the right to abstain from participation in the study or to withdraw consent to participate at any time without reprisal. After ensuring that the subject has understood the information, the physician should then obtain the subject's freely-given informed consent, preferably in writing. If the consent cannot be obtained in writing, the non-written consent must be formally documented and witnessed.'

This is, I'm sure, a counsel of perfection. I doubt very much that consent is obtained in this way in every trial. The declaration does elsewhere allow research without consent when patients are too sick to give it.

The study that the *BMJ* published on 'stroke family care workers' would not, I think, be acceptable with the revised declaration.[264] It does not allow researchers to avoid consent in order to improve the scientific quality of their study. It might perhaps be argued that the introduction of the care worker was part of routine practice (see below), but I think not. The study of the patients infected with HIV in intensive care in South Africa might perhaps be allowed under the revised declaration.[267]

Those who drafted the new declaration (and did it well, I judge) clearly had difficulty drafting the section on the point where practice and research merge. As the following passage shows, doctors can when necessary venture into the unknown when treating a patient—but they must get informed consent and would need to make the uncertainty clear. The declaration also urges that doctors try to make the exploration research. Again, this is a counsel of perfection. Doctors are regularly in the unknown and usually do not share their uncertainty with patients. Even less often do they turn their uncertainty into research.

> 'In the treatment of a patient, where proven prophylactic, diagnostic and therapeutic methods do not exist or have been ineffective, the physician, with informed consent from the patient, must be free to use unproven or new prophylactic, diagnostic and therapeutic measures, if in the physician's judgement it offers hope of saving life, re-establishing health or alleviating suffering. Where possible, these measures should be made the object of research, designed to evaluate their safety and efficacy. In all cases, new information should be recorded and, where appropriate, published.'

Together with Iain Chalmers, one of the founders of the Cochrane Collaboration, I have described a way in which what the Declaration of Helsinki advises could begin to become a reality.[280] All doctors (and perhaps all patients) would be supplied with information on what the evidence says on medical problems. Doctors in many countries already have access to such information—for example, through the Cochrane Library or *Clinical Evidence*. If no evidence is available then the doctor and patient would look to see if a trial was underway. Already there are registers of trials underway. If a trial was underway, the patient might decide to enter the trial. There is evidence that patients in trials do better than patients receiving routine treatment, even if they receive a placebo. If no relevant trial could be found then the doctor would inform a central database of questions arising in practice. In this way research could then be concentrated on the questions arising in practice. This too is a pipedream—but an achievable one.

Interestingly, the revised declaration now puts duties onto authors and publishers (but not, surprisingly, editors):

> 'Both authors and publishers have ethical obligations. In publication of the results of research, the investigators are obliged to preserve the accuracy of the results. Negative as well as positive results should be published or otherwise publicly available. Sources of funding, institutional affiliations and any possible conflicts of interest should be declared in the publication. Reports of experimentation not in accordance with the principles laid down in this Declaration should not be accepted for publication.'

So publishers who allow editors to turn down negative studies as 'boring' are now in breach of the Declaration of Helsinki. I doubt if you could find a single publisher who is aware of this responsibility.

The revised declaration is a very progressive document, although it ran into problems by suggesting that placebo controlled trials were often unethical. I will discuss this further in chapter 15 on medical journals and the developing world. The progressiveness of the declaration is shown by the following short paragraph: 'The subjects must be volunteers and informed participants in the research project.'

Patients, although somewhat confusingly called 'subjects' in the first part of the sentence, are to become 'informed participants'. The declaration doesn't explain what it means by this, but it is, I think, the future of medicine and medical journals. Perhaps the next revision of the Declaration of Helsinki will be drafted not by an organization of doctors but by one that has a much broader representation.

'Nothing about me without me', is the slogan of those who believe that patients must become partners in healthcare. Wherever decisions are being made that will affect patients they must be there. It applies at every level—the interaction of individual doctors and patients, the setting of clinical policies, the planning of healthcare, and every aspect of research.

There are broadly three ways in which doctors and patients can make decisions. First, the patient might describe his or her symptoms, and the doctor will then decide what should be done. This is how medicine has been mostly practised. Second, the doctor and patient will decide together the best thing to do, or, third, the doctor could offer advice but the patient will decide. During a morning's work when a doctor might see 20 patients decisions will probably be made in all three ways. Clearly if the patient is unconscious then the doctor will decide (although relatives might well be involved or the patient might have left an advanced directive, 'a living will'), and different patients like different ways of making decisions. The same patient will want different sorts of decisions made in different ways: if I'm sick and weak I might prefer the doctor to decide; but if I'm deciding whether or not to take a drug for high blood pressure for the rest of my life then I'd either like to decide myself or to decide with the doctor.

The current trend is very much in the direction of doctors and patients making decisions together, which is not always easy for either the patient or the doctor. After a professional lifetime of taking decisions on behalf of patients it isn't easy for doctors to change.

Doctors like to think that they fully understand the needs of patients, and they resent any suggestion that they and their practices are not 'patient-centred' in the new jargon. But there is a growing mountain of evidence that doctors and patients do not see the world in the same way. Let me illustrate with four stories.

'For doctors Parkinson's disease is mostly above the neck, something to do with the substantia nigra. For patients it's mostly below the waist. Can they walk? Can they get their knickers on? Are they continent? Can they have sex?' These are the words of Mary Baker, former chief executive of the Parkinson's Disease Association and once the patient editor of the *BMJ*. It's the same, much evidence suggests, for other conditions. Doctors and patients think differently and have different concerns. This theme is further illustrated by personal accounts of doctors of their own illnesses. Stereotypically, they read: 'Until I had X I never knew what it was like to be a patient. Now I do. This illness has changed me for ever as a doctor.' My thought is that it doesn't. After a while they are back to being doctors again. This not a fault. It is the way of the world.

Or consider the story of a colleague Rhona (told with her consent). She is a doctor in her early 30s and has a severe and unusual form of scleroderma. Rhona has had the fingers amputated on both hands. Her bowel is also severely affected. She is very thin and needs repeated blood transfusions.

The specialists who look after Rhona were shocked by the severity of her disease. They thought that everything possible must be done if not to cure her then to hold back her disease. She's so young. They have tried aggressive, experimental treatments— with little success, it has to be said—and they want to try more. Rhona is far from keen. For her work is very important, and she doesn't want to lose time from work undergoing poisonous treatments. To Rhona quality of life is more important than quantity.

Despite Rhona being a determined person and despite her doctors being caring, she has had the greatest difficulty getting this message across to her doctors. To them she has a serious disease that must be fought. She is much too young to be giving so much emphasis to work and putting quality before quantity of life. Her doctors, I'm sure, consider themselves patient-centred, but they are not—at least in her case at the moment.

My third and fourth stories are about the system rather than individuals. Consider parking in hospitals, always a contentious matter. Usually there is restricted and expensive parking for patients. Often they have to walk past the cars of hospital staff in order to reach the hospital. This would be inconceivable in a supermarket. Or consider doctors' letters about patients. These traditionally are written from one doctor to another in language that the patient cannot understand. It has been for them to transport the letter not read it. Now an increasing number of doctors write to the patient and copy the letter to the other doctor, but it's still not the norm.

So a profound change—of patients becoming partners and equals—is happening. But what does this mean for medical journals? They are, I think, following not leading—and they are following slowly.

There have always been some patients who read medical journals, and with the arrival of internet journals there are many more. Increasingly patients have access to the same information as doctors, and all doctors have had the experience of patients arriving with printouts from the internet. Journals are usually willing to consider for publication articles by patients, and sometimes publish them. Sometimes journals even commission patients to write pieces. Some journals—particularly American journals—publish 'patient versions' of their studies. But mostly, I think it would be true to say, medical journals are written by doctors for doctors. Patients appear mostly within the pages rather than on editorial boards. They have been tolerated not encouraged.

We made an attempt to change this at the *BMJ*, but it is still at the beginning—and considerably behind what is happening in other places in healthcare. When we first appointed an editorial board—in the mid-1990s—we included a patient representative. Later we appointed two when it was pointed out to us that to be one— token—patient in a room of 30 professionals is hard. In 2002 we appointed a patient editor—Mary Baker. She came one day a fortnight, and her remit was to remind us constantly of the patient perspective. Then we appointed a board of patient advisers, and in the spring of 2003 we published a theme issue of the journal that was designed for an imaginary, future world where doctors and patients are equals and work in partnership. Some doctors liked it; others cancelled their subscriptions immediately.

The aim was not to make the *BMJ* a publication for patients. Nor was the aim—although it might be in the longer term—to create a journal that was intended for both doctors and patients. The aim was to help doctors understand how the world has changed, how patients have different perspectives from doctors, and how to be the best possible doctor you need both to understand the perspective of patients and know how to work with them. 'It's very hard for doctors,' says Mary Baker, 'they need help.'

Some other journals have taken such initiatives, but they are still rare. Medical journals remain cocooned in a world where doctors are dominant while most of healthcare has moved on.

So in about 40 years medical journals have tried to move from a world where they included abusive experiments conducted on patients without their consent to a world where patients are equals and partners in both healthcare and research. Progress is at best 'patchy'.

►14

Medical journals and the mass media: moving from love and hate to love

Medical journals are the main conduit by which medical research reaches the public, and the public seems to be ever more interested in medical stories. Consequently the mass media pay ever more attention to medical journals. In Britain Friday morning is '*Lancet* and *BMJ*' morning. Virtually every week the morning's media will include stories from one or the other or often both, and, although editors may sometimes be critical of the media, they love the attention. But is this passion for publicity corrupting the journals? Should the journals far from courting the mass media be keeping them at a distance?

I have experienced the vicissitudes and power of the mass media at first hand. For six years I was a 'television doctor'—for four years on BBC Breakfast Time and two years on TV-AM. I've also made a few television programmes. These experiences taught me some things about the media that it may be useful briefly to share.

Very scared, I appeared first on a live programme broadcast late at night in Newcastle—'a programme made by drunks for drunks'. As I came off the set, the producer said to me, 'You were wonderful, a natural television personality.' Three hours and a few drinks later she said, 'You were awful. I couldn't understand a word you said.'

Lesson one: Beware the flattery of the media.

When it came to the first programme on BBC Breakfast Time, the producer asked me what we might discuss. 'What about heart disease?' I suggested. 'It kills half the population.'

'But is there enough to talk about for three minutes?' the producer asked.

Lesson two: Time is very short on television and becoming shorter, but 15 seconds talking to 10 million people is the same amount of time as 10,000 people spending four hours reading the book of which this chapter will form a part, which is unlikely to happen.

One week in the early 1980s the *Lancet* published a complex study that suggested that certain sorts of contraceptive pill were associated with breast cancer. This was the first time that most people, including me, had heard of the link. It was hard to make sense of the study, and the *Lancet*—unfriendly in those days to the media (and perhaps readers)—had no press release and no editorial discussing the possible importance of the findings. I had to explain the findings at the peak spot on the programme with Dame Edna Everidge, a famous female impersonator, in bed beside me. When asked about the safety of the pill, she said, 'As long as I keep the pill between my knees it's safe and it works.'

Lesson three: Those of us who work in calmer circumstances should recognize the difficulties faced by those working in the mass media.

On Thursday afternoons I would tell the producers about stories emerging from that week's *Lancet* and *BMJ*. 'Too boring', they would often say. But then they would ring me at 4 o'clock in the morning about a 'fantastic story' that they'd read in the morning's papers. It was often the story they'd pronounced too boring.

Lesson four: The media are like lemmings. They want to break stories but they are confident that a story is a true news story only when they see it somewhere else.

I was keen to discuss both AIDS, then a new disease, and testicular cancer on the programme. The producers were unwilling to discuss either—because AIDS was a disgusting disease and the British couldn't tolerate talk of testicles over breakfast. A friend working at the time on the *Guardian*, Britain's most liberal national newspaper, was told he couldn't use the phrase 'anal intercourse'.

Lesson five: The mass media can be very prudish.

One morning, prompted by a strange episode, I told the presenter that you had to be ready for anything in medicine. 'What strange things have you seen recently?' he asked.

I didn't see patients, and the only thought that came into my mind was that I'd had two letters from women who were worried that they might be pregnant by dogs (probably, in retrospect, spoofs). I wondered whether to mention this but then did. Feeling obliged to answer the question, I said: 'Of course, you can't be, although,' I added, trying to be interesting, 'you could perhaps be pregnant by a gorilla.' Afterwards the producer asked me if I was aware that this was live television.

Lesson six: Live media can lead you to some very strange places.

Finally, I remember the day when a woman rang me from Leeds Station to say that she was about to get on a train to bring her blind daughter to see me. 'I'm sure, doctor, that you can cure her. I've seen you on the television.' With difficulty, I dissuaded her.

Lesson seven: The media can have remarkable power.

The world of live, mass market television is very different from the world of medical journals, but some medical journals are getting close to the mass media. Most major journals employ at least one press officer and put out a press release with each issue. The *BMJ*, for example, puts out a press release each week that usually describes four or five 'stories' from the *BMJ*. The press release is faxed or emailed to hundreds of journalists around the world, and is placed on websites accessible only to journalists, one of which is owned and run by the American Association for the Advancement of Science.

What should be included in a press release? It's tempting to include studies that are 'important' in that they describe new evidence on common and important diseases. These are the things in which the media ought to be interested—and sometimes they are. But often they are not. 'Worthy but dull' is the withering judgement from newspaper editors. The media are interested in things that are new, exciting, amusing and likely to appeal to the public's interest (quite a different thing from the public interest). They are particularly interested in 'counterintuitive stories'—'man bites dog' rather than 'dog bites man'. Sex, alcohol, food (especially for some odd reason garlic—perhaps an atavistic link with vampires), and alternative therapies are perennial favourites. The media are increasingly a branch of the entertainment industry, competing desperately with a thousand other interests for people's attention. (This is true as well of journals.)

At the *BMJ* we thus tended to press release what we thought would interest the media rather than what we judged ought to interest the media. Was this wrong? Some would argue that we were shirking our responsibility to the public health, succumbing to the degraded values of the media. Our line was that it is a waste of everybody's time to press release the worthy but dull. In addition, we tried to make the worthy less dull. For example, we conducted a vote on our website on whether I should resign my unpaid professorship in Nottingham because the university had taken £3.8m from British American Tobacco to fund a centre for the study of corporate responsibility? The university condemned the vote as a 'cheap publicity shot', but it succeeded in provoking a worldwide debate that hadn't happened when the grant was first announced. (The vote was that I should resign, and I did.)

What should be the style of a press release? One option is to write a complete story that could be placed straight onto the page by penurious publications, of which there are many. This is what some journals do, but the *BMJ* chose not to. We saw the press release as a taster. We wanted the journalists to read the paper and speak to the authors and perhaps others. In other words, the journalists would 'add value', enrich the story and move it on. Another view is that journals should energetically try to help journalists make sense of the story in order to avoid 'scares'. So journals might, for example, give various ways of presenting risk. They might, for example, explain not only that a pill causes a 50% increase in risk but also that the risk goes up from two in a 1000 per year to three in a 1000 per year. There are other ways to present risk, and people are actively researching how best to do it. This information can usefully be presented in a press release, but I argue that it should also be in the paper in the journal or in an accompanying editorial—because most doctors are little better than most members of the public at understanding and interpreting risk.

The *BMJ* press release was usually distributed on a Tuesday, with the stories embargoed until 11 pm on Thursday evening London time. The new issue went up on bmj.com at exactly the same time. Increasingly original research papers, which are the source for most media stories, are placed on bmj.com as they become available. This opens up the possibility of journals receiving media coverage every day of the week. The paper version of the *BMJ* is dated Saturday. The American journals tended to have longer lead times—because it takes that bit longer to distribute the paper copies of the journal around the United States. *JAMA* also puts out a video release, providing pieces of video that television stations can use. This makes sense in a country where many more people watch television than read newspapers and where there are so many small television stations. Major British channels like the BBC are reluctant to use videos provided by others.

Journalists can get electronic access to the studies under embargo before they are released to the rest of the world. One argument for an embargo is that it gives journalists time to interview people and prepare a clear and accurate story. It's the opposite of my experience with the *Lancet* study suggesting that the pill might cause breast cancer when I had almost no time to contact people and interpret the study. Another argument is that the embargo prevents an unseemly scramble, with journalists trying to outdo each other. The embargo also means that doctors will be getting their paper copies of the journal at the same time that stories are appearing in the media. If a study evokes a 'scare'—as the *Lancet* pill study did, with tens of thousands of women stopping the pill—then doctors have full information for advising patients.

Many doctors would prefer to have the full information before a media blitz occurs. They would then be prepared. Unfortunately this is unachievable in a world of instant electronic communication. The moment a publication is publicly available it circles the world. The embargo is a compromise, which journalists accept because it makes their lives easier—but it would be impossible to enforce an embargo that was even hours after doctors got their copies.

Some journalists also object to embargoes, on the grounds that journalists are being manipulated and that journalistic values are being undermined. Important stories shouldn't in the public interest be held back for even a few moments, let alone two or three days. Independent Television News (ITN) took this line with the *BMJ* a few years ago, and we threatened not to provide them with a press release. They pointed out that this was an empty threat because they had links with dozens of news organizations around the world and would have no difficulty getting our press release. We argued that the embargo worked in everybody's best interest and that they would drive us back to a world of the mad, midnight scramble. I'm not sure if they agreed, but something stopped them breaking our embargo.

In a global world of 24-hour media the time of the embargo works well for some people and badly for others. For years both the *BMJ* and the *Lancet* had the same embargo of 00.01 am on Friday morning, ideal for a gentlemanly world where journals had limited coverage in the *Times*, the *Guardian* and other 'quality dailies'. But there are now tens of thousands of media outlets, and most are electronic—not only radio and television but also web-based. ITN argued to the *BMJ* that Britain had now followed the United States in television being everything. The newspapers, they told us, are giving yesterday's news. They would like an embargo that was 6 pm Thursday evening—then they could break the stories first. But that would upset the doctors: patients would be getting information 12 hours before they did. It's a world of uneasy compromises, but at the *BMJ* we moved our embargo back to 11 pm on Thursday to catch the evening broadcasts in the United States, the world's only superpower as readers will hardly need reminding.

Journals used to be very proprietorial over their studies. The *New England Journal of Medicine* had something called 'the Ingelfinger–Relman rule', named after two of its editors.[281] The rule said that if the journal saw even a whisper of one of their studies in the mass media then they would decline to publish the study. This was very threatening to authors—because getting published in the *New England Journal of Medicine* was supremely important. The journal's argument was that material should not be released until properly peer reviewed. Another argument, a much better one to my mind, was that the world needed access to the full study in order to be able to decide whether or not to believe the results. Simply presenting the conclusion of a study could be very misleading. The journal also wanted a reward for investing so much time and energy in a study. It didn't want its thunder stolen.

Many journalists objected strongly to the rule, arguing that journals were holding back information, much of it funded with public money, that was important for public health, and interfering with the free flow of information. Surely journals should be promoting the dissemination of information, not impeding it. There was also a problem in that the rule impeded scientific discourse. The rule might have worked acceptably in the days when scientists met in closed meetings, but increasingly journalists attend scientific meetings. Indeed, the major societies that hold the meetings increasingly employ public relations companies to publicize the meeting and the studies being presented at them. Authors became very confused. Could they not present their studies at meetings? If not, didn't that mean that journals were standing in the way of scientific debate, something essential to the scientific process?

The *BMJ* operated a dilute version of the Ingelfinger–Relman rule and would explain to authors that we didn't mind them presenting at meetings but that they shouldn't give any data to journalists or talk to them. But this seemed to be a formula for encouraging stories that are misleading. Slowly but surely the rule collapsed, and the *BMJ* gave up worrying about where material appeared before it was in the *BMJ*. Everybody tends to agree, however, that it's best if media stories and full scientific reports can appear simultaneously—otherwise, the world may be left wondering whether it's true that 'porridge cures (or causes) cancer'.

Journals have responded to the criticism of holding back information that is important for the public health by creating fast track systems of peer review and by posting studies on their websites as soon as they are peer reviewed. But who decides what's important for the public health? This often seems to be a political rather than a scientific processes.[123] Powerful voices achieve rapid release. So there tend to be early release of lots of studies on AIDS and breast cancer or studies that are of interest to pharmaceutical companies but fewer studies of ageing and mental health problems.

The problem of medical journals being slow to publish could potentially be ancient history. Various journals, including the *BMJ*, have created websites where authors could post studies the minute they are complete. This has happened routinely in high energy physics for some years, but it hasn't proved attractive to medical researchers. The websites are largely unused, and one factor seems to be anxiety about premature reporting of results in the media. High energy physics rarely makes it into the mass media, but studies linking lifestyle factors—perhaps coffee drinking—with some dreadful disease are a staple diet of the media.

Despite the electronic possibilities that are open to the journals the first that most people, including most doctors, know of a study that appears in a weekly journal is when they hear about it through the mass media. Some groups—for example, medical directors of pharmaceutical companies—resent this greatly. I became embroiled in an argument with them after we published a short paper describing the serious side-effects of minocycline, a drug used to treat acne, together with an editorial that argued that minocycline should not be used as the first drug when treating patients with acne.[282,283] Perhaps because it was a very quiet news day, the paper was reported on the front page of a very popular British newspaper. One response was a huge number of calls to the company on the day of publication—for which it was unprepared. Another effect was a dramatic drop in prescriptions for minocycline.[284] (Would this drop have happened without the media coverage, I wonder. Probably not.)

The company was annoyed, and the medical director joined with other medical directors to ask that they be given access to our press releases before the embargo. I declined. My argument was to ask where we draw the line if we extended beyond journalists. They, I argued, are an extension of the dissemination process. We can logically draw a line between them and everybody else. But if we were to alert medical directors why not regulatory authorities (worldwide, not just in Britain), charities, pressure groups, governments, royal colleges, public health authorities and so on? Where could the line be drawn?

I did point out, however, that the authors are free to contact whomever they want and that with drug side-effects the *BMJ* requires authors to contact the manufacturers—to see if they have had other reports of the side-effect. The medical directors were unconvinced.

The same issue arises with material that might cause a public health scare. Should journals notify public health authorities so that they are prepared? Again the *BMJ* tended to leave it to the authors, but perhaps this is not enough.

One group whom the *BMJ* thought should be informed before anything appears in the mass media is participants in studies. This issue became prominent after women with breast cancer who had participated in the Bristol Cancer Help Centre study found out from television news (wrongly, as it turned out) that having been to the centre made them more likely to die prematurely (see p 20). This was clearly a poor way to reward people for having participated in studies. Ideally participants should be given the results of the study by the researchers and should have the chance of questioning them on the implications of the results. This is a tradition in occupational research on workforces, and one to be encouraged. The *BMJ* had the unfortunate experience of publishing research that described increased risks of those working in the nuclear industry—and then hearing afterwards that the workforce knew nothing of the results.

Producing press releases may create various problems, but they seem to be effective in producing coverage of studies from journals in the mass media. The table below shows the results of a search that I did on Google in July 2003 and then repeated in

Journal	Google news hits 2003	Google news hits 2006	% change
JAMA	1620	3070	87
New England Journal of Medicine	1550	3060	97
Lancet	580	2100	262
BMJ	412	1240	200
Annals of Internal Medicine	179	190	6
Journal of the American College of Cardiology	165	28	489
British Journal of Psychiatry	18	38	111
Canadian Medical Association Journal	17	139	718
Public Library of Science Medicine	n/a	115	n/a
Medical Journal of Australia	22	71	223
Archives of Disease in Childhood	0	3	Infinity
Annals of Rheumatic Diseases	0	0	0

April 2006 to see how many times various journals had been quoted in some 4500 internet-based news outlets from around the world in the last four weeks.

As with all data it's fascinating to try and draw meaning from them. These are the messages I draw. First, there is considerable coverage in the mass media of material from medical journals. Second, the vast majority of the coverage comes from the major general medical journals. Third, the American weekly medical journals dominate. Fourth, the coverage received by the journals seems to correlate with their prestige and their impact factor. Fifth, the non-American general journals have seen the biggest percentage increase in coverage. This is probably the result of the internet making the non-American journals much more available to the American media, which tend to dominate. The huge percentage increase in coverage of the *Canadian Medical Association Journal* is largely caused by the controversy surrounding the recent sacking of its editors.

Why do journals want this coverage? The editors of the *New England Journal of Medicine* used to give the impression that they saw coverage in the mass media as a necessary evil. This was ironic in that the journal's pre-eminent position was closely linked with its extensive coverage in the mass media.

Indeed, the journal published a clever opportunistic study in 1991 that looked at how coverage of studies in the *New York Times* affected citation in scientific journals.[285] Those studies from the *New England Journal of Medicine* that were reported in the *New York Times* received more citations for every year of the next 10 years than those not reported. In the first year after publication they received roughly 80% more citations. Thoughtful readers might think that this is simply because the *New York Times* reported the most important studies. But during the study the *New*

York Times went on strike for three months. The journalists continued to produce a newspaper of record, but it wasn't distributed. Those articles that were selected from the *New England Journal of Medicine* during those three months did not receive more citations. So it seemed to be the coverage itself that increased citations.

The result is probably not surprising. Scientists pay attention to the mass media just like everybody else. The studies selected will thus be brought to their attention, and almost certainly being reported in the *New York Times* would be closely related to being reported in other media, including international media. Several studies have also shown that doctors get much of their new medical information from the mass media. They are overwhelmed with information. It's very convenient to have studies selected and professionally presented by the mass media, particularly television. Instead of tired doctors having to struggle through the complexities of a scientific study they can slump in front of the television and have the story told to them attractively—and often by the authors—in two minutes.

So one reason to seek media coverage is to increase citations to your journal— something that obsesses many editors in this age of academic accountability based on the impact factors of journals. Next, ironically, you may reach your own readers more effectively through the mass media than through your own publication. Certainly you will reach a huge audience of researchers and doctors who you will not reach directly through your journal.

Then for many journals—and certainly the *BMJ*—it is a desirable end in itself to reach the public. Much of the research journals publish is funded with public money and all of it is intended to improve the health of individual patients or the public. The logic of the age of patient partnership is that patients and the public should have access to research.

Dissemination of journal material through the mass media is also part of the political process. Improving health is in many ways a political activity, and journals are much more likely to have a political impact if their contents—and not just research but also editorials—are covered in the mass media. Politicians pay much more attention to the mass media than they do to medical journals.

Coverage in the mass media is also very gratifying for all those involved in journals. Some may pretend to be too high minded to care, but almost everybody loves the coverage. These days authors may find themselves doing 50 interviews in a day. They rub shoulders with celebrities that they otherwise only see in *Hello* magazine, and their words, wise or otherwise, may be broadcast across all six continents. Their research reaches not just a few buddies but millions. Their mothers are excited. Old friends from Australia that they haven't heard from for years email them. And their universities and funders—hungry for prestige and cash—love it, which is why they employ public relations companies to get authors into as many media as possible. Many authors find a day or two being fêted by the media very exciting after years of careful and unglamorous analysis of data. Because authors and their institutions like media coverage they are more likely to submit their studies to journals that receive much coverage, providing another reason for journals to pursue the mass media.

Playing with the media—particularly the more downmarket media—is, however, playing with fire, and it can get very rough. Jim Drife, a professor of obstetrics and gynaecology and one of the *BMJ*'s columnists, discussed the case for women at high risk of breast cancer having bilateral mastectomies as a preventive measure. He was then depicted as a monster in the media. Various doctors in prominent positions played down the idea that bovine spongiform encephalopathy could cross from cows to man and then were ridiculed when it did. But mostly authors presenting research in the mass media are given an easy ride. The presenters and journalists simply want to tell the story as clearly as possible. They rarely challenge it.

Editors and the staff who work on journals also like media coverage. It feels like a public affirmation of their work. Then the business and marketing people like it too. Coverage in the mass media is a highly cost-effective way to get your journal known, and some journals have broken into new geographical markets by targeting the media. So there is probably a long-term financial return for coverage, but these days there is also a short-term return. Many journals have a 'pay per view' facility on their websites. People can pay about $10 with their credit card to get instant access to an article. Unsurprisingly, studies covered in the mass media are the ones that attract most of this income.

So if editors are so attracted to media coverage are they more likely to accept studies that will attract such coverage? Did the *Lancet* accept the infamous study that linked the measles, mumps and rubella (MMR) vaccine with autism because of its taste for publicity?

If medically and scientifically important studies were also the studies most likely to get media coverage, then there would be no problem. But they aren't quite the same thing. 'Skateboarding duck stories', as we called them at the *BMJ*, will get coverage but are not medically and scientifically important. But then again the media select such stories because they think their readers will like them, and the readers of the *BMJ* are not a completely different population: they will probably enjoy them too. Medical journals like the *BMJ* are poised somewhere between academia and journalism and have some journalistic values. The *BMJ* wouldn't, I like to think, take a piece of research that was scientifically ridiculous but journalistically exciting, but journalistic value is a factor it considers.

I remember a debate over a paper we published in our Christmas issue, an issue traditionally devoted to slightly strange, wacky and amusing material. A long-term follow-up of a population in Wales showed that men aged 40 who had 50 orgasms a year lived longer than those who had fewer.[286] There would inevitably be doubts over the data. How honest are people about their sex lives? Perhaps the fact that the men had more orgasms was simply a marker of other characteristics that made them likely to live longer. Or maybe healthier men were capable of more orgasms. This study was neither medically nor scientifically important, but it would interest our readers and get lots of media coverage. I decided that we would publish the study—and it did get lots of coverage.

I see it as largely beyond the scope of this chapter to discuss how the mass media cover medical stories, some of which come from medical journals, but I want to make a few comments. There is no doubt that coverage of health issues in the mass media is increasing, and it may be that the increased coverage is contributing to patients becoming as smart as their doctors, changing forever the relationship between doctors and patients. Knowledge is power, and increased knowledge must be a good thing.

Increased information does not, however, equal increased knowledge. Ann Karpf, a journalist and sociologist, has argued that the increased coverage is leading to more confusion.[287] People are often misinformed. The mass media do a mostly competent job of reporting on new studies, although the complexities, the 'ifs and buts', are inevitably left out. Feature articles on health are, however, less good. Certainly in the British media, health is mixed together with beauty and fitness, and there is a great enthusiasm for alternative treatments. The *Observer*, one of Britain's oldest newspapers, has for years run a column by 'the barefoot doctor'. He publishes amiable and perhaps helpful tosh. Probably people, including my wife, who read his columns understand the nature of what they are reading, but I find it hard to believe that the postmodern mishmash served up by the media is helpful.

Then there are the recurrent 'scares', many of them it has to be said started by medical journals. The scare over the MMR vaccine is familiar to everybody, but we have had scares over whooping cough vaccine, brain death, the contraceptive pill, toxic shock syndrome, 'mad cow disease,' total allergy syndrome, the 'flesh eating bug,' and many other issues. Mostly these scares contain some genuine cause for worry, but the 'flesh eating bug' scare was a classic scare story. A journalist somewhere discovered a case of necrotizing fasciitis, a rare but well recognized condition caused by a bacterium. A subeditor added the sobriquet of the 'flesh eating bug,' and editors around the country began a search for cases. Even with a rare disease you will find cases if you don't restrict yourself in time and space. Suddenly the media were full of accounts of cases of a dreadful disease that nobody had heard of before. It seemed as if a new disease was rampant. Knowledgeable health reporters tried to explain to editors that there was nothing new, but they were swept aside. Eventually the story fizzled out, but many people must have lain awake at night worrying that the disease would soon strike them.

Stories in the media can always get out of control, and the mass media are probably even more prone than medical journals to manipulation by those with vested interests. The *San Francisco Chronicle*, for example, carried a piece extolling the virtues of prostate specific antigen (PSA), a marker for prostate cancer. The article suggested that every man who was middle-aged or older should know his PSA. The editors of the *Western Journal of Medicine*—friends of mine—wrote a letter to the newspaper saying that its piece had overstated the case for testing men. Screening all men for prostate cancer is not recommended by public health authorities, and mass testing might well create more problems than it solves—partly because many men will be made unnecessarily anxious and partly because many older men have prostate cancer and yet will not be troubled by it. The *Chronicle*—to its credit—liked their letter and asked them to write a full article. They did, and within moments of publication they were subjected to a firestorm of abuse. They were accused of 'geriatricide', and several people wrote to their employers—in one case the University of California— demanding they be sacked. Urologists, many of whom stand to benefit financially from increased PSA testing, led the charge.

I am an unapologetic populist, and I believe that medical and health issues should be debated in the mass media, but we would probably all benefit from there being more places where there could be a higher level of debate. Perhaps medical journals have a role here and perhaps they should consciously try to appeal more to non-doctors.

Medical journals are moving, I believe, from being rather offhand about—or even sometimes hostile to—media coverage to liking it. Doctors and academic institutions are moving in the same direction. My hope, however, is that journals' engagement with the mass media will enhance not debase the value of what they publish. I have to say that I'm much less worried about journals' involvement with the mass media than I am with their involvement with the pharmaceutical industry.

►15

Trying to stop failing the developing world

Most sickness, disability and premature death happens to people in the developing world. Yet only 2% of the 3000 medical journals listed on Medline are from the developing world, and those journals struggle. Furthermore, until very recently doctors and health workers in the developing world have been starved of up to date information. All the major medical journals, including the *BMJ*, aspire to be global journals of medicine and health, and yet publish little from and relevant to the developing world.[288–290] They also have become very confused over the ethics of publishing research from the developing world. Why are medical journals doing so poorly in relation to the developing world and what can be done?

Some parts of the developing world—for example, India and China —have many medical journals, but they struggle and make little impact internationally. In some ways this is true as well with journals from developed countries. Little is heard internationally of the Scandinavian, French, German and Italian journals. Nor is much heard from English language journals published in Australia, Canada and New Zealand (indeed, the *New Zealand Medical Journal* has just ceased to exist in paper form, which I fear is a prelude to extinction). The world is dominated by the major general journals and a few major journals from each specialty. These journals are usually American and sometimes British.

National journals should probably do a job that is different from international journals. Too many journals simply ape the major journals, but what is the point of having a fourth rate version of the *Lancet* filled with research that has been rejected by five other journals? I experienced this when as a student I became editor of *Synapse*, the Edinburgh Medical School journal. The journal comprised mostly boring and largely irrelevant research. So nobody read it. I thought that if the journal had any purpose it was to cover the issues that were important to the medical community in Edinburgh but uninteresting to the rest of the world. Isn't that the point of national journals? The Norwegian medical journal should be covering the issues that matter in Norway and be the place that Norwegian doctors decide what they think about the issues of the day.

Samiran Nundi—an Indian surgeon and the first editor of the *National Medical Journal of India*—and others analysed the contents of Indian medical journals and discovered that they contained little on the problems important in India.[291] He started the *National Medical Journal of India*, with support from the government, to be a uniquely Indian journal that concentrated on Indian issues. In many ways he succeeded, producing a lively journal that covers Indian issues well but has also made it into *Index Medicus*. [*Index Medicus* is compiled by the United States National Library of Medicine, and it's a mark of respectability to be included in the index.] Friends from other parts of India tell me, however, that the journal is too much of a Delhi journal and doesn't have enough input from the other major centres in India.

Journals in developing countries have problems that are not terribly different from smaller journals in developed countries. They are often edited by a lone editor who does everything, don't receive enough articles, are desperately short of resources and go unnoticed by the rest of the world. Often they are not even read by the people they are published for.

I once judged a competition among some 40 journals from India at a conference on editing in Delhi organized by the *National Medical Journal of India*. The journal that won—a paediatric journal—was impressive: full of energy, insight and material that would be useful and interesting not only to paediatricians in India but to all paediatricians, particularly those in other parts of the developing world. But many of the other journals were terrible, and I couldn't avoid the thought that it would be better to pool resources and produce fewer, better journals. The same would be true in the developed world, and after three centuries of expansion in medical journals we are beginning to see mergers of journals.

(Not only medical journals but also medical institutions seem to proliferate. The Royal College of Physicians, for example, has split into colleges of pathology and of paediatrics and child health, and various faculties. One driver, a Cambridge don, told me is that 'there is no kingdom too small for a doctor to be king of'. And an editor is a very lowly king.)

While India may have too many journals some parts of the developing world—like West Africa—have effectively none. There was the *Nigerian Medical Journal* and there is the *West African Medical Journal*, but these journals hardly ever appear. The *Nigerian Medical Journal* hasn't been published for years. The only African journal outside of South Africa that has come out consistently is the *East African Medical Journal*. It has been published for over 75 years, developing into an important journal from a frankly racist journal full of pseudoscience that first appeared in colonial times.

But in most of Africa it's proved impossible in recent times to produce journals regularly. The difficulties are not only a lack of resources but also war, political upheaval and corruption. Plus many countries now have medical cultures that set little store by reading journals and publishing. This may be partly because most doctors in countries like Nigeria have been starved of high-quality material. If you can't get it you learn to live without it, and you are then not much interested even if it does become available. A downward spiral is established. I travelled regularly to West Africa and watched with great interest as medical leaders tried to revive cultures of reading and publishing.

The case hardly needs to be made that the major journals contain little from and for the developing world, although I think that there may have been an important change very recently (which may be a triumph of hope over experience or ascertainment bias—seeing what you want to see). Obuaya surveyed the five leading general medical journals in 2001 for research articles relevant to the diseases of poverty.[289] It was zero for *Annals of Internal Medicine*, 2% for *JAMA*, 4% for the *New England Journal of Medicine*, 6% for the *BMJ* and 16% for the *Lancet*.

These analyses of content are tricky to do because people have different ideas on what constitutes 'research…relevant to the diseases of poverty'. Asad Jamil Raja and Peter Singer looked at four of these general journals in January 2002 and again in January 2003 for material 'partially or wholly related to developing country research priorities'.[290] Among original research articles it was 35% of those in the *BMJ* in 2002 (20% in 2003), 18% in the *Lancet* (5% in 2003), 10% in the *New England Journal of Medicine* (9% in 2003) and 6% in *JAMA* (0% in 2003). Among editorials it was 37% for the *BMJ* in 2002 (25% in 2003), 50% for the *Lancet* (75% in 2003), 7% for the *New England Journal of Medicine* (0% in 203) and 0% for *JAMA* in both 2002 and 2003. Overall, they found that in 2002 24% of 234 pieces published in the *BMJ* were relevant to developing countries and 22% of 234 pieces published in the *Lancet*, compared with 8% of the 86 pieces in the *New England Journal of Medicine* and 7% of the 182 pieces in *JAMA*.

All of these figures have to be treated with caution. They cover only short time periods and are sensitive to how the authors interpret the relevance of the articles. Nevertheless, there is some evidence that the British journals have more material relevant to the developing world. This is not perhaps surprising as both the *Lancet* and the *BMJ* have specifically been targeting the developing world in a way that the American journals have not. The data on editorials and reviews are particularly important because as they are largely commissioned they express intent.

One very obvious reason why these journals publish little research from the developing world is that only 10% of medical research is undertaken in the developing world.[292] Furthermore and tragically, much of the research conducted in the developing world is intended to benefit those in the developed world. Such research may be undertaken in the developing world because the disease prevalence is much higher (with AIDS, for example), ethical constraints are less and the cost is lower.

There are many reasons both why relatively little research is undertaken in the developing world and why it is hard to get the research that is undertaken published, but a useful summary comes from the survey Richard Horton, the editor of the *Lancet*, undertook among African academics.[293] He sent out 33 letters and received 22 replies (67% response rate). The barriers to undertaking research include medical schools and hospitals being in disarray. This is more true in some African countries than others and is a greater problem in Africa than many other parts of the developing world. The shortage of money (particularly foreign exchange) means not only that little is available for funding research but also that the hospitals are short of drugs and equipment. In addition, academic salaries are low and career structures poor, and many potential researchers may be driven into the private sector. Those who are left are often forced to put service work and teaching before research. There are thus few mentors available for those who want to pursue research, and it can be hard to get training. In short, there is no research culture.

There is also a tendency—in the developed as well as the developing world—to see research as a 'luxury', something that can be afforded only by those who are rich. But research is actually an important engine of development. We also understand now from the Commission on Macroeconomics and Health set up by the World Health Organization (WHO) that investing in health may be the very best way to promote development, and the commission emphasized that an essential part of investing in health is to invest in health research.[71] If resources are short it becomes still more important to undertake research to ensure that resources are employed effectively. Only the rich can afford the luxury of wasting resources on the ineffective, as they do on a massive scale.

International journals may publish little research from the developing world not only because there is little of it but also because it is of low quality. I don't have data on this, but it would not be surprising if some of the research was of lower quality. Good research may be expensive and may demand good facilities, and resources are lacking in the developed world. More important, however, is probably lack of training. Research is increasingly a complex, professional business that demands good training. There may also be a problem with the writing up of research, particularly if the authors' first language is not English—but journals can fix the language, whereas they can rarely fix the research.

Another obvious reason why the major journals have published little relevant to the developing world is because until recently most of their readers have been in the developed world. The *BMJ*, for example, had no electronic version until 1994. The weekly paper edition of the journal had a print-run of 115,000, and about 100,000 of those were circulated in Britain. Of the 15,000 that went overseas only a small fraction went to developing countries—partly because they couldn't afford it. We did circulate some copies for free, and we did have a South Asian edition of the journal. But the vast majority of our readers were in the developed world. This didn't mean that we shouldn't publish anything relevant to the developing world—because some readers were in the developing world, and if we cared at all about the health of everybody in the world (and we liked to think that we did), then it was essential to publish on the problems of the developing world and draw them to the attention of those in the developed world. But editors obviously have to avoid a gross mismatch between what they publish and what their readers want and need.

Economics are also important. Journals need a sustainable business model, and often their owners want them to make substantial profits. The vast majority of the income to journals—subscriptions, advertising and reprints—comes from the developed world. Special attention thus has to be paid to the rich world. This is somewhat analogous to pharmaceutical companies creating 'me too' drugs (a drug similar to one already available) for those in the rich world rather than new drugs for largely untreatable conditions seen most commonly in the developing world. Doctors in the rich world are drowning in journals and newspapers, most of which come to them free, while those in the developing world have, until very recently, been starved of information.

In many ways it is unfair to blame pharmaceutical companies and commercial publishers for this state of affairs. They are obliged to make profits for their shareholders, and that is much easier to do by producing drugs and publications for the rich world. Special steps need to be taken for encouraging the production of new drugs for the developing world—and some have been taken. Similarly special steps have been taken to increase the availability of publications in the developing world—and again progress has been made.

Could the bias of journals be caused by something analogous to institutional racism, asked Richard Horton, editor of the *Lancet*, in a provocative editorial?[288] Institutional racism has become a familiar concept in Britain, and seems to exist in most of our institutions, including the National Health Service.[294] Institutional racism is when an institution unwittingly behaves in a racist way even though nobody within the institution is overtly racist or intends to be so. A good example is when institutions appoint people to new positions without advertising externally: if the organization is predominantly white then this introduces bias against non-whites, even though nobody explicitly intended that to be the case.

It does seem likely that institutions like journals that have been published in rich, predominantly white countries for well over a century take time to learn new ways. Prompted by a study that showed severe under-representation of people from developing countries on the editorial boards of 10 leading psychiatric journals,[295] Horton looked at the composition of the editorial boards of the major journals.[288] The boards of the *Annals of Internal Medicine*, *JAMA* and the *New England Journal of Medicine* didn't include anybody from the developing world, and 94%, 74% and 53% of their boards respectively came from the United States. The *Lancet* had three members from the developing world and 25% from Britain. The *BMJ* had five members from the developing world and 35% from Britain.

Horton didn't analyse the editorial staff, but if he did I suspect that he'd find almost nobody from the developing world and that virtually everybody came from the home country. And when it comes to editors I think that all the editors of the British journals have been British and all the editors of the American journals American. The *BMJ* is the only one of the two British journals to have had a woman editor (Fiona Godlee, my successor), and every editor of the *BMJ* for a century bar one came from one medical school—St Bartholomew's Hospital Medical School. That's how insular journals are.

The *BMJ* didn't have an editorial board until nine years ago, and when we set it up we carefully selected people to represent different parts of the world, different specialties and patients. We were keen to have people from Africa, Asia and South America, recognizing that these continents contain predominantly developing countries. But how was it that we ended up with three people from Australia and only one from Africa? And how come we didn't have anybody from the Middle East? Some sort of bias must be at work. Partly it's whom we know, who publishes in the *BMJ* and where we travel.

I think of it less as being biased against those from the developing world and more of us struggling to rise above our origins. Is a global journal really possible? I know that many people in Scotland thought of the *BMJ* as the English Medical Journal, and our North American editor kept spelling out to us how the *BMJ* felt very British and very unAmerican. CNN employs people all around the world and has offices in London, but it feels American to me. I'm sure that to people in the developing world media from the rich world do not reflect or understand the realities of their world.

Being global is much more an aspiration than a reality at the moment, but I feel that if the *BMJ* and our other journals have a future it's a global future. Sticking to Britain would mean severe retrenchment and probably death. The BMJ Publishing Group's journals have long been global in that one-half of their papers were submitted from outside Britain and two-thirds of their subscriptions were from outside Britain—but as recently as 10 years ago the editors, editorial board and reviewers were all British, not even American. The journals were more colonial than international. Now more than half of the editors are from outside Britain—but none is from a developing country.

How does a journal like the *BMJ* or a publishing company like the BMJ Publishing Group become truly global? I thought a lot about this question but never found the answer. If we were a huge company we would have made sure that we had staff in every country and that our senior management came from all around the world. But we were 250 people, most of us living in London and most of us British. One answer might have been that we should have become much more of a virtual organization and employed people around the world. Another answer might have been to form partnerships and strategic alliances.

I'm straying from the point here, but I'm trying to suggest that journals' bias against the developing world—although it can legitimately be described as institutional bias, racism, elitism, nationalism—is not the result of negativity towards the developing world but more a case of them being bound up with their origins. The glass is one-quarter full rather than three-quarters empty and is filling not emptying. Or is this complacency?

Medical journals have perhaps illustrated their ignorance of the developing world by tying themselves in knots over the ethics of trials conducted in the developing world. Marcia Angell, deputy editor of the *New England Journal of Medicine*, famously compared a trial of treating pregnant women infected with HIV with a short course of zidovudine to try and stop the virus infecting their babies with the Tuskegee study, the infamous study in the United States where black men with syphilis were left untreated.[296] The problem was that some pregnant women were getting a placebo when there was a treatment available—albeit a treatment that was unaffordable in Africa.[297] For Angell this was wholly unethical, but those who carried out the research took exactly the opposite view—and because they had difficulty getting heard in the *New England Journal of Medicine* they argued their case in the *BMJ*.[298]

Angell, who had many supporters particularly in the mass media, argued that such research would not be allowed in the developed world and that it cannot be acceptable to have different ethical standards for the developed and developing world. Those conducting trials should test the new treatment against optimal treatments. Those who argue that such research can be acceptable point out that the expensive treatment will be unavailable to most in the developing world.[298,299] Thus to test the new treatment against the complicated regimen would not produce a useful answer. Most women in the community get no treatment at all. Indeed, most women who are infected are not even identified. The women had given fully informed consent, and the studies were approved by local and international ethics committees and complied with international standards.

These debates have been heated, but there is, I suggest, much that we could agree about. First, nothing should be hidden. Everything should be disclosed to participants, ethics committees, funders of the research, and eventual readers and consumers of the research. Second, properly constituted local and international ethics committees should approve the research. Third, the care received by those in the trial should not in any way be poorer than that received by people in that community. Fourth, it should be possible to see how the research might benefit the community where it is conducted. Fifth, all participants should give fully informed consent. Sixth—and this is hard to judge—the possible benefits to that community should outweigh the benefits to researchers (academic status, publication credit, etc).

Such conditions were met in the trial of short-course zidovudine against placebo in pregnant women infected with HIV. But they would probably not be met by a trial of a new expensive treatment for hypertension. It could, however, be argued that even such a trial might meet the criteria: the benefit to the community would come not perhaps from the drug being widely available but from the short-term improvement in healthcare and from the economic benefit that would accrue to the community. Indeed, some might argue that it would be patronizing to ban such a trial (or refuse to publish its results) so long as nothing is hidden, participants give fully informed consent and a fully competent local ethics committee approves the research.

The World Medical Association (WMA) has in revising the Declaration of Helsinki addressed this problem of using placebos in trials in developing countries when an established, albeit unaffordable, treatment is available. It would be fair to say that things remain confused: the WMA initially took the same line as Marcia Angell but then retreated. Professor James Whitworth from the Medical Research Council said: 'It seems a strange sort of logic to stop doing trials in Africa that are trying to help improve the health of poor people so that people in rich countries can have peace of mind.'[300]

Discussions about ethics, medical journals and the developing world often focus on the ethics of publishing trials from the developing world, but the much bigger issue is how can medical journals do a better job of meeting the needs of the developing world. How can research capacity be increased? How can local journals be helped to flourish? How can better information be made available in the developing world? How can the major journals make themselves more useful to those in the developing world?

The gap between the rich and the poor worlds has been increasing not decreasing in recent years, and there have been a great many initiatives to improve health and health research in the developing world that have come to nothing. Nevertheless, there are currently genuine reasons to be optimistic. Global health has risen up the agendas of international organizations and the rich countries. First, as mentioned before, the WHO's Commission on Macroeconomics and Health made it clear that investing in health is essential for development.[71] Second, there is an increasing recognition that global health and global security go together. One consequence is the Global Health Fund, which has large sums for investing in health.

There is also increasing recognition that investment in health research must accompany investment in health services and public health. There is now a Global Forum for Health Research, which meets regularly and aims to encourage governments to think more about health research and to build research capacity.[301]

The *BMJ* published a theme issue on promoting research in the developing world, and as part of the exercise we ran a vote on our website on the best ways to promote research. The proposal that got the most votes was strengthening national research institutions and networks. Second was to give local researchers incentives to resist the brain drain. The third proposal was to improve telecommunications and internet access in developing countries, which is happening—and at dramatic speed in some countries. Fourth was to promote North–South partnerships between researchers and research institutions. This is happening increasingly and is a means of not just getting research done but also of training. Fifth was to ensure that developing countries allocate 2–5% of their health budgets to research. This is a level of expenditure that many developed countries don't manage, but there are very strong arguments for doing so in a 'knowledge-based' enterprise like healthcare.

An increase in local research capacity might be the single biggest boost to local journals—not just because it will provide material to publish but also because it will provide people to serve as editors, reviewers and authors of editorials and reviews. But those concerned to develop local journals should not, I believe, simply copy journals that exist in developed countries. Journals are likely to change dramatically in the next 20 years. Original research—including research from the developing world—will probably appear on the web and be available to everybody. The difficulty that researchers in the developing world have in getting their material to each other and to people in the rich world may disappear. The job of editors of local journals will be less to peer review research and more to find research and other material important to their audience and present it in as attractive and useful a way as possible.

Experienced editors from the developed and developing world have a job to do in training and supporting others, and the World Association of Medical Editors (WAME) is the most important step in this direction.[302] The WHO has become steadily more interested in encouraging the flow of information to, from and within the developing world.

The *BMJ* had many local editions, and some of these were in developing countries. In particular, the West African edition of the *BMJ* was almost the only journal that appeared with any regularity in West Africa. But was it right for the *BMJ* to be publishing this? Should we instead have been supporting a local journal? Was what we were doing re-inventing colonialism in some way?

The South Asian edition supported itself and allowed doctors from India, Sri Lanka, Nepal and Malaysia to read *BMJ* material that was particularly relevant to them and at a price that is a fraction of the price of an international selection. The edition didn't compete head on with the local journals. But the BMJ Publishing Group supported the West African edition financially, although most of its support came from Nigerian doctors in Britain. The editors-in-chief of the journal were some of the most distinguished doctors in Nigeria and Ghana, including a former deputy director general of the WHO. A strength of the West African edition of the *BMJ* was its independence. This was a major benefit in countries where political pressures can be extreme. The journal also avoided corruption, which is not easy in West Africa.

When it comes to those in the developing world being able to access research journals there has been a dramatic change in a very short while.[303] As recently as September 2000 a scientist from the WHO wrote that global inequity in access to the internet was greater than any other inequity.[304] Less than six years later more than 2000 health institutions in 106 developing countries have free or low-cost electronic access to over 3200 journals, access that is equal, and sometimes better, than in institutions in New York, London and Paris.[305]

This has happened because of a WHO initiative. In July 2001 Gro Harlem Brundtland, the director general of WHO, announced the launch of HINARI (Health Internetwork Access to Research Initiative), a voluntary partnership between WHO and 28 publishers to provide free or nominally priced access to health information to institutions in the developing world. The first phase launched on 31 January 2001, supplying 68 countries with free access to 1400 journals. All the major weekly medical and scientific journals could be accessed for free. On 31 January 2003 access was extended to another 42 middle income countries. Institutions in these countries had to pay $1000 for access to all the journals (which would buy subscriptions to about three journals at normal prices), but the publishers donated the revenue to WHO to use for training librarians in using HINARI. The network plans to include electronic books, bibliographical databases and continuing education programmes. The project was deemed so successful that there are plans to copy the programme for information on agriculture and the environment.

HINARI has transformed information access in a very short time, but it is no panacea. Access to the internet in the developing world is still limited, expensive and far from robust, although it is increasing exponentially in many poor countries. HINARI is aimed at researchers and policy makers. Further steps—perhaps using paper—need to be taken to reach front line health workers. Librarians and others need training in how to find the best information.

The programme is also primarily about supplying information from the rich world to the poor world. It's equally important to increase the flow of information in the developing world and from the poor world to the rich world.[306] Most important of all is to create cultures of reading, questioning, debating, researching and publishing. An improved information supply is a necessary but not sufficient condition for creating such cultures.

I am critical of publishers in chapter 17 on the business of publishing, but publishers have behaved admirably in this exercise. They have not had to be dragged in kicking and screaming as have some pharmaceutical companies, but the cost of supplying this information to the developing world is close to zero—and publishers had very few subscriptions from these countries.

What now might international journals do to make the material that is being delivered free to those in the poor world more useful to them? They could commission more material from developing world authors on developing world topics, use more reviewers from the developing world (which is now infinitely easier with web-based peer review systems), build more contacts, add more people from the developing world to editorial boards and recruit staff from the developing world. The *Public Library of Science Medicine*, which was launched in October 2004, has done many of these things—and is probably a more truly global journal than any of the long-established general journals.

A project that particularly excited me was the *BMJ* handing over a whole issue of the journal to editors from South Asia and later to editors from Africa.[307–310] Other issues are planned for the Middle East and China. Editors from all the countries in South Asia produced the issue of the *BMJ* that described health problems in South Asia and discussed solutions. Some 70% of all deaths of children under five happen in South Asia, and yet the two major countries in the region—India and Pakistan—are spending billions on nuclear weapons. The very act of having a journal edited jointly by an Indian and a Pakistani was hugely symbolic in a region with bitter divides.

The question is often asked about whether or not journals should adopt lower standards for publishing research from the developing world, but a better question is whether or not journals should have different standards. We didn't, for instance, have one standard for everything at the *BMJ*, and we all the time traded off against each others' originality, importance and methodological validity. The ideal paper scores highly on all three criteria, but there are few if any ideal studies. Many questions that are important in healthcare are hard to address. It wouldn't make sense to have the same methodological standard for a trial of the 23rd versus the 24th beta blocker for hypertension as for a trial of an intervention to encourage sex workers in Kinshasa to use condoms.

It was a dozen years ago that the *BMJ* developed different standards for general practice research, and in the early days we devoted resources to encouraging and developing primary care (general practice) research in a way that we didn't find necessary for research from disciplines with a long tradition of research. Now some of the best research the *BMJ* publishes comes from primary care. We did something similar for research on quality improvement, education and information technology in healthcare. We even tried (with little success) to introduce special standards for surgical research. Surgeons think, with some justification, that general medical journals are unsympathetic to their research—particularly because they do few randomized trials.

Steps to make journals more understanding of different categories of research are to involve the relevant researchers in producing guidelines on the category of research and to educate editors on the research. Journals should do this with research from the developing world.

Until very recently doctors and other healthcare workers in the developing world were largely failed by medical journals—both locally and internationally. Now— thanks largely to the arrival of the internet—substantial improvements are underway. The world is shrinking fast.

►16

Medical journals and pharmaceutical companies: uneasy bedfellows*

One of my first experiences of the relationship between medical journals and medical companies occurred in May 1982 after the *BMJ* had published papers suggesting that a new drug, benoxaprofen, a drug for arthritis, might have serious side-effects.[313–315] We were visited by three stern men from Eli Lilly, the company that manufactured the drug. Tony Smith, the deputy editor, conducted the meeting as the editor was away. He asked me to join him. The men, whom I remember (probably wrongly) as having gold teeth, threatened us with legal action, at which point Tony said: 'In that case we'll see you in court.' They backtracked hastily and asked simply for a prompt response to the papers. Later that day a competitor of Lilly rang and asked if we could get one hundred copies of the *BMJ* containing the papers on benoxaprofen to New York at once for a press conference they were holding to launch a competitor drug to benoxaprofen. I can't remember how we responded.

Those papers and other reports of side-effects led eventually to benoxaprofen being banned, but the drug's rapid demise may well have been caused by its rapid ascent. The summer before the meeting with the men with gold teeth I had visited the world headquarters of Eli Lilly in Indianapolis. I had won a prize from the Medical Journalists Association, and the prize money had to be spent on a journalistic investigation. I was interested in compensation for medical injury, including injury from drugs, and decided to visit the United States to look at its system. The prize money came from Lilly, and as Lilly had been involved in one of the biggest cases of drug injury—from diethylstilboestrol—it seemed to make sense to visit them. My wife and I were put up in a grand hotel at the company's expense and treated exceptionally well.

(Some years later I supported a motion proposing that the Medical Journalists Association cease to take money from the pharmaceutical industry for prizes and introduced a policy at the *BMJ* that we didn't go anywhere paid for by anybody else. The Indianapolis experience taught me something about conflict of interest: your opinion may not be bought, but it seems rude to say critical things about people who have hosted you so well.)

While at Lilly's headquarters I was shown films that were to be used to promote benoxaprofen when it was launched. They seemed to me wildly over the top. Patients

---

*This chapter has been published in part in much shorter forms in both the BMJ[311] and Public Library of Science Medicine.[312]

were shown with severe arthritis before they took the drug and then shown afterwards dancing without any problem. The message was that benoxaprofen didn't simply relieve the symptoms of the disease—like other similar drugs—but actually reversed the disease. I was sceptical of this claim, and even if it had some truth I thought the films excessive.

When the drug was later launched in Britain Eli Lilly held a press conference at which extravagant claims were made. The *Liverpool Echo* carried a report of 'a miracle drug'. Heavy marketing meant that the drug began very rapidly to be widely prescribed. This meant—ironically—that reports of side-effects also appeared rapidly, culminating in the papers in the *BMJ*. Research published later suggested that benoxaprofen probably didn't cause any more side-effects than other similar drugs. But nor did it reverse the process. Benoxaprofen may have died from being overhyped. As Stephen Lock, the *BMJ* editor, said to me at the time: 'Those who live by the sword shall die by the sword.'

The banning of benoxaprofen prompted the media to look at the relationship between doctors and the pharmaceutical industry, suggesting that doctors were being bought too easily. The documentary programme, Panorama, filmed a group of doctors being taken on the Orient Express to Venice to be 'educated' on another anti-arthritis drug like benoxaprofen. The doctors were put up at the very best hotel in Venice and left most of the time to do what they wanted. The 'education' was far from onerous. The company was inept enough to try and stop the television team from filming on the train, suggesting that they had something to hide. But the team got onto the train and interviewed a group of drunken doctors. The interviewer from the television team asked a doctor if he'd found the trip satisfactory.

'Yes,' he answered, 'apart from when the train jolted and I spilled my champagne.'

The interviewer then asked whether or not the company had paid for everything. 'Of course not', snapped the doctor.

'Well,' said the interviewer, 'the company has paid for the train, your flight, and your hotel and meals in Venice, all very expensive. What did you pay for?'

'My bus fare to Heathrow.'

I have perhaps overdone this story, but the benoxaprofen story had a formative influence on me and caused me to fret about the relationship between doctors and the pharmaceutical industry. There is a tendency to see the industry as the villains and the doctors as the innocent victims, but that's horribly oversimplified. It may even be the opposite. The industry clearly has a duty to its shareholders to market its products as powerfully as it can, staying on the right side of the evidence and the law. Doctors have a duty to do their best for their patients. They will of course need to use the products of the industry, and it's reasonable that the industry should have an opportunity to promote its products to the doctors. But surely doctors should be looking as well to independent sources of information, and how did we get to the point where so many doctors won't attend an educational meeting unless it's held in an exotic venue and accompanied by free and luxurious food and a bag of 'goodies' that would be acceptable even to a film star nominated for an Oscar? Something's wrong, and medical journals are part of what's wrong.

The pharmaceutical industry has unequalled power within healthcare.[316–318] Virtually every new drug in the past 50 years has been produced by the industry, and even those not produced by the industry need the industry to manufacture them. These new drugs have transformed medicine from a process—in Voltaire's words—of amusing the patient while nature took its course to something that can make a real difference to patients, albeit with increased risk. Even surgical innovations have depended on new drugs—such as better anaesthetic agents, antibiotics and drugs that suppress the immune system allowing transplantation of organs.

Because of its success—and because it has taken big risks—the industry is immensely profitable. Year after year it was until recently the most profitable industry in the United States. It thus has immense financial power, and it has great political power. Many politicians in the United States, particularly in the Bush administration, are heavily beholden to the industry. It can afford the best lobbyists and the best lawyers. And the industry has a global reach within a sector that is mostly not global. Most healthcare systems and organizations are nationally bound. The World Health Organization is global but has nothing like the financial and political clout of the pharmaceutical industry. Some medical journals, including the *BMJ*, are global, explaining in part why medical journals matter to the companies.

Although the pharmaceutical industry is immensely powerful, it currently has something of a productivity crisis. Companies succeed and grow rich by producing 'blockbuster' drugs that have huge worldwide sales. These are usually drugs that are genuinely innovative, producing real benefits to patients. Unfortunately such drugs are rare and becoming rarer, but to stay successful companies must keep producing them—because once existing drugs come off patent other companies produce them at a fraction of the cost. The industry hoped that the revolution in molecular biology would lead to a new golden age when 'cures' would be discovered for the chronic and degenerative diseases that cause most illness in the rich world. So far this hasn't happened, and the number of new drugs approved by the Food and Drug Administration in the United States in 2002 was 15 compared with an average over the past five years of about 30. And many of the new drugs that are produced provide small benefits at high cost.

One 'rational' response to this productivity crisis is to concentrate more on marketing. Sell as hard as you can the drugs you have. Try to capture market share. Encourage doctors and (in some countries patients) to use your drugs. The industry in the United States is estimated to have spent $15.7bn on promotion in 2000. Since 1995 research staff in American research-based drug companies have fallen by 2%, whereas marketing staff have increased by 59%. Currently, about one-fifth of staff are employed in research and development, while two-fifths are in marketing. Nevertheless, the industry still spends more on research than promotion. A congressional inquiry that reported at the end of 2002 said that in 2001 companies spent $30.3bn on research and development and $19.1bn on all promotional activities. About $10,000 a year is spent on average marketing to each doctor in the United States, and around $2.5bn were spent on advertising to consumers in 2000. Increases in the sales of the 50 drugs most heavily advertised to consumers were responsible for almost half (47.8%) of the $20.8bn increase in spending in 2000.

Finding it increasingly difficult to discover new drugs the industry has turned its attention to inventing new diseases. The journalist Lynn Payer called this disease mongering,[319] and another journalist, Ray Moynihan, has built on her work citing the examples of female sexual dysfunction, baldness, the menopause and social phobia.[320-323]

Medical journals are of great interest not just to research people within pharmaceutical companies but also marketing people. Advertising in journals can increase the prescribing of drugs, but even more powerful can be favourable material on editorial pages. The marketing people in pharmaceutical companies are becoming steadily more sophisticated in knowing how to use journals effectively. They are not doing anything wrong, but journals have to be very careful. They may be used both to create diseases and to market drugs.

Advertising is the most straightforward and least deceptive way in which pharmaceutical company marketeers use medical journals. In most countries—with the United States and New Zealand being exceptions—pharmaceutical companies are not allowed to advertise to the public but only to doctors (and some others who can prescribe). This creates a lucrative market for publications to doctors, and in many countries there are many publications that are sent free to doctors paid for by advertising. In Britain, for example, general practitioners receive three free weekly newspapers—*Doctor*, *General Practitioner* and *Pulse*. In addition, they receive many other publications for free less frequently. General practitioners receive many more free publications than hospital doctors because they prescribe most of the drugs in Britain. About three-quarters of the perhaps £35m spent on pharmaceutical advertising each year in Britain is spent to reach general practitioners.

These free publications are entirely driven by advertising. They exist in order to capture the advertising market and generate profits for their owners. If the advertising market shrinks they die. But in order to attract advertising they have to be read by the doctors at whom the advertisers are aiming. This means that they work hard at making themselves attractive, relevant, interesting and easy to read—in contrast to journals, which are often delivering complex, difficult to read material of limited relevance. In some countries—for example, New Zealand—the free newspapers have captured almost all of the advertising from journals, so putting some of them out of business. In the United States several journals that published original research for family physicians have either gone out of business or stopped publishing original research because they can attract neither advertising nor subscriptions (it's hard to get doctors who are sent 50 publications for free to pay for anything).

Journals compete with three free publications for advertising. Doctors in Britain receive the *BMJ* free in part because of the support the journal receives from pharmaceutical advertising. They receive it as part of their membership of the BMA, and most imagine that most of their subscription to the association goes to the journal—because that's what they see—but in fact none of it does. *BMJUSA*, which circulated monthly to 90,000 doctors in the United States, was paid for entirely by advertising, as are other local editions in some other countries. The *New England Journal of Medicine* is circulated free to many hospital doctors in Britain paid for by advertising, and *JAMA* is sent free to many doctors in the United States paid for by advertising.

Often journals are sent to doctors who are of particular interest to advertisers. This may be because of their specialty or geography, but often in the United States journals are sent to 'high prescribers'—doctors who are known to prescribe more drugs than the average. Influencing these doctors to prescribe your drugs will obviously bring a richer return than influencing those doctors who prescribe fewer drugs than the average. Pharmaceutical companies in the United States have a great deal of information on doctors, and marketing is becoming steadily more sophisticated. Journals and newspapers have joined in the sophistication by allowing advertisers to reach particular audiences. *American Family Physician*, which is read by more family physicians in the United States than any other publication and has one of the largest incomes from advertising, has up to 8000 different editions: they are editorially the same but carry different advertising. The advertising can be targeted precisely.

Although there are reasons to bemoan free newspapers, there are also reasons to celebrate them. They have provided competition and inspiration for traditional journals, obliging them to become more attractive, relevant, readable, useful and even entertaining. I have written that journals are on a long march from being dense, dry, unreadable and (it has to be said) unread to being more like popular magazines.[67] This understandably gives rise to anxieties about 'dumbing down', but I believe that with the arrival of the internet journals can be simultaneously more scholarly (on the web) and more readable (on paper and the web).

There seems little doubt that pharmaceutical advertising does affect prescribing; a congressional inquiry concluded just that at the end of 2002.[324] There are no randomized trials, and most doctors will say that they are not influenced by advertising. Nevertheless, publishers have calculated a return on investment of drug advertising and argued that it produces a better return than spending money on drug company representatives or 'detail men'. Publishers, of course, wanted such a result and are always worried that companies will cut back on advertising (always easy to do in a recession) and shift money to representatives. The advertising market is cyclical, but it might be that advertising to doctors will fall steadily because of a shift to direct to consumer advertising, the decline in the number of new products, the fact that doctors must increasingly follow formularies, or some other reason. If the market is permanently down there will be a shakeout of publications, which may be no bad thing.

Companies are also keen to spend money on 'educational activities'. Probably what companies want is a mix of promotional methods. Different doctors will respond to different methods, and with many a mix of methods will be most effective. A journal advertisement will get the drug into the doctor's mind; the representative can follow up with more of a sell. One of the ways we sold advertising space in the *BMJ* was through data showing that the *BMJ* was more likely than any other publication to be read by doctors who would not see drug representatives. (These were, I suspect, also the doctors most likely to object to advertising, and they might well have been appalled to learn that they were a selling point for *BMJ* advertising.)

We have good evidence to show that much drug advertising is misleading.[226,324,325] The congressional inquiry reported that between August 1997 and August 2002 the Food and Drug Administration (FDA) issued 88 letters accusing drug companies of advertising violations: 44 concerned broadcast advertisements, 35 print advertisements and nine both types. In many cases, the agency said, companies overstated the effectiveness or minimized the risks of the drug.[324]

These violations pursued by the FDA are almost certainly, however, the tip of the iceberg. The 1992 study that contributed to the departure of the editors of the *Annals of Internal Medicine* found many more problems.[226] The authors took all the full page advertisements from 10 leading medical journals, which turned out to be 109. They also tried to track references cited in the advertisements and found four-fifths of these. They then sent the advertisements and the references to reviewers—two physicians in the relevant clinical area and one academic clinical pharmacist, asking them to evaluate the advertisements using criteria based on FDA guidelines. In one-third of cases two or more reviewers disagreed with the advertisers' claim that the drug was the 'drug of choice'. The reviewers felt that information on efficacy was not balanced with that on side-effects and contraindications in 40% of advertisements. Overall, reviewers would not have recommended publication of 28% of the advertisements and would have required major revisions in another one-third before publication.

The authors of a Spanish study looked at whether or not cited references supported the claims made in 264 different advertisements for antihypertensive drugs and 23 different advertisements for lipid lowering drugs selected from six Spanish medical journals.[325] They found 102 references, and two reviewers concluded that in 44% the promotional statement was not supported by the reference—most commonly because the slogan recommended the drug in a patient group other than that assessed in the study.

In some countries the problem is much worse. India, for example, has no regulations on what can appear in drug advertisements, and a study of drug advertisements appearing in the South Asian edition of the *BMJ* found some highly misleading advertisements.[326,327] In one case an advertisement for a drug that dilated blood vessels was copied from an American advertisement. The American version specifically said that the drug should not be used for brain problems, but the Indian advertisement was for brain problems.

As advertisements influence prescribing and yet are often misleading the question arises as to whether or not medical journals should publish them and whether or not they should peer review them if they do. The editor of one of the *BMJ* journals—Mike Docherty, the editor of the *Annals of Rheumatic Diseases*—took the position that he wouldn't publish any advertisements—which was interesting for us, the managers of the journal, caught between editorial freedom and our need to maximize income for the owners. The editor of the *studentBMJ* also decided that she didn't want to publish a drug advertisement. I persuaded her to publish it on the condition that we would debate the issue in the journal. She wrote a piece arguing against advertising.[328] I wrote a slightly patronizing piece arguing the case for.[329] The vote on the *studentBMJ* website went overwhelmingly her way.

Nevertheless, few editors (and even fewer owners) take the position that they won't publish advertisements at all—although many journals have no advertisements because nobody wants to advertise, usually because their circulation is so small. Many more editors, however, choose to review advertisements and turn down those that they think are making misleading claims. They have many systems for doing this, but often, I suspect, the editor simply scans the advertisement. The South Asian edition of the *BMJ* started a system of reviewing advertisements after the study showing how many were misleading, and the editors turned down advertisements—something that was seen as extraordinary in India.

At the *BMJ* we didn't attempt to review the claims made by advertisements, a declared position that many found extreme. We did review advertisements for taste but rarely turned any down. This was the logic of our position. First, there are strict British and European laws on claims that can be made in advertisements. Second, the industry has a code regulating advertisements, and this seems to be a case where self-regulation is more effective than government regulation in that companies are quick to report each other for breaking the code. It's clearly disadvantageous to a company if a competitor can get away with breaking the rules. Third, we knew that readers discount advertising—although I concede that this conflicts with evidence that advertising changes prescribing. Fourth, we thought that it made sense for us to concentrate our resources on improving editorial not advertising pages. Fifth, we encouraged readers to criticize advertisements just as they criticized editorial pages, and we also encouraged readers to make complaints to the authorities if they thought the offence serious enough.

This was all against the backcloth that we wanted the income from advertising. Like many editors, we believed it bought us independence. Advertisers have no power to influence what is published—partly because there are many of them. But if owners have to support a journal financially then they are likely to want the journal to promote its view of the world. We also know that if readers are given a choice of paying for a journal without advertising or receiving a journal with advertising for free they will almost always opt for the free journal.

Advertisers would always prefer favourable editorial coverage to an advertisement—because they too know that readers discount advertising. So, most crassly, advertisers will offer to buy advertising if it can be accompanied by favourable editorial mentions of their products. I've no direct experience of this, but I suspect that it happens. Next, advertisers will seek to publish 'advertorials', advertising that is mostly words and that they hope may not be distinguishable from editorial material. The *BMJ* allowed 'advertorials' only if readers can see at a glance that they were advertising—meaning that they were not really advertorials.

What happens most commonly is that advertisers want to know what material is to be published in the journal. They would then like to position their advertising alongside editorial material that is favourable to their products. Many journals seem to sell advertising space on this basis. The weekly *BMJ* didn't, but some of the local editions of the *BMJ*, which are published in countries around the world, did. Our argument for not doing it with the weekly journal was less that it will affect our selection of articles (although unconsciously it might) but more that readers might perceive our independence to be compromised. And in some sense perception is reality.

The *BMJ* had a policy of a Chinese wall between the editorial and advertising departments. The advertising department didn't know what would appear on editorial pages. The editorial department approved advertisements but did not know when and where (in which section of the journal) they would be published. This policy meant that sometimes there would be 'hits', where by chance advertisements and related editorial material would be published alongside each other. The editorial might either favour or disfavour the product being advertised. Other journals—like the *New England Journal of Medicine*—had a policy of looking for 'direct hits' and removing the advertisements.

The *BMJ* also had anxieties about where it positioned advertisements. In the United States the major journals publish advertisements only at the beginning and the end of the journal. Readers can read the articles without being disturbed by advertising. At the *BMJ* we published advertisements in the middle of articles, but we used to refuse to back editorial pages with advertisements. Then we did, but we did not allow editorial and advertising material on the same page. This was a game of us playing hard to get and the advertisers tempting us. Advertisers love innovation for its own sake. Once every few months somebody from our advertising department would call me with a new wheeze—gatefolds, pop ups, post it notes and so on. I was rather sanctimonious about it all, feeling that I was being tempted. But increasingly I would say: 'Let's try it and see if we get complaints.' Usually we didn't. Doctors are so awash with advertising and other forms of promotion that they were inured to the *BMJ*'s rather tame experiments.

Other issues that arise are the number of advertisers and the proportion of advertising in the journal. The weekly *BMJ* had many different advertisers so the number was not an issue, but some of the local editions had far fewer. We—somewhat arbitrarily—insisted on three, the logic being, to use a common analogy, that you have more independence as a whore than as a kept woman. With volume, we—again arbitrarily—set the limit on advertising at 35%, but then we relaxed it for the *BMJ USA* on the grounds that 40% was normal in the United States. Most of our local editions had difficulty getting advertisements, so the limit was not a problem. But *BMJ Middle East* became very popular and attracted large amounts of advertising. Again we relaxed the limit—partly because a higher number of advertisements seemed normal in the market and perhaps even signified success.

This problem of imposing Anglo Saxon values on cultures that think differently arises constantly. We used to have an Italian edition of the *BMJ*, which looked much more beautiful than the weekly edition produced in London. The publishers kept breaking our rules, selling advertisements next to articles and including advertorials that were indistinguishable from editorial pages. We flew to Milan to explain our anxieties, but the Italian publishers couldn't understand our anxieties. In the end, we had to cancel the contract. The same thing happened with the Spanish and Latin American editions. Were we being culturally insensitive? Perhaps not too much—as I'm now regularly asked to speak on conflict of interest in Italy. It's become a major topic, perhaps because their last prime minister—who owned many media outlets and other businesses—was the most conflicted person in the world.

Problems of positioning advertisements and selling them against particular articles arise as well with advertising on the web. Should journals have exactly the same rules, or is the web different? So far advertising has not been very successful on the web. The money is still in paper advertising. Banner advertisements (at the top or side of the screen) are hard to design and easy to ignore. What's more, the web provides advertisers with data on just how many people 'click through' on their advertisements. The answer is very few and falling. My feeling is that the same would be true of paper advertisements, but the data are not available. I regularly read a whole issue of a paper journal and not register one advertisement—but nobody can record that.

We were less anxious about the positioning of advertisements on the web. We had collections of articles on many subjects. Why shouldn't we sell advertising for an asthma drug in a collection of articles on asthma? It was no different, we thought, from if we had a journal on asthma. Similarly people signed up to receive emails on particular topics. Again we sold advertising messages to go on the bottom of these emails. So a reader would receive a message about a paper on asthma together with an advertisement for an asthma drug. Was this a step too far? We thought not—but we were perhaps not being logical and consistent. It might be argued that the perception argument applies just as strongly on the web as on paper, but we thought that the web was different. One piece of evidence to support this idea was that I never received a single message about poor spelling and grammar with the *BMJ*'s rapid responses (electronic letters to the editor) despite them being full of errors, whereas about once a month I received a letter from somebody upset by an infelicity in the paper journal.

Ultimately medical journals are probably more useful to pharmaceutical companies for publishing trials than they are for advertising. The companies know that many of the free newspapers are better read than journals, and those newspapers are driven primarily by the needs of the advertisers. They are much less ethically precious than medical journals and will be happy to oblige if the price is right. What the newspapers cannot provide, however, is the worldwide approval that accompanies a major trial in an international journal.

The randomized trial, as I discussed in chapter 6, was one of the greatest scientific inventions of the 20th century, and a large, well done randomized trial provides some of the best evidence on the effectiveness of a treatment, although a well done systematic review is better. A major trial that is favourable to a drug can cause its worldwide sales to rocket. Such a trial is a major step in creating the 'blockbuster drug' that all companies desire. This means that the marketing people in a pharmaceutical company will often be more interested in clinical trials than researchers—because many trials are scientifically uninteresting. So what is happening is that this major scientific invention—the randomized trial—is being debased for marketing reasons. The same thing is happening with other methodologies—systematic reviews and economic evaluations—as they become more important. And medical journals are very much part of this process because they are the outlets for these trials—and the impact of a trial is much magnified if it is in a major journal.

The best trial asks a simple, medically important question, is properly randomized (to avoid bias), and is conducted on a very large scale (to avoid getting the wrong answer by chance). Unfortunately, there are many ways to debase the process for marketing purposes.[116,330,331]

Sometimes companies will conduct trials for no other reason but to get doctors to prescribe their drug. These are called 'seeding trials'. Often they are scientifically meaningless. There is no clear question and no controls. But they are conducted on a large scale, and 'investigators' (often ordinary doctors not researchers) are paid substantial sums to enter patients into the trial. A variant is a 'switching trial' in which a doctor is paid to switch patients from their usual treatment to the new treatment. These sorts of trials will rarely make it into major journals, but many may be published somewhere—and then used to promote the drug with doctors, most of whom are scientifically naïve.

Yet another variant—with more scientific justification—is called 'postmarketing surveillance'. Many adverse effects of drugs do not emerge until after they are put onto the market. This may be because the side-effect is rare and so doesn't become apparent until the drug is widely prescribed. Or the adverse effect may be apparent only in certain sorts of patients—who perhaps have another condition or are taking another drug and who were not included in the original trials. Or the adverse effect may emerge only after prolonged use of the drug. For all these reasons it makes scientific sense to gather data on patients taking new drugs, but it can also make marketing sense as a means to get many doctors prescribing the drug. Again doctors may be paid substantial sums 'for expenses'. My guess is that they rarely explain this to patients. Instead, patients may be flattered to think that they are getting the newest (with a false implication of best) treatment. These trials will often be published and sometimes in major journals—because they give important data on adverse effects.

Pharmaceutical companies are usually required to conduct a trial of their new drug against a placebo in order to get a licence for the drug. This requirement may conflict with the Declaration of Helsinki in that it is deemed unethical to give patients a placebo if there is an evidence-based treatment available. As most new drugs are not completely new but rather what are known as 'me too' drugs (a drug similar to one already available) then this conflict arises often. What patients and doctors want to know is whether the new drug is better than existing, evidence-based treatments not whether it is better than placebo. But pharmaceutical companies have a horror of what are known as 'head to head' trials, where treatments are tested against each other in trials that are big enough to give a clear answer on which treatment is best. The clear implication of such a trial conducted with, say, five drugs is that four of them will not be as good as the fifth. This would be a dreadful result for a company that had spent hundreds of millions of dollars bringing a drug to the market and perhaps tens of millions on the trial.

Companies thus prefer a trial against placebo or a trial that will simply show that their drug is as good as another. These 'equivalence' or 'non-inferiority' trials are particularly hard to interpret. In essence, the trial is not big enough to be able to show that one treatment is better than another but not so small as to be meaningless. The majority of trials funded by pharmaceutical companies are in these categories, which is why, as I described in chapter 11, it is possible for not one of 56 trials of non-steroidal anti-inflammatory drugs (like benoxaprofen used mainly in arthritis) funded by pharmaceutical companies to come up with a result unfavourable to the company.[213] It's less a matter of suppressing unfavourable results but more a (less dishonest?) matter of making sure that you don't fund a trial that will work against you.

There are other ways to make it more likely that results will be favourable to you. One is to use a dose of the competitor drug that is lower than the optimal dose. Or, alternatively, if you are trying to argue that your drug is better because it has fewer side-effects then you might use the competitor drug in a dose that is higher than optimal and so will have more side-effects. This may have happened with trials of new antipsychotic drugs used for treating schizophrenia, where the selling point is not that they are more effective but rather that they are less toxic.[332] When the *BMJ* published systematic reviews suggesting that this may be the case we were accused of being in the pay of the government—in that it doesn't want to be obliged to pay for newer and (always) more expensive drugs. The government, which is much more often criticized than praised by the *BMJ* (as we are on the side of the governed not the governors), would find this idea laughable, but the accusation was made by those with close ties with the companies that make the drugs.

I'm sure that I have not produced an exhaustive list of ways to get the results you want, and there are a similar array of methods of getting favourable results from systematic reviews and economic evaluations. Indeed, economic evaluations, which are relatively unfamiliar to editors and readers of medical journals and highly complex, may be particularly easy to manipulate. It's very difficult with all of this to sort out dishonesty, honest bias and clever use of legitimate methods, but journals need to try and do so—not least because three-quarters of randomized trials in the major general journals are funded by the pharmaceutical industry.[186] Often too the trials are conducted not by academic researchers (who at least in theory will not be beholden to the industry) but by contract firms who are paid a fee to get the job done. These firms will not object—as academics might—if the company chooses not to publish the results, perhaps because they are unfavourable.

A recent systematic review found 30 studies that compared the results of studies funded by the pharmaceutical industry with results of studies funded from other sources.[187] Five of the studies looked at economic evaluations and in every study the results were favourable to the pharmaceutical company. Sixteen studies looked at clinical trials or meta-analyses, and 13 of these had outcomes favourable to the companies. Overall studies funded by companies were four times more likely to have results favourable to the sponsor than studies funded by others.

Importantly, 13 of the studies examined the quality of the research, and none of the studies found the quality of drug company sponsored studies to be inferior; four of the studies, indeed, found that the research funded by the industry was of superior quality. This is not surprising as drug company trials are tightly regulated. There are explicit high standards, and companies can afford to hire the best.

Why then do companies usually manage to fund research that is favourable to them? The authors of the systematic review considered four possible answers. First, companies might selectively fund research on drugs that they are confident are better than those of competitors. The authors thought this explanation unlikely. Second, the quality of the research might be lower—not in the methods that are used but more in the questions asked. Third, the companies might make inappropriate comparisons— comparing their drugs with poor drugs or drugs used at the wrong dose. Fourth, there may be publication bias in that favourable studies are more likely to be published—

because the companies push them or suppress unfavourable ones or because editors are biased.

The same problem seems to arise with systematic reviews. Veronica Yank, Drummond Rennie and Lisa Bero presented at the 2005 Conference on Peer Review and Biomedical Publication in Chicago the initial results of a study looking at whether or not sponsorship of systematic reviews was associated with bias.[333] They studied 71 systematic reviews of antihypertensive drugs, 23 (32%) of which were sponsored by pharmaceutical companies. They found no difference between meta-analyses with or without pharmaceutical sponsorship in the proportion of positive results. But the conclusions in sponsored reviews were much more likely to be positive. Sponsored reviews were positive in 91%, unclear in 4%, neutral in 4% and negative in none, whereas conclusions in unsponsored reviews were positive in 72%, unclear in 2%, neutral in 17% and negative in 8%. As with the study of trials the mean quality scores for each group were similar.

This result is particularly disturbing for journals because it represents a failure of peer review. The editors and reviewers had let the authors of sponsored studies get away with exaggerating the conclusions of trials—despite the evidence to the contrary being in front of their eyes.

Another paper presented at the same congress showed that cost-effectiveness studies were highly likely to produce results that suggested that new interventions should be funded by health systems—especially if the study was funded by industry. The researchers found that about 712 of 1433 studies produced results that the cost of the intervention would be less than $20,000 a year for a quality adjusted life year—and industry funded studies were twice as likely to produce such results. [A quality adjusted year is a measure that combines number of years lived and the quality of life during those years. If a person is fully healthy then the number of years lived equals the quality adjusted years, but if a patient is less than fully healthy then the number of quality adjusted years will be less than the number of years lived.] The figure of $20,000 is important because it's roughly the cost that will lead bodies like the National Institute for Health and Clinical Excellence to recommend that the intervention be made widely available.[334]

Particularly nasty fights can arise when companies try to suppress results that they don't like. The most famous case in recent years concerned Nancy Olivieri, a Canadian doctor and expert on hereditary blood diseases.[335] Her case was used by the thriller writer John Le Carré in his novel *The Constant Gardener*, in which a fictional pharmaceutical company conducts unethical research in Africa and murders various people who discover what it is up to.[336] The book became a highly successful and evocative film.

The real case doesn't feature murder (although there are anonymous poison pen letters) and is not quite so dramatic (although not so far off) but is more complex. Olivieri conducted trials in patients with thalassaemia with a drug called deferiprone in the Hospital for Sick Children in Toronto. The research was funded in part by Apotex Incorporated, a company that acquired the commercial development rights for the drug. There were two contracts for the research, and one contained a confidentiality clause that gave Apotex the right to control communication of the data for one year after the trial ended. Such a clause was normal for the University of Toronto at the time. Apotex also had the right to terminate the trials at any time.

In 1996 Olivieri noted a problem. In some of the patients the drug ceased to work. She decided that she needed to inform patients of the risk. Apotex disputed the risk and said that there was no need to inform the patients. The hospital's research ethics board agreed with Olivieri that she did need to inform the patients. Apotex then terminated the two trials and issued a legal warning to Olivieri not to inform the patients or anybody else.

Some patients did benefit from the drug, and an arrangement was made for them to receive the drugs. Meanwhile, another researcher—Gideon Koren, whose research was funded by Apotex—went ahead and published re-analysed data from the terminated trials. He reported that the drug was safe and effective.[337] He did not disclose Apotex's support for the research, Olivieri's worries, or her role in the research. Koren was later disciplined for gross misconduct for writing anonymous poison pen letters to Olivieri and others.

In 1997 Olivieri noticed another, even more serious, problem with the drug—that it caused progressive liver fibrosis in some patients. Apotex again threatened her, but she notified the patients and the regulatory authorities—and a report was published in the *New England Journal of Medicine*.[338] The story then becomes impossibly complicated, but far from supporting Olivieri the university and the hospital acted against her—blowing the whole dispute into an international story of drug companies acting improperly with the craven support of a university. The dispute still rumbles on and has damaged the university.

A story of equal complexity and even greater length concerned a researcher Betty Dong from the University of California San Francisco who with others looked at whether or not four different preparations of thyroid hormone were equivalent to each other.[339] The research was commissioned in 1987 by Flint Laboratories, who manufactured one of the preparations and was confident that it was more effective than the other three. The manufacturer had promoted its preparation on those grounds, and it dominated the market. It commissioned the work to demonstrate the superiority, but unfortunately from its point of view the research, which was completed by 1990, showed that the four preparations were essentially the same.[340]

Boots Pharmaceuticals Inc—who had taken over Flint Laboratories while the research was underway—immediately set about discrediting not only the research but also the researchers. They made complaints of misconduct to the university, which conducted two investigations but found only trivial problems. In 1994 the research was submitted to *JAMA* with an explanation that Boots was very critical of the study. *JAMA* peer reviewed the study and accepted it for publication.

The study was about to be published when Dong suddenly withdrew it. Boots was threatening legal action, pointing out that Dong had signed a contract in 1988 to the effect that the research could be published only with written consent from Flint Laboratories. Boots did not give permission, and the university lawyers advised her against publication—despite the university being committed to doing only research that could be published. The pharmaceutical arm of Boots was now itself about to be taken over, and any damage to its most important drug could have serious consequences. The company was bought in March 1995 for $1.4bn and became part of Knoll Pharmaceuticals.

In a parallel to the Olivieri case employees of Knoll went ahead and published the research without acknowledging the researchers who did the work and who reached opposite conclusions.[341] The work was published in a new journal called the *American Journal of Therapeutics*. One of the authors of the revised study was an assistant editor on the journal.

In 1996 the whole sordid story was told in the *Wall Street Journal*,[342] and the Food and Drug Administration took an interest. Eventually under pressure the company agreed to publication of the original paper, and it was published in *JAMA* in 1997 together with a letter from Knoll apologizing for blocking publication.[340,343]

It's hard to know how often companies block research that they don't like or persuade the researchers that they have misinterpreted the data. Both Olivieri and Dong fought prolonged battles and came under terrible pressure. Both must have paid a considerable personal price. It seems to me likely that most people would not be so persistent. Most cases probably never reach the public's attention. One small piece of evidence to support this suspicion is an estimate from the head of the sponsored research office of Massachusetts General Hospital that about 30–50% of contracts submitted by companies have unacceptable clauses on publication that must be renegotiated.[344]

As I described in chapter 9, the International Committee of Medical Journal Editors has made a small stand against such practices by saying that journals should publish papers only if the authors control the right to publication.[345] This is of course tokenism because it means they will not receive for publication papers where the sponsors controlled publication and didn't like the results.

The major journals try to counterbalance the might of the pharmaceutical industry, but it is a very unequal battle—not least because journals themselves profit so much from publishing studies funded by the industry. Major trials are very good for journals in that doctors around the world want to see them and so are more likely to subscribe to journals that publish them. Such trials also create lots of publicity—partly because the companies work heavily to create them—and, as I discuss in chapter 14, journals like publicity. Finally, as I described in chapter 11, companies purchase large reprint orders of these trials. Sometimes they will spend more than a $1m on reprints of a single study, and the profit margin is huge. These reprints are then used to market the drugs to doctors, and the prestigious name of the journal on the reprint is a vital part of that sell.

Another way in which journals become entangled with pharmaceutical companies is through the publication of supplements to the journal. The big weekly journals do not publish supplements, but many specialist journals do and it can be very profitable. Some journals have a supplement with every issue, and—to be blunt—the worse the supplement the bigger the profit. If a journal is willing to publish every paper presented at a symposium that was funded by a single company and dealt with one drug then it can charge a very substantial fee. Often these papers will be set pieces by, to be crude for a moment, 'paid industry hacks' and will have been published many times. If, however, the journal wants to peer review every study in the usual way and take only those that are original and pass review, then the fee and the demand will be smaller.

Studies have shown that the quality of papers published in supplements is poorer than those published in the main journal.[346,347] The importance of this finding is amplified in my mind by the knowledge that journals that publish many supplements are poor journals in the first place.

Some journals have been bought by the industry and exist primarily to publish drug company research that cannot get published in better journals. I mustn't sound too snooty about this—as I have argued that it is misconduct not to publish (chapter 10). Companies will say that they can't get their studies into more respectable journals and that therefore journals that are willing to publish their studies are needed. I hope that this problem can be solved by publishing such studies on the web not on paper.

I wrote the first draft of this article in 2003, and I was shocked by how much I convinced myself that medical journals were much more than I had realized creatures of the pharmaceutical industry. I was long familiar with the arguments over advertising, but it was the realization that so many of the studies that journals publish are biased. In 2004 I was given a prize for promoting independence in medical journalism by an organization called Healthwatch—and I had to give a lecture. I chose a polemical title, 'Medical journals are an extension of the marketing arm of pharmaceutical companies', and set to work.[312] I convinced myself—and perhaps some others—that the argument had validity. The piece was published in *Public Library of Science Medicine* and attracted a lot of attention.

In the piece I floated the idea that journals should stop publishing trials—because these highly biased fragments of information would bias doctors' prescribing and threaten public safety. Again what seemed like a radical idea seemed more and more true as I thought about it, and I've now published—with researcher Ian Roberts—an argument that journals should stop publishing trials and that instead the totality of evidence should be made available on the web.[348] The job of journals would be to discuss, digest and report—not publish partial evidence.

I conclude with the sad thought that there is a sense in which all journals are bought—or at least cleverly used—by the pharmaceutical industry. The industry dominates healthcare, and most doctors have been wined and dined by the industry. It's not therefore surprising that medical journals too should be heavily influenced by industry. But healthcare, doctors, journals and—I believe—the pharmaceutical industry would all benefit from relationships being less grubby and more arms length and businesslike.

►17

The highly profitable but perhaps unethical business of publishing medical research

'All publishing is theft', the BMA librarian used to joke. I was arrested by the phrase when I first heard it in the 1980s but thought it nonsense. In reality, I simply didn't understand. By the time I stepped down as the chief executive of a publishing group as well as editor of a journal I recognized that the librarian was right in many ways. Many other academics and librarians think the same, which is why a major effort is underway to make all medical research available free to everybody everywhere. Sooner or later, I believe and have for some time, it will happen. When is much less clear.

Publishing scientific research is a highly profitable business—unsurprisingly because publishers are given the research, which is highly valuable, for free. Robert Maxwell—a notorious British business bully who fell off his yacht and drowned after robbing the pension fund of his employees—got rich not through publishing the *Daily Mirror* but through publishing science.

Reed Elsevier, the world's largest publisher of scientific research, publishes over 1800 journals. In 2005 it made an adjusted operating profit of £1142m on a turnover of £5166m. The scientific part of the company contributed 39% of the profit (£449m) from 28% of the business (£1436m). In other words, the scientific part of the company (which is predominantly medical) makes a large part of the profits and in some ways supports the non-scientific parts. Reed Elsevier's profits for the past five years have been around £5bn, much of them extracted from science and particularly from journals.

It's hard to come by the accounts of an individual journal, but I have seen many over the years. There are many comparatively minor journals that have an annual income of £1m. (I've never seen the accounts of the *New England Journal of Medicine*, but its annual income will be tens of millions of dollars and probably close to $100m.) The million pound journal might well have a gross margin (income minus direct costs like paper and printing) of £600,000. After subtracting the overheads the profit might well be £350,000. By no means all journals are so profitable, but this is a much more profitable enterprise than most.

I want to illustrate why publishing research journals is so profitable by considering who does what and the value of their contribution. I should make clear that I am describing the classic research journal, which is comprised almost entirely of original research. Many of the world's 10,000–20,000 biomedical journals (nobody knows the true number) still take this form, although many are now adding other features, such as review articles.

Of all the value that resides in a journal the vast majority is in the research itself. Many randomized trials, for example, cost millions, even tens of millions of dollars, to conduct, but more than the cost it's a difficult undertaking. Comparatively few people have the skills and competence to undertake major trials. Patients of course must give their bodies, time and commitment. They take risks, albeit with the chance of reward. They are not paid. Research ethics committees must examine and approve the research, again without financial reward. So the research paper that is submitted to a journal is very valuable. I've used the example of a randomized trial, but other kinds of research can be equally valuable. Sometimes the research depends on a profound creative insight. It will be impossible to repeat—and so in some ways is as unique as a Titian painting and perhaps as valuable. Indeed, a rationalist might say that it's more valuable than a Titian painting because people can benefit directly from the results, whereas the benefits that flow from a Titian painting are less easily measured.

When authors submit a paper to a journal they must usually agree both not to submit elsewhere and to transfer copyright (for no fee). Why, I often wonder, do authors agree to these requirements? Many journals have huge numbers of papers submitted, but all journals would like more high-quality papers. There is intense competition for the best papers. Why don't authors announce that they have an excellent paper and then ask journals to bid for them? Various authors have thought of this idea, but it requires concerted action to break the stranglehold of the journals. And why do authors hand over copyright? Some publicly funded organizations—like Britain's Medical Research Council—do not, and the journals have to accept it. When they do hand over copyright authors have to ask permission from publishers in order to reproduce their own material—perhaps in a lecture. This seems an extraordinary state of affairs, and increasingly journals do allow authors to do what they want with their own material—including placing it on their own or their institution's website.

Once submitted to a journal the study will be registered. The process of registering a paper is not complex, and the administrative tasks associated with a journal can be carried out with comparatively little training. Publishers do pay such editorial assistants, but they pay them little—and one assistant might look after several journals. Increasingly these administrative processes are carried out on the web. There are costs in buying such systems, but in the longer term there should be savings. Indeed, a free open source publishing system will soon be available. This means that any individual or organization might start a journal at a very low cost—rather in the way that anybody can create a website or blog.

Next the study will be scrutinized by an editor. I am, of course, hopelessly biased, but I believe that good journals depend first on good editors—albeit that their main job is to assemble an excellent team to do the work. The work of editors may therefore be valuable, but as I'm primarily concerned with the contribution of the publisher we don't need to be detained by an argument over the exact value of an editor—because in the classic research journal they are paid nothing. (Some, perhaps an increasing number of publishers, do pay editors, and certainly the editors of the journals published by the *BMJ* Publishing Group are paid.) They do it for the honour of the position and the good of the discipline. I've met many editors who labour long and hard over the journals and yet who receive no payment. Indeed, they forego income—

because they could be spending the time doing something for which they are paid. They work weekends and nights for the good of the journal. Many of these naïve (and it's hard to avoid the word) academics have no idea that they are working for free for a journal that may be bringing the publisher a 60% gross margin. The academics are, of course, paid a salary by a university or similar institution. It might be that they do all their editorial work in their own time, but often they don't and can't. This is an example of theft. Worse, the academic's secretary might also do some work for the publishers without payment. Nor often is there a payment for office space or overheads.

Yet many of these editors have unique knowledge and skills. Many also have famous names that bring lustre to the journal. Their 'market value' could be huge, but luckily for publishers academics have not thought in such terms (although increasingly they do). The editors do, of course, get something important from being an editor. It's fun and gives a sense of being at the centre of a community. Editorship often brings academic credit, and so may bring promotion and financial rewards. These rewards come, however, from the academic community not the publishers. This might be described as the 'secret ingredient' of the publishers: they have so entangled themselves in the system of academic credit that it's hard for the academic world to 'uncouple' publishing from credit.

The editor then sends the paper out for peer review. To produce a good review of a study is time consuming and difficult. Almost by definition, only a few people are capable of the task. Yet peer reviewers are very rarely paid and are never paid the market rate. (The *BMJ* did pay £50, but this was a token and has now stopped.) So the value injected by the reviewer, which could be considerable, is injected at no cost to the publisher. Reviewers don't even get credit—because most peer review is still conducted anonymously.

If the study is accepted then it must be technically edited. This is a process that can add considerable value if well done, but publishers often pay for only the most minimal editing—correction of the grossest errors. The technical editors are poorly paid, work from home, and are often expected to edit several papers in a day, obliging them to edit only lightly. Sometimes the unpaid academics do the technical editing as well. I've encountered surgeons—who could earn well over a £1000 an hour doing operations in the private sector in Britain—doing technical editing unpaid. This is economic madness: the surgeons should do the operations and then pay technical editors well to edit papers carefully.

The publishers pay for the design of the journal, but it's usually minimal. They also pay for the typesetting, paper, printing, online hosting and distribution. These comprise most of the direct costs, but they are all something that anybody could go out and buy. The publishers sell advertising space, but many research journals do not contain any advertising. The marketing and selling are also done by the publishers, but some of these journals are 'must have' journals with very small circulations. Almost all the copies go to academic libraries—and these libraries have had to buy them.

Recognizing that some academic libraries cannot do without these journals, publishers have charged huge prices. *Brain Research* famously costs $23,617 for a year, the price of a car. Furthermore, the publishers have for around 20 years been following a business model that I call 'less for more'. Recognizing that libraries will cancel subscriptions—partly because of shrinking budgets and partly because of rising journal prices—publishers have put up prices by substantially more than the rate of inflation to compensate for the cancelled subscriptions The *reductio ad absurdam* of this policy would be a single subscription at a vast price.

This business model was clearly unsustainable, and it created anger among librarians and the academic community, particularly in the United States. They were angry because the publishers were sucking money out of the academic community and adding little or no value. Indeed, I argued in a submission to the Competition Commission in Britain over the takeover of Harcourt by Reed Elsevier that far from adding value publishers were subtracting value. They have 'Balkanized' research information so that it becomes very difficult to do the systematic reviews that are essential in modern research. Doing a systematic review means finding every relevant study on a topic, but this is very hard to do because there are so many different journals and different databases that it's hard to find the studies. And then it's hugely expensive to pay for them. This argument was not popular. Derk Haank, the former chief executive of Elsevier Science, whom I met a few days after making my submission made it clear that what I'd written was nonsense and insulting. He was not amused.

The fact that publishers make money by restricting access to information is unfortunate for the world economy—because trade in information and ideas is quite different from trade in physical objects. As George Bernard Shaw pointed out: 'If you have an apple and I have an apple and if we exchange these apples then you and I will still each have one apple. But if you have an idea and I have an idea and we exchange these ideas, then each of us will have two ideas.' Ideas breed. The more people who have access to information and ideas the more ideas we will have—and ideas are a major source of wealth in the information age.

I have perhaps in my arguments against the present practices of scientific publishers insufficiently acknowledged the complexity of the process of publishing a journal and all the support processes—finance, information technology, legal, human resources and so on. Perhaps too I have not recognized adequately that publishers often took the initial financial risk in starting journals and are entitled to a return on their investment. In addition, in the days before the internet the process of distributing research was time consuming and tiresome. Academics didn't want to waste their time with the business of publishing.

These arguments have some weight, but my response is that the processes of producing research journals is straightforward and that often the publishers did not take the initial risk with the journals: either they don't own them at all but publish them on behalf of medical societies who own them, or they bought them as going concerns and then bumped up the prices dramatically. I should also make clear that it isn't just commercial publishers who make high profits. There are many society publishers who make big profits. It's some consolation to the academic community that these profits instead of ending up in the pockets of shareholders often re-enter the academic world as research or training grants.

But if my overall argument is right—that publishers of research journals are making unjustified profits from the academic community without adding value—then the usual rules of economics do not seem to be working. Competitors should emerge to capture the excessive profits by reducing costs or adding more value. Because there is no traditional monopoly: although there are some very large publishers, there are many small ones. Antitrust authorities like the Competition Commission have not so far stopped mergers and takeovers.

Publishers are now being found out and challenged, as I will discuss below, but why hasn't it happened sooner? The first answer is that academic credit depends so much on publishing in particular journals. Academics need to publish in them in order to progress, and academic libraries have to have them. It would be a bold or foolish academic who declined to publish in the top journal because it was too expensive or owned by a rapacious publisher. I happened to be at Mill Hill, the main research centre of the Medical Research Council which may have Britain's greatest concentration of biomedical researchers, just after the initial announcement of PubMed Central, the free database of research. We discussed the case for changing the publishing model. The reaction of the researchers was: 'There's much we don't like about the present set up, but we are nervous of change. We know how to play the present game well. If the game is changed we mightn't do so well.'

Perhaps the second answer to the question of why change hasn't happened sooner is that nobody has hurt quite enough. The academics didn't have to pay for the journals themselves. The librarians had to pay but became increasingly clever at getting papers from journals they didn't subscribe to themselves. And those running the whole academic and research system had much to think about apart from the excessive prices of journals.

A third factor may have been that many academics were in some way associated with societies which were making generous profits from their journals and using them to underwrite the costs of the societies. Many academics also benefited personally from the largesse of the publishers. I went and spoke in Amsterdam at the editorial board meeting of a journal published but not owned by Reed Elsevier. The board had all been flown from America, and the hospitality was spectacular. My cynical mind thought that the profits flowing to Reed Elsevier would be even more spectacular.

Making money through restricting access to research is, I believe, ethically very questionable for academic societies. The British Society of Lumpology (which I have, of course, imagined) exists to raise standards in and promote lumpology and reduce the mortality and morbidity that results from lumps. Its journal, the *British Journal of Lumpology*, publishes much of the most important research in lumpology. Much of that research is funded with public money. The point of the research is to 'raise standards in and promote lumpology and reduce the mortality and morbidity that results from lumps', exactly the mission of the British Society of Lumpology. So doesn't restricting access to that research conflict with the mission of the society? To my mind, it clearly does.

The British Society of Lumpology responds to this ethical challenge first by refusing to see it. It publishes an excellent journal full of important information on lumpology. It's been doing so for years. When challenged the society says that the profits of the journal are important because they support the society and fund some research. The existence of the society might be threatened if the profits disappeared.

Many societies have become dependent on the profits from their publications. My answer is that if the society and the research have value then other ways will be found to fund them. If they don't, then they shouldn't be funded anyway. I worry too that some of the profits go on the dinners and ceremonies of which such societies are usually fond.

Whatever the reason, the traditional business prospered for many years, but the arrival of the World Wide Web is changing everything. It opens up the possibility of authors communicating directly with readers without any intermediary. Publishers, librarians, peer reviewers and editors could potentially all be swept away. They are all still there at the moment, but rather as in a balloon debate they may have to justify their existence.

We are still, I'm sure, at the beginning of the electronic revolution—the 'paradigm shift' from the industrial to the information age and from a paper world to a paper and electronic world. Ten years ago almost no journals had electronic versions. Now virtually every journal does. We may think that that is a big change in a short time, but at the moment we are largely copying the old paper world in electronic media. The change to doing everything completely differently is just beginning, and it's hard to see the shape of the future. Thomas Kuhn, who invented the idea of paradigm shifts, says that those stuck in one paradigm cannot see the next. We are entering a phase of what the Austrian–American economist Joseph Schumpeter called 'creative destruction'. New technologies allow new ways of doing things but destroy the old at the same time.

We can, however, see drivers of change, and in the business of publishing money is one. Academics are fed up with being ripped off and are proposing different ways of making research available. A second driver is abhorrence of the 'Balkanization' of medical research that I've described above. A third is the slowness of the paper world, but the fourth—and perhaps ultimately most powerful—driver is the power of a new vision. It has been expressed best by Stevan Harnad, a prophet of the digital age:

'It's easy to say what would be the ideal online resource for scholars and scientists: all papers in all fields, systematically interconnected, effortlessly accessible and rationally navigable, from any researcher's desk, worldwide for free.'

Ten years ago this would have seemed a fantasy, but the appearance of the web has made it achievable. Every word in this pithy quote is important for the vision, but it's the last two words—'for free'—that sends a tremor through publishers. Harnad expresses the vision of what is called 'the open access movement', those who believe that research should be available for free and that people should be free to republish it with the only conditions being that they cite the original source and credit the authors.

Just as the appearance of the World Wide Web has allowed Harnad's vision so it has allowed publishers to break out of the 'less for more' business model. The electronic world allows a very different business model because the marginal cost (the cost of supplying one more customer) is effectively zero, whereas in the paper world it costs about £60 to send somebody else a copy of the paper *BMJ*. Publishers are now linking together all their electronic copy and trying to persuade librarians to buy more material for more money. So if a library previously purchased 80% of your journals for £X it can now have electronic access to all your journals for £X plus perhaps 10%. So it's a 'more for more' model.

There are problems with this model. First, the librarians may not want the other 20% of your journals—particularly as the other 20% may be very poor quality (which is why they didn't buy them in the first place). A second problem is that most librarians still have static or shrinking budgets. So if they spend more money on your collection of journals (the 'bundle' in publishers' jargon) then they will have to cancel other journals, and these are journals that they did want to buy. So big publishers may be pressurizing librarians into reducing the quality of their collection.

Perhaps—despite antitrust authorities not taking any action—the market is anticompetitive. Mark McCabe, an economist who worked for the US Department of Justice's antitrust division for seven years and is now an assistant professor at the Georgia Institute of Technology, concluded that the market for scientific and medical journals is suffering from 'true market failure'. That's why prices for journals have risen around 200% in the past 10 years, but the number of journals has fallen by only 5–10%. Although no publisher has what seems a monopolistic share of the market, it's important, he says, to understand that libraries purchase not individual titles but portfolios, collections of journals. Then it becomes clear that the market is anticompetitive. The problem, says McCabe, will get worse as publishers sell not individual titles but bundles of electronic journals. Reed Elsevier's bundle, *Science Direct*, includes over 1800 journals. If a publisher managed to reach more than 50% of the market then it would have 'supermarket power'. 'Effectively,' says McCabe, 'the publisher could say, "Either spend all of the budget…on my 60%. . .or you can go and spend your entire…budget on the 40% of stuff out there that is not in my bundle."' The shift to digital bundles is likely to 'precipitate the exit of smaller publishers'.

'Antitrust enforcement alone is not going to fix the market', says McCabe. Instead, organizations like the National Science Foundation ought to invest some of their funds in a new journal initiative. 'Unlike most markets the non-profit sector does a better job than commercial publishers in almost all dimensions of performance.'

This is exactly what is happening. The academic community is creating alternative ways to disseminate research that cut out traditional publishers. But before I discuss those initiatives I want to consider further how publishers might respond. Derk Haank's argument is that it is silly for the academic community to waste its time worrying about publishing. Publishers, he says ingenuously, are stupid, not clever enough to do important research. So they should get on with building wonderful databases and delivering material to the desk of every researcher while academics do Nobel prize winning research. Plus building electronic databases is expensive and risky.

One obvious flaw in this argument is that the academic community doing more of its own publishing doesn't mean Nobel prize winners abandoning their labs to start worrying about disseminating research results. Some other part of the academic community can take on the work, which is exactly what has happened with HighWire Press, a subsidiary of Stanford University Library (and electronic publishers of the

BMJ's journals), with PubMed Central, which is supported by the National Library of Medicine, and with the Public Library of Science, a not-for-profit organization founded by academics. It has to be said as well that their electronic creations are superior to those produced by Reed Elsevier. (While writing this book I had regularly to access the websites of the *Lancet*, which is published by Reed Elsevier, and those of the *BMJ* and *New England Journal of Medicine*, both of which are hosted by HighWire. The superiority of HighWire is immediately apparent, as the editorial staff of the *Lancet* were some of the first to acknowledge.)

Another potential flaw in Haank's argument is the financial one. How is he going to make bigger profits, which his shareholders want him to do, and release money for the academic community? He has an answer. He observes that most of the money spent on academic libraries is not spent on journals. It is spent on staff and buildings, and neither may be necessary. The buildings could be replaced by access to a computer, which has already happened in many places, and the staff could be replaced by stupendous searching, which again has happened to some extent—when did you last ask a librarian to find you something? Google, which I'd never heard of when I started this book, has delivered stupendous search powers to the desk of anybody with internet access, and no doubt something even more powerful will arrive soon. So maybe the librarians will be the first to be thrown out of the balloon, but it could be a messy fight. As illustrated by HighWire Press, librarians can reinvent themselves and take over at least some of what publishers used to do. And they have the great advantage of being within the academic community.

I wouldn't buy shares in Reed Elsevier, but readers might be wondering whether or not I—once the chief executive of a publishing group—see any future for publishing or whether or not I plan to retire to Venice and write ever longer and crazier books (a hugely tempting idea). My answer is 'add value'. It's the traditional and boring way to make money. Create something that people want more cost effectively than your competitors and you have a business. I believe that eventually research material will—and should be—free. But most of the customers of medical journals—ordinary doctors and other healthcare workers—don't want to read original research anyway. They want digested, actionable, readable and even entertaining material that they can easily access and use—call it knowledge, and before I left the *BMJ* we were slowly turning the *BMJ* from 'an information business' to 'a knowledge business'.

But let me return to the alternatives being created to traditional publishers and journals. The Public Library of Science has a vision very similar to that of Harnad, and it has some very powerful and clever supporters—including the Nobel prize winner Harold Varmus, who was previously head of the National Institutes for Health. (Since I first wrote that sentence I've joined the board of the Public Library of Science, meaning that on average the organization is less clever than it was.) It wants all medical and scientific research to be available free on the web for everybody, and it has an embryonic model—PubMed Central. PubMed, a forerunner, is an electronic database of the titles and abstracts of research articles produced by the National Library of Medicine in Washington, funded by the American taxpayer, and used by hundreds of millions of people. (I often describe it as one of America's two great gifts to the world: the other is jazz. Perhaps Google is a third.) PubMed Central is an extension of PubMed in that it has the full text of the research. It started with relatively few articles—because most publishers, including society publishers, refused to allow their material to be included. Most publishers do, however, allow their articles to be placed on PubMed Central after a period of time (often a year), and so the repository of free material is beginning to grow. (It's also possible to find on the web a high proportion of material that is supposedly behind access controls.)

So the problem of the Public Library of Science is how to get from where it is now to where it wants to be. It first tried a boycott of journals that wouldn't play ball. Researchers were invited to sign the following pledge:

'To encourage the publishers of our journals to support this endeavor, we pledge that, beginning in September 2001, we will publish in, edit or review for, and personally subscribe to, only those scholarly and scientific journals that have agreed to grant unrestricted free distribution rights to any and all original research reports that they have published, through PubMed Central and similar online public resources, within 6 months of their initial publication date.'

Some 30,000 researchers from 180 countries signed this pledge, but it didn't have much impact. Now the library is trying another tack. It has started its own journals. Importantly it also has what may prove a workable business model—'author pays'. It reverses the present model, whereby authors pay nothing (although they do actually have to pay page charges for some journals) and publishers get their money back through subscriptions, to a model where authors pay for peer review and their material being placed on the web but their material is then available free to everybody.

The idea that authors might pay to have their research published at first thought sounds like vanity publishing. But if you have had a grant of $5m for your research why not take $2500 of it to pay for peer review. Your research will then be available worldwide for free. An increasing number of research funders—including the Wellcome Foundation—are willing to pay these fees and, indeed, require their researchers to publish in open access journals. Furthermore, the model has already evolved so that your institution will pay. The National Health Service (NHS) and the universities in Britain have done deals with BioMed Central—a commercial publisher that uses the author pays model and then provides open access—to allow all NHS funded research to be processed by BioMed Central and made available free. Traditional publishers—like Oxford University Press and the BMJ Publishing Group—are also experimenting with the model.

There is potentially a substantial saving here for the academic community. It's been calculated by Andrew Odlyzko (with the calculation updated by Jan Velterop of BioMed Central) that the academic community currently pays around $5000 to be able to access a peer reviewed article—so a payment of $2500 for everybody in the world to have access is a huge saving as well as an improvement in access.

The author pays model also has the potential to allow the power of the market to operate where it has not operated before. The model currently advocated is that authors pay for peer review and the posting of their article only if it is accepted. This seems to me to create an uncomfortable conflict of interest. Editors and publishers will be rewarded financially for accepting material. Another model might be that every author pays a little on submission, meaning that those who have their papers rejected in some ways support those who have their papers published. This might mean that inexperienced authors support experienced ones, a regressive measure. All of this is of course irrelevant if institutions simply pay a flat fee to have all papers submitted by their employees reviewed—although a snag with this model might be that publishers cut costs in order to make a profit.

To some extent this happens already. The *BMJ*—like other major journals—has around 6000 papers a year submitted to it. Yet it publishes only about 600. I used to tell our editors that we should invest our resources in the papers we were going to publish, not in those we rejected. This means that we were quick and brutal with many of our rejections.

I can imagine a model in which authors have a choice in paying for various services. They might pay $50 for a rapid rejection, $150 for a detailed rejection with ideas on how to improve the study for submission elsewhere, $250 for external review (more for more reviewers) with the journal passing on some of the money to the reviewers, and $450 for a detailed report from our editorial committee. They could then choose whether or not to pay to have their paper technically edited, perhaps even with a choice over how extensively, and choose whether or not to pay for us to prepare a short version for the paper journal. Subsequently they might pay for press releases, media support, or even a dissemination and change programme—funders fund research to achieve change not just a publication in a journal.

The beauty of a properly functioning market is that resources will flow to where they add most value. I imagine too a hybrid model where authors pay for what matters to them and readers pay for what matters to them. So research papers—which matter more to authors than readers—might be paid for by authors and made available free to everybody, whereas material that editors produce—by writing themselves or commissioning—would be paid for by readers. This would mean that editors would have to make sure that they were meeting the needs of readers, not indulging themselves.

At the moment the market functions poorly. Publishers make money from value they do not originate and by restricting access to ideas that will breed more ideas if shared. They make bigger profits by keeping their costs to a minimum and by pleasing authors not readers. By bundling their products they promote the importance of quantity not quality, and the anticompetitive nature of the market works against the smaller publishers, many of whom have the potential to perform best.

A move to a market where authors and readers pay for what they value should produce a much healthier market, but authors tend to react negatively when they first hear about the author pays model. Their first thought is that it is a move to 'vanity publishing', but importantly authors pay not for publication but for peer review—and for publication only if the paper passes peer review. The next worry is that the poor will be disadvantaged. This is a legitimate worry, but publishers might want to make their services free to those from the poor world (as at the moment they make access free). The Public Library of Science allows authors to decline to pay a fee without the need to give any reason. Only about 20% do so. Plus this problem would be avoided if institutions rather than individuals paid—just as it's mostly institutions rather than individuals who currently pay for subscriptions.

People feel passionately about open access—both for and against it. At the *BMJ* we had many intense debates where people's emotions ran high. Meetings between open access enthusiasts and traditional publishers are often intemperate. The open access enthusiasts think that traditional publishers are so against open access publishing because it threatens their livelihoods. The more I've reflected on the debate the more I've come to realize that it has a strong religious flavour: it's like the reformation.

This thinking led me to develop what I believe are the credos of the two sides, and here they are.

The 'central dogma' of the open access movement is that 'research should be available free to everybody everywhere'.

Proponents believe:

- Exposure to the ideas of research creates more ideas, and the world needs ideas.
- Most research is publicly funded, and the public shouldn't have to pay twice for research results.
- The vast majority of the value of a piece of research lies in the research itself. The processes of peer review and distribution add some value but it's very small compared with the value of the research. Much of the value added by, for example, peer review comes from academics anyway—and usually they are not paid.
- Openness is intrinsically good: 'Whatever isn't transparent is assumed to be biased, corrupt or incompetent until proved otherwise'.
- Publishers have for too long been ripping off academics by making substantial profits from value added not by them but by researchers.
- An open access model of publishing—perhaps the author/institution pays model—should release substantial sums back to the academic community.
- 'Academic credit' and 'place of publication' should be uncoupled.
- Peer review is largely 'an empty gun': it's slow, expensive, biased, ineffective, largely a lottery, hopeless at spotting errors and fraud, and easy to abuse.
- Most research does not need to be published on paper but should simply be available through the web.
- A new model of publishing could open a market for peer review, copy editing, etc in a way that the traditional model doesn't allow—meaning both that the value of those activities could be established and competition introduced as a driver to improve those activities.

The 'central dogma' of traditional publishers is that 'the traditional way of publishing science has served science well and should not be disrupted'.

Proponents believe:

- Publishers add a great deal of value to the process of publishing science and are rewarded for the value they add.
- Any other mode of publishing is untested and moving away from the traditional model may lead to a collapse in the communication of science.

- Traditional journals are of great value, and researchers will want to continue to publish in them even if access to their research is restricted for some time.
- Most researchers can access most research under current arrangements.
- Many 'researchers' do not have grants and so would find difficulty in publishing through author/institution pays models.
- The author pays model is essentially 'vanity publishing'.
- Many journals are owned by scientific and professional societies, and the journal profits are used by worthy causes.
- Traditional publishers are highly efficient and so moving to a new system might increase overall costs—even allowing for the profits of publishers.
- Shifting payment to researchers would be a tax on research intensive organizations.
- New journals started by open access publishers may well not last, leaving lots of important science 'lost in space'.

Writing this in April 2006 I feel that author pays and open access will be a workable model for the future, but immured in the old paradigm I may be wrong. I may also be wrong in thinking that the business of publishing research will change from something that seems to me almost unethical to something much more ethical where the whole world has access to research. I don't think here though that I will be wrong: the drivers for change are too strong. It will not be possible to resist them forever. More difficult than predicting the direction of change is predicting the rate of change.

Section 6: Ethical accountability of researchers and journals

►18

Relations between research ethics committees and medical journals: guarding the probity of research

Research ethics committees (or institutional review boards as they are called in the United States) are the main guardians of the probity of medical research. But they have many problems. The committees don't exist everywhere, and where they do exist there are usually far too many. Most are overworked and under-resourced, and yet the demands on them are increasing. Many lack the full range of skills needed to properly assess research proposals. Few are equipped to deal with misconduct. Most committees are conflicted between the interests of their institutions and patients. And for many of them approval of the research protocol is the end of the process. What happens thereafter is not monitored.

So there is a need for others to help maintain and guard the integrity of research, and journals have a crucial role to play. Journals can ensure that all research has approval from an ethics committee (and often it doesn't) and can provide a back up to and check on the committees. At the *BMJ* we certainly didn't assume that ethics committee approval automatically means ethical acceptability. We often challenged committees.

Many forces came together to make the establishment of research ethics committees inevitable.[348–352] Before the Second World War much medical research was carried out without the consent of patients. Austin Bradford-Hill, a researcher of huge influence and one of the originators of randomized trials, wrote in the *BMJ* as late as 1963: 'I have…no doubt that there are circumstances in which it [informed consent] need not—and even should not—be sought…Surely it is often quite impossible to tell an ill-educated and sicker person the pros and cons of a new and unknown treatment versus the orthodox and known?…Can you describe the condition so that he does not lose confidence in you…'[353] An editorial in the *BMJ* did not agree: 'No-one who conducts experiments on human beings can really free himself from all bias in forming an ethical judgement of what he does.'[354]

The Nuremberg trials of Nazi war criminals were central in raising consciousness about human experimentation, and the Declaration of Helsinki has its origins in the trials. Crucially important in the United States were experiments that caused widespread horror. In the Tuskegee study of untreated syphilis in the Negro American male, poor black men with syphilis were left untreated to see what doctors coyly call 'the natural history' of a disease—what would the disease do to the men? In the Willowbrae State School Experiments young people with learning disorders (the modern phrase for what had been called mental handicap) were deliberately exposed to hepatitis. And in experiments at the Jewish Chronic Disease Hospital in New York patients were injected with cancer cells.

An important spur in Britain to the creation of research ethics committees was the publication in 1967 of a book called *Human guinea pigs: experimentation on man.*[355] It was written by a physician, Maurice Pappworth, and described research on patients conducted by doctors that was dangerous and for which no consent had been given. The doctors were well known, and the research was published in peer reviewed journals. At about the same time as Pappworth's book was published in Britain, a paper describing similar research in the United States was published in the *New England Journal of Medicine.*[356] It is clear that research that today would be considered unethical was routine in medicine in the decades after the Second World War. Ideas on what is acceptable change, and in particular it is now unacceptable to leave it to doctors alone to decide what is ethical.

Although Britain and the United States were alerted at the same time to unethical research, Britain took considerably longer than the United States to establish research ethics committees. The scandals in the United States led to the formation of the National Commission for the Protection of Human Subjects of Biomedical and Behavioural Research. By 1981 the United States Department of Health and Human Services produced regulations for the protection of human subjects.

In Britain the Royal College of Physicians recommended in 1967 that research should be approved by a committee of doctors.[357] The *BMJ*, illustrating the inconsistency of medical journals, took a different line from its earlier editorial and declared that, 'In the final reckoning the decision about a particular project is one for the doctor concerned, and for him alone.'[358] Perhaps because of such opposition the college did not publish guidelines on ethics committees until 1984. The committees began to appear but were very variable in their quality, composition and ways of working. Some worked only by post. In 1991 the Department of Health gave responsibility for local research ethics committees to health authorities, and their composition was broadly standardized.

In the United States, Britain and most other countries researchers wanting to do research on humans must have approval from a research ethics committee or institutional review board. The American regulations identify eight basic elements of properly informed consent:[352]

- A written statement that the study is research and an account of what will be involved.
- A description of any foreseeable risk or discomfort.
- A description of benefits expected to flow from the research.
- Disclosure of alternative treatments.
- A statement on the extent of confidentiality.
- An account of compensation for possible problems.
- Information on whom to contact for further information on research and the rights of participants.
- A statement that participation in the research is voluntary and can be stopped at any time without detriment.

In the United States, Britain and the rest of Europe there is evidence of inconsistency among committees and of them being overworked and under-resourced.[359–362] Researchers doing multicentre research in Britain had to apply to over 150 committees, leading to huge delay and high cost.[363] Worse, the multiple applications showed great variability in the decision-making.[363,364] The last issue of the *BMJ* that I edited included five spontaneous reports of researchers being driven close to despair by Kafkaesque experiences with ethics committees.[365]

Members of the committees received little or no training, and many committees were ill equipped to deal with the technical and legal aspects of research. Yet most people would agree that research that is 'unscientific' in that it will not allow confident conclusions is inevitably 'unethical' in that it is wasting resources and may pointlessly expose patients to risk.

Multicentre research ethics committees were established in Britain in 1997, but local committees still kept control over 'pertinent local issues'. Inconsistency remained. A chairman of one of the multicentre research ethics committees describes the inconsistency of local committees: 'One will oppose informing patients that the research has been approved by the research ethics committee (because it is 'coercive'), the next insisting this information be given; one will oppose any payment to research subjects, the next will support it; one will accept family members as translators for the non-English speaker, the next insist on accredited professionals only.'[350] The president of the Royal College of Physicians suggested in 2000 that 'the cure [of creating multicentre ethics committees] was worse than the disease.'[364]

John Saunders, the chairman of a multicentre ethics committee, at the end of 2002 identified five reasons why the British system was untenable.[350]

First, the remit of the committees was expanding. They were required or were about to be required to consider research on health staff, research in social services, schools and the private sector, research in complementary medicine, and even market research. Some also argued that committees should help researchers with protocols not simply approve or disapprove their research.

Second, there were increasing difficulties with recruitment of members for the committees, particularly among doctors. This was not surprising when the workload was heavy, the work difficult and the rewards scanty.

Third, many members of committees had little or no training. Many don't have the time for training even when training was offered. Furthermore, Britain had seen a torrent of new documents and advice aimed at research ethics committees, and yet many members of the committees were unaware of the new advice.

Fourth, the increasing workload was leading to more committees being created, which despite advice on standardization was likely to lead to more inconsistency.

Fifth, more and more members of committees were saying they required to be paid. Statisticians argued they should be paid, and so did pharmacists. Those members of the committees who were employed in the health service would have time for work on the committees written into their contracts, but this then divided them from the lay members who received no pay.

Saunders's conclusion was that professional committees were needed, and Julian Savulescu, then a professor of medical ethics in Oxford and editor of the *Journal of Medical Ethics*, reached the same conclusion.[366] He examined the deaths of two participants in research in the United States and concluded that failures of the institutional review boards had contributed to their deaths.

In particular, he argued that ethics committees should require a systematic review of all research that had gone before. This has been argued not only for ethics committees but also for bodies funding research. Sometimes a systematic review will show that the question has been adequately answered, in which case the research is not needed. Always a systematic review will provide context for the new research, sharpening the research question and methods. Sometimes a systematic review will reveal important information on safety in the research being proposed.

Such information would have been revealed in the case of Ellen Roche1, who died after being given the drug hexamethonium wrongly. The authors of the study that gave hexamethonium to 20 healthy patients cited four previous studies in which there had been no adverse events. But an inquiry after the death discovered many reports of the drug causing serious lung problems. If the institutional review board had asked for a systematic review, then perhaps Ellen Rochel would still be alive.

But neither the researchers nor the ethics committee were negligent because it is by no means usual to perform a systematic review before starting on a piece of research. The argument is that it should be and that research ethics committees should be competent to appraise such reviews.[366] Somebody with such skills might be much more important than somebody representing one religion, particularly in cultures like Britain where there are many religions.

The death of Jesse Gelsinger in an early trial of gene therapy was also partly because of failure of the institutional review board, argues Savulescu.[366] It approved the therapy being tested on an adult who was mildly affected when it would have made much more sense to test the treatment on a severely affected baby who would inevitably die without treatment. This emphasizes the point that an ethics committee should not simply approve the research presented to it but should also think about alternatives, something that requires considerable scientific competence.

Savulescu concluded that there should be fewer ethics committees, that they should perhaps be suprainstitutional, and that the members should be paid, well resourced, guided and trained.[366] Members of the committees should include experts on systematic review, ethics, research methodology and communication skills.

Saunders too believes that ethics committees need to be 'professionalized'.[351] He believes that there should be fewer committees meeting weekly not monthly. Members should be paid, trained, guided and accountable through a contract. Their performance would be audited, and they would be expected to be familiar with all relevant developments. Proper recruitment procedures should be used.

The Institute of Medicine in the United States has also concluded that current arrangements are inadequate.[367] It advocated replacing institutional review boards with a 'human research participant programme'. Research proposals would be reviewed by not one committee but by three—one for scientific methodology, one for ethics and one for conflicts of interest.

These arguments have had some impact. In 2004 the British government announced a review of ethics committees, and a report was published in June 2005.[368] It proposed fewer committees that would sit more often and include paid members. In contrast to

Savulescu's proposals, the government review suggested that the committees should leave scientific review to others and concentrate on substantive ethical issues. A *BMJ* editorial thought it unlikely that this rushed report would solve the severe problems of ethics committees.[360]

Until recently journals did a poor job of ensuring that the research they published met the highest ethical standards.[369,370] Often they didn't consider the ethical aspects of the research they published and failed to ensure that researchers did have ethics committee approval for the research they had conducted.

Drummond Rennie and Veronica Yank discovered that about one-third of clinical trials published in the five main general medical journals between July 1995 and December 1996 did not report ethics committee approval and one-third did not report informed consent.[370] About one in six reported neither. This improved after 1997 to about one in five not reporting ethics committee approval, about one in five not reporting informed consent and about one in 10 reporting neither. The *BMJ*, I have to confess, had one of the worst records.

Studies in other specialist journals have often found poorer results, and the study by Yank and Rennie reported only on clinical trials. These trials are often major studies conducted by highly experienced researchers with substantial resources. The results might well be worse for smaller studies.

The *BMJ* now uses a checklist to ensure that researchers have ethics committee approval for their research. Often they don't. This may be because they didn't think that their research needed approval from an ethics committee or because there was no ethics committee. Britain, for example, does not have an ethics committee for research in private practice, and some countries have no ethics committees.

I remember vividly some research submitted to the *BMJ* in the 1980s before there was a system of ethics committee approval for research conducted in primary care. As I described in chapter 8, in one case a general practitioner had become convinced that electroconvulsive therapy was an effective treatment for not only severe depression, which it is, but also for a great many conditions—including many non-psychiatric ones. He had given the therapy to dozens of his patients and had submitted the results to us. We were aghast. The doctor must, we thought, be mad. We rejected the paper, and—interestingly, viewed from 2006—we didn't think that we had any duty to take any action.

In another case a general practitioner who had been a trainee in psychiatry took all the patients in his practice who were on antidepressants off their drugs and conducted an elaborate test on them. We thought the research very poor. It was not important, clear, new or even interpretable. Patients had been put unnecessarily at risk. Again we did nothing, but such research would never be allowed by a research ethics committee.

Research in primary care in Britain is now covered by a system of research ethics committees, but some areas of private practice are not. We had a study submitted to us at the *BMJ* by a private practitioner who had been 'experimenting' on his patients with combinations of drugs, including Viagra, to try and find optimal treatment for middle-aged men with sexual problems. We thought the research very poor because there was no clear question being asked and the methods—simply trying different drugs on different patients—would not allow any confident conclusion. We asked the private practitioner whether or not he had ethics committee approval and whether or not the men had consented not only to take the treatment, which they must have done, but also to be part of an experiment. He responded that he could not get ethics committee approval because there was no ethics committee for private practice and that the patients didn't need to consent to an experiment because they weren't in an experiment.

This question of where legitimate clinical innovation ends and research begins is extremely difficult. Partly because I thought it good to have guidance on this question and partly because I thought the practitioner guilty of research misconduct, I referred the case to the General Medical Council. It accepted that there was no research ethics committee and so the practitioner could not have got approval. It also agreed with the practitioner that this was not research and so he didn't need consent from his patients to be part of an experiment.

I was unimpressed. It seemed to me that the practitioner must have considered the study research in order to have written it up and submitted it to a scientific journal. I wondered too what sort of consent he had got from his patients. Were they aware of the degree of uncertainty?

This question of where research begins arises repeatedly, particularly with authors from some countries where research ethics committees either don't exist or exist in only a rudimentary form. An author from the Middle East sent us a huge series of patients whom he had treated for migraine with an operation on blood vessels outside the skull. He had complete success in every case, something that's always hard to believe in medicine. We challenged him on the research, asking about research ethics committee approval. He said simply that the patients had consented to the treatment. In another case from the Middle East surgeons had done elaborate operations on the genitalia of women to treat sexual problems. We gained the impression that it was the husbands of the women who had asked for the treatment, which—with our Londonocentric view of the world—we thought unacceptable. There was no response to our questioning of the research.

Similar problems arise as well in Britain. A private cosmetic surgeon sent us a series of cases of enlarging women's breasts by implanting fat removed from another part of the body. The surgeon had no approval from an ethics committee. We were worried by this, and a reviewer advised us that such a process might be dangerous because it could lead to calcium forming in the breast, making it difficult to detect possible cancers if the woman went for mammographic screening. We challenged the author, who disagreed that the technique was dangerous and said that he didn't need research committee approval because this was not research and that there was evidence to support the technique. He sent us some very unconvincing reports from American cosmetic surgery journals that we'd never heard of. We asked for guidance from an official body of plastic surgeons but heard nothing. They perhaps wisely decided to stay out of such a tricky dispute. We did not publish the paper and gave up pursuing the surgeon.

Another area of difficulty is whether or not authors of improvement or audit studies need approval from a research ethics committee. Part of modern health is to try and continually improve. This usually means measuring how you are doing with, say, managing the patients in a hospital or practice with diabetes. Always there will be imperfections and room for improvement. So a change would be introduced—perhaps a new record system or a nurse designated to work with such patients—and then further measurements made. Sometimes the changes will lead to improvement. Sometimes they won't. Sometimes what seems like an innovation likely to lead to improvement will make things worse. Further changes will then be tried, and this cycle of audit or improvement will continue indefinitely.

But isn't this research and shouldn't it therefore be approved by a research ethics committee? Some medical journals have taken the line that it is and therefore will not publish reports on such activities without ethics committee approval. An experiment is being conducted, they argue, which means the results are unknown. Harm could result. At the very least resources will be used, and if they are wasted—on, for example, an experiment that will be uninterpretable—then that seems 'unethical'.

Many healthcare workers involved in improvement projects and many members of research ethics committees think that such projects do not need approval from an ethics committee. They are part of best practice. Indeed, it would seem wrong not to try to improve what you do. They are also part of routine practice, and much of routine practice includes actions with uncertain outcomes. It would be completely impossible for research ethics committees to consider every action with an uncertain outcome: they would be overwhelmed and improvements in healthcare would stop. Plus there is little chance of patients being harmed.

The *BMJ* did not have an explicit policy on this issue, but our implicit policy was that we were willing to publish quality improvement reports (and we actively encouraged their submission) without approval from a research ethics committee. One obvious problem, as with clinical innovation, was deciding where routine work ends and research begins. Research is sometimes defined as 'finding the right thing to do', whereas audit or improvement is 'finding how to do the thing right'—but these are not completely different enterprises. They exist on a spectrum, and if it is decided that improvement activities do not need ethics committee approval then somebody has to decide where to draw the line and separate the two. This is not easy.

Eventually the *BMJ*'s ethics committee did consider this question, and one member of the committee, Derick Wade, produced a very thoughtful paper.[371] His starting point was that 'ethical considerations should apply to all medical practice'—not just research. He then argued that research and audit could never be neatly separated. Rather than trying to decide whether an activity was research or ethics the question should be whether or not the activity needed 'additional ethical scrutiny'. The following questions, he argued, would help decide whether additional scrutiny was required:

- How much does this activity deviate from current normal (accepted, local) clinical practice?
- What is the (additional) burden imposed on the patients (or others)?
- What (additional) risks are posed to the patients (or others)?
- What benefit might accrue to the patients (or others)?
- What are the potential benefits to society (future patients)?

These questions are important in research, practice and audit. Wade's view is that the lead investigator or clinician should consider these questions and decide whether or not additional ethical scrutiny is merited. If it is, the ethics committee is consulted, but Wade believes that many minor research projects would not need ethics committee approval.

I feel somewhat anxious leaving the decision on the need for ethics committee approval entirely to the lead investigator—because he or she will hope to gain honour and recognition from the research and may thus have a bias towards deciding that the research doesn't need additional ethical scrutiny and so avoiding delays and possible interference. I agree, however, that we have to try and avoid grappling with ethical difficulties by replacing moral debates with bureaucratic debates on whether an activity is research or audit.

Moral debates often don't have clear answers, and sometimes journals take different views from research ethics committees on what is ethical. In chapter 8 on research misconduct I told the story of a journal that decided that a chairman of a research ethics committee had been wrong to allow researchers to conduct an experiment of exposing children with known allergies to substances that might cause them to have a major allergic reaction that could possibly kill them.

The *BMJ* experienced a somewhat similar case of a randomized trial in which children with an allergy to food were rechallenged with the food. We had accepted the study for publication before we realized that the authors—who came from a major British hospital—did not have approval from an ethics committee. The authors argued the treatment was part of routine management, no drugs were involved and that ethics committee approval was not necessary. One author added: 'I discussed this informally with a member of the ethics committee who felt that this was a reasonable decision.' Neither we at the *BMJ* nor the Committee on Publication Ethics agreed. We declined to publish the paper and reported the authors to the chief executive of their hospital. After an investigation requirements to seek ethics committee approval were tightened.

In another case we had again accepted for publication a study of an innovation that helped with making a microbiological diagnosis in a clinical condition before we discovered that the authors did not have ethics committee approval and had got only verbal not written consent from patients. The authors said that the chairman of the ethics committee knew about the study and said that 'written consent might have reduced the numbers in the study and caused unnecessary distress'—both wholly unacceptable responses. We rejected the study. We didn't report the authors or the chairman of the ethics committee to their employers, but in retrospect we probably should have done.

Sometimes we disagreed with the judgement of an ethics committee but—recognizing legitimate grounds for disagreement—would publish the study with a commentary. We did this with a study in which the authors exposed the siblings of babies who died from cot deaths to very low levels of oxygen.[372] This could help answer the question of whether or not it was safe for these babies to fly. The hospital research ethics committee approved the research, and the parents gave written informed consent. Our editorial committee (this was before we had an ethics committee) worried, however, that this was research on healthy children and that it might be difficult for the parents of children who had died to refuse to participate.

So we published the paper with a commentary written by Julian Savulescu, in which he argued that the research should not have been approved.[373] The chairman of the ethics committee wrote that the committee had started from the same position as us but changed its decision after hearing all the arguments.[374] The authors justified themselves.[375] Some critics thought it odd that we should publish research that we judged unethical—despite accompanying it with a commentary. (Some thought that we were simply indulging a weakness for publicity, rather as we did when we published a series of articles on sexual health with a warning on the cover about the journal containing sexually explicit pictures. The warning guaranteed high readership.) Our position was that ethical issues are often complex and uncertain and that there is room for debate both to deepen understanding of issues and to raise consciousness about them.

As I described in chapter 13, the *BMJ* published two trials in which ethics committees had given approval for trials to be conducted without informed consent. We accompanied each paper with a commentary arguing that the ethics committees were wrong to approve the studies together with defences from the committees. The debate that followed was rich and productive.

I cannot remember an example of where we have agreed to publish research that an ethics committee had judged to be unethical. This is not surprising as it would be a bold researcher who went ahead with a study refused by an ethics committee. Nor can I remember examples of research ethics committees criticizing journals, although there could be many circumstances where it would be legitimate for them to do so— for example, if a journal declined to publish a study simply because it had negative results.

One of the reviewers of the proposal for this book wrote that he or she didn't see any point in a chapter such as this. Research ethics committees and journals have, he or she wrote, nothing to do with each other. I can see why somebody might take that position, but I hope that I might have convinced readers that what the committees and the journals have in common is that they are part of the apparatus for trying to ensure that research is of high quality and ethically sound. Sadly, the apparatus is still inadequate, and there is almost certainly room for research ethics committees and journals to work more closely together, not least in keeping an eye on each other's performance.

► 19

Ethical support and accountability for journals: an ombudsman, an ethics committee, and next?

Ten or so years ago I sat in a seminar for editors run by Raanon Gillon, then editor of the *Journal of Medical Ethics*, and he asked each editor in turn about his or her ethical problems. 'None', said editor after editor. 'I don't have any.' I was shocked. I had begun to feel that ethical issues were presenting themselves every day in my editorial work. Now editors have followed doctors and begun to recognize the ubiquity of ethical problems. The next step is to recognize the need for help with these ethical problems. This kind of thinking led the *Lancet* to set up an ombudsman, the *BMJ* an ethics committee, and editors in general organizations like the World Association of Medical Editors (WAME) and the Committee on Publication Ethics (COPE). In this chapter I want to discuss these forms of ethical support for editors.

Several of the best newspaper around the world had appointed ombudsmen (this is a Norwegian word that, I'm assured, cannot be converted to the inclusive ombudsperson—although *JAMA* could not resist doing so[376]) and readers' editors, but the *Lancet* was the first medical journal to do so. A few other journals—but very few— have followed.

Richard Horton, the editor of the *Lancet*, in his editorial announcing the appointment of the ombudsman, says that the idea arose from the call for an international scientific press council.[377] The call came from Doug Altman, Iain Chalmers and Andrew Herxheimer in a paper that described three cases of editorial misconduct (see chapter 12).[237] But I think that Horton may also have had in his mind the problems that arose from the *Lancet* publishing the Bristol Cancer Help Centre study that suggested that women who attended the centre for complementary treatment died sooner than those who didn't (see chapter 2).[17] The interpretation of the study was later withdrawn, but the women involved in the study had many grievances with the *Lancet* that were never satisfied. Perhaps if the *Lancet* had had an ombudsman at the time the dispute could have been defused.

The *Lancet* ombudsman deals primarily with maladministration. He (the two so far have both been men) is required 'to record and, where necessary, to investigate episodes of alleged editorial maladministration when a complainant remains dissatisfied with the journal's first response to criticism'. He specifically does not deal with 'complaints about the substance (rather than the process) of editorial decisions'. It's easy to see why the *Lancet* made this exclusion: otherwise, authors might potentially appeal to the ombudsman on every rejected paper—something around 8000 a year at the *Lancet*.

But at the same time this exclusion means that the ombudsman does not become involved in some of the major disputes involving the *Lancet*. This is why the ombudsman has made no comment on the *Lancet* paper that suggested that the measles, mumps and rubella (MMR) vaccine might cause autism (see chapter 2),[1] and the ombudsman was involved only informally, he reports, in the dispute around the *Lancet* paper that suggested that genetically modified potatoes might have damaged the stomach lining of rats (see chapter 2).[39,378] In other words, there is a feeling that the *Lancet* ombudsman is not 'where the action is.' He may be more decorative than effective.

The remit of the ombudsman includes dealing with delays in handling submitted manuscripts, discourtesy, failures to follow procedures outlined in 'writing for the *Lancet*', and failure to take reasonable account of representations to editors by authors and readers. He can also deal with 'challenges to the publishing ethics of the journal— for example, accusations of editorial dishonesty, favouritism, victimization or conflicts of interest; matters of taste; and the editorial handling of complaints about author misconduct'. In addition to not considering complaints about the substance of editorial decisions the ombudsman does not consider criticisms of editorial content or accusations of scientific misconduct.

The model for the *Lancet*'s ombudsman is Britain's Parliamentary Commissioner for Maladministration.[376,379] He investigates complaints against government departments and is independent and unpaid. Investigations are confidential, and if he upholds a complaint he recommends redress. The *Lancet* ombudsman deals only with complaints that have already been considered by the editorial team. If complainants are dissatisfied with the editorial response then they write directly to the ombudsman without the letter being seen by the editors. He investigates by reading correspondence and background papers and sometimes by interviewing editors. Complainants receive a written response from the ombudsman, and he may ask for redress from the editors. Each year an annual report of the ombudsman's inquiries is published in the *Lancet*.

The first ombudsman—Thomas Sherwood, a former dean of the medical school in Cambridge and former member of the *Lancet*'s international advisory board— involved himself very much in the processes of the journal. He attended editorial meetings, talked to editors and 'dug through deep filing cabinets'. The idea to have an ombudsman seemed to be very much that of the editor, Richard Horton, and the other editors were initially suspicious. They felt that they were being watched and that their independence was compromised. 'Slowly,' wrote Horton in 1998, 'a phase of grudging acceptance was entered, and now we have begun a period marked by polite approval, if not joyous enthusiasm, at his presence.'[376] Horton has told me that the biggest benefit from the ombudsman may well have come from him observing the *Lancet*'s processes and prompting improvements.

There have now been eight annual reports from the ombudsman,[378,380–386] and he seems to deal mostly with rather trivial complaints. Horton published an analysis of the 20 complaints received in the first 18 months.[376] Sixteen of the complaints were about editorial issues, but four were excluded because they were primarily about editorial judgement. Seven of the remaining 12 complaints were upheld, but most were about delays. One embarrassing but hardly very serious case involved a contributor to a multi-author book reviewing the book. (I find it extraordinary that he or she should agree to review the book.) A 'failure to respond appropriately to an allegation of misconduct' sounds more serious, but we have no more details. To my amusement, an 'improper attack on a national medical association' (could this have been an excoriating editorial by Horton on the all round uselessness of my former employer, the British Medical Association [BMA]?) was rejected. Four of the complaints were about the business side of the *Lancet*—two about advertising and two about subscriptions—and despite these not being in the original remit of the ombudsman he took them on and upheld all four. I imagine that this has made the editor very popular with the business people.

Sherwood was replaced after four years by Richard Carter, a professor and cancer researcher. The new ombudsman was appointed after open advertisement. Carter has produced four reports,[383–386] and his 2002 report describes four new cases and one continuing case. Two complaints of delay were upheld as was a case of a 'badly defective copy of journal sent to a subscriber in Sri Lanka'. (There does seem to be something faintly ridiculous about this being investigated by an ombudsman and reported on the editorial pages of the *Lancet*.)

The other two cases deal with things that are potentially much more serious, but the ombudsman's report is cryptic. In order to have some understanding of the significance of these findings you would need background information. The ombudsman upheld 'Complaints from reviewer directed towards editorial processing (and subsequent editorial decision) of paper on mammographic screening [and]…additional complaints about handling of an Editorial, commissioned from the reviewer by the *Lancet Oncology*, which was eventually withdrawn from publication by authors.' The *Lancet* published a systematic review of mammography that suggested that it was ineffective and may have caused many women to have unnecessary operations to have their breasts removed.[387] This review gained worldwide publicity and was strongly attacked by enthusiasts for mammography. The *Lancet*'s study was accompanied by an editorial that described internal difficulties of the Cochrane Collaboration which produced the review.[388] Several years afterwards the controversies continue, and we should perhaps have been told more about what went wrong at the *Lancet*. It's not even clear whether the problems were serious or not.

The continuing case described a paper published in the *Lancet* in 1995 that investigated whether or not children with cystic fibrosis might be running into problems because of drugs they were prescribed. A researcher who had been involved with the study was anxious about the results, and his anxiety was increased when the pathologist involved in the case was found to have stored, without consent from the parents, huge numbers of specimens from babies who had died. This happened at Alder Hey Hospital in Liverpool and led to a major investigation. This time the cryptic comments of the ombudsman are less of a problem because several letters were published in the *Lancet* telling the story.

The great day for the *Lancet* ombudsman came in 1998 when he was asked—by the editor not an author—to look at front page stories in the British newspapers alleging that a *Lancet* editor had been in the pay of the tobacco industry.[381,389] I remember reading the story on the day it was published and thinking it implausible. The story originated in tobacco company documents placed on the internet in the United States.

A memo to the tobacco company, Philip Morris, from its lawyers was the source of the information.

The ombudsman asked the editors of the time, 1990, whether or not they knew anything about the allegation. They denied it. A cynic would inevitably observe that 'they would, wouldn't they?' Further reports then suggested that the 'editor' was Petr Skrabanek, a famous and gifted iconoclast who scoffed at political correctness and died in 1994. One of his famous aphorisms was to observe that the World Health Organization's definition of health—complete physical, psychological and social wellbeing—was achieved only at the moment of mutual orgasm. Skrabanek had never been on the staff of the *Lancet*, but he had contributed 14 unsigned editorials. The *Lancet* ombudsman decided to break anonymity to disclose that none of the editorials was on tobacco. Skrabanek had, however, contributed two letters on tobacco and an essay entitled 'Smoking and statistical overkill'.[390] We don't know whether Skrabanek was paid by the industry, but it's not inconceivable that he was. Sometime after this episode it was revealed in a similar manner that another iconoclast—Roger Scruton, a philosopher and columnist—was paid by the industry. He was sacked from his job as a columnist on the *Financial Times*.

The ombudsman concluded that the *Lancet* was innocent, that its independence was illustrated by the fact that the story originated in the *New Scientist*, which was owned by the same company that owned the *Lancet* (clever that, to pull a positive message from a negative story), and that it would be a good idea for editors and members of the editorial board to be required to declare any conflicts of interest.[381] I've no doubt that the existence of the ombudsman was very helpful in these circumstances. How else could the journal have investigated? An internal investigation would have been less convincing, but to set up an independent investigation would have been difficult, time consuming and expensive (the ombudsman, remember, is not paid).

The *Lancet* is convinced that its experiment with an ombudsman is a success. I too think it a step in the right direction, and I hope that those who have read chapter 12 on editorial misconduct will be convinced that something needs to be done. The world at large doesn't, however, seem to have been much impressed, and few journals have copied the initiative.

We at the *BMJ* debated several times whether we should have an ombudsman, and our editorial team eventually decided that we should. But I put the case to our editorial board, and they advised against it. My argument was that introducing an ombudsman would help us improve our processes and provide an outlet for complaints. Members of the board argued that a better way to improve processes was to introduce systems of continuous improvement. They also argued that there did need to be a clear complaints system but that the *BMJ* was different from the *Lancet* in that it was owned by a medical organization, the BMA, whereas the *Lancet* is not (it's owned by the huge listed company, Reed Elsevier). Readers should be able to complain to the owners of the *BMJ*, and to open a new route for complaints would create confusion. Instead, the *BMJ* should make clear its complaints system.

Here I must confess that I had 'write an editorial on how to complain' on my 'to do' list for several years but didn't ever write it before I left. Somehow there's always something else to do, which illustrates, yet again, how we are much keener on the accountability of others than our own accountability. I did get as far as posting the draft code of conduct for medical editors produced by the Committee on Publication Ethics on the *BMJ* news pages and inviting comment.[154] One thing that the code stated was: 'Editors should respond promptly to all complaints and should ensure that there is a way for complainants who are dissatisfied with the response to take complaints further. Ideally this mechanism should be made clear in the journal.' The 'ideally' was a let out, but the *BMJ* never did make clear how you should make a complaint—and still doesn't as far as I can tell. Nor could I find anything on how to complain on the *Lancet* website—or (on 30 April 2006) any mention of how to complain to the ombudsman.

Believing strongly that 'every defect is a treasure', we assiduously collected all complaints at the *BMJ*—and once a quarter we analysed and debated them. One editor thought it too negative to concentrate just on complaints so we also collected compliments. I'm nervous of compliments because they may lure you into complacency, something that terrifies me and that I believe can destroy a journal as termites will destroy a house. But sometimes compliments were useful: if we had five complaints from readers outraged by a cover then it was good to know that four people liked it enough to contact us to say so.

But generally complaints are more useful—because they provide a direct route to action. We usually had around 30 or 40 a quarter to analyse, but every so often we hit the jackpot. We had over one hundred when we got Mozart's birthday wrong, around 150 when our imaginative Irish columnist seemed to advocate running over cats, and almost 200 when we produced an issue of the *BMJ* as it might look in 20 years' time. 'It was like a favourite aunt turning up drunk and in drag', wrote one complainant. We would of course in the last case have been disappointed not to receive complaints. 'The more you alienate the more you reach', said 1960's revolutionary Jerry Rubin.

When we had repeated complaints about refusing to publish obituaries of doctors who had died more than three months previously we decided to rescind the policy. Obituaries are a common cause of complaint, and I looked in every quarter to see how many complaints we had. As with the 'dog that didn't bark' in the Sherlock Holmes case, I paid attention to the absence of complaints. Repeated complaints on the long time we took to publish paper letters joined with our own dissatisfaction to force us to find ways to improve. People regularly complained that we seemed to have a different policy for pictures derived by doctors from their patients (where we wanted written consent) and for pictures from news agencies (where we didn't ask for any more consent than for any other publication). We thus asked our ethics committee to advise us.

I tried to respond to all complaints myself, particularly because I discovered that it wasn't difficult to turn a complainant into an enthusiastic supporter with a considered and polite response. Usually complainants were satisfied with such a response, but sometimes they wanted to go further. The main route of complaint was to the BMA, the owners of the *BMJ*. These were sent to various officers but usually found their way to the chairman of our board. Sometimes his response was enough, but rarely was the full board asked to consider the complaint. The process was not clearly laid down—but should have been.

People could also complain to the Press Complaints Commission, a body that regulates the British press. We paid for the privilege. People did complain to the commission about the *BMJ*, but as the commission spends much of its time on newspapers paying prostitutes to provide stories on celebrity clients or actresses being photographed naked without consent it tended to find the complaints about the *BMJ* both quaint and trivial. The commission did, however, take very seriously a complaint about the obituary we published of David Horrobin, as I described in chapter 2.

In addition to complaining to the Press Complaints Commission, people can also complain to the Code of Practice Committee about pharmaceutical advertisements in the *BMJ* or to the Advertising Standards Authority about any advertisement, and if people wrote to me to complain about advertisements then I usually urged them to complain to these authorities. Quite often the Code of Practice Committee would rule in favour of the complainant, and we would carry a piece in the journal. People can now complain to the Committee on Publication Ethics (COPE) about editorial misconduct (although it has very limited systems of redress, as I explained in chapter 12), and people can of course resort to the law if they think that they have been libelled (as I will describe in chapter 20).

Whether or not our ethics committee would consider complaints was one of the first things we had to discuss as we were setting it up. The conclusion of the committee was that it would be unwise to have two committees that could consider complaints. The BMJ Publishing Group Board should be the body that considers complaints, but if it wanted advice on an ethical complaint the ethics committee could be asked to advise.

We set up our ethics committee for two mains reasons.[86,391,392] First, we recognized that ethical problems were common in our work and that we needed regular expert advice. Second, we thought it important that we had a clear process of examining ethical issues that included independent advisers. We hoped that the committee would not just consider cases where we asked for its advice but would also review our existing policies and suggest ones that we need but don't have. The committee would also prompt us with our coverage of ethical issues. Interestingly, when we asked readers what they wanted, more of ethics comes second only to education.

We set up our ethics committee in 2000, three years after COPE was established, and one question that arose commonly was why we needed both. One reason was that COPE has to consider cases anonymously to avoid libel. The *BMJ* ethics committee, in contrast, has access to all the papers. Next, COPE was purely advisory, whereas the ethics committee took decisions. The editors might choose to ignore the advice, but if we do so then we had to justify in writing in the journal why we were ignoring the advice. This hasn't yet happened, and I suspect that it never may because the advice is very carefully considered and editors are part of the discussion. The *BMJ* ethics committee can also concentrate on the *BMJ*, advising on all its policies, in a way that couldn't happen at COPE which has a membership of around 200 journals.

The editorial team, the management of the BMJ Publishing Group and the board all approved the setting up of the ethics committee. One issue was whether or not the committee should cover business as well as editorial issues. The business people were anxious, worrying that the committee might get in the way of efficient and business-like decision-making. I didn't agree, but as the whole thing was an experiment it seemed sensible to begin with editorial issues and perhaps extend later to business issues. As I've described above, the *Lancet* ombudsman found himself dealing with some business issues—on subscriptions and advertising—straight away. So far the *BMJ* ethics committee has only dabbled in business issues—with a debate over whether or not it was acceptable to advertise skeletons for sale. (The committee decided it was unless there was any suggestion that the skeleton was an aboriginal skeleton, raising the possibility of theft and religious problems.)

Once everybody had agreed that we should have an ethics committee we wrote a job description for a chairman and advertised. We had many high-quality applicants, and an appointment was made by the chairman of the BMA ethics committee, one of our editorial board, an assistant editor and me. We appointed Sandy McCall Smith, professor of medical law in Edinburgh—and subsequently a world famous author. Once we had a chairman we debated further the role and composition of the committee and advertised for members. Like the *Lancet* we paid expenses but not a fee—to avoid compromising the independence of the committee. Again we had many high-quality applications.

We appointed three practising doctors, one of them from Canada, a journalist with a particular interest in ethics, a medical writer who had worked in the pharmaceutical industry, and the secretary of the BMA ethics committee (for her very wide experience of practical ethical issues rather than to provide a formal link with the BMA committee). We later invited a doctor from the developing world to join the committee. I attended the meetings, and we provided a secretary. Other *BMJ* editors attended from time to time. The meetings were roughly quarterly, and anonymized minutes were posted on the *BMJ* website.

It's no exaggeration to say that ever since the first meeting I wondered how the *BMJ* got through 160 years without such a committee (and, as far as I know, every other journal in the world manages without one). The discussion was deep, useful and fascinating. As editors, we learnt a lot. The discussions also changed what we did.[392]

At the first meeting we discussed a paper submitted to us from China that described the first step in giving people malaria as a possible treatment for infection with the human immunodeficiency virus (HIV). We, the editors, had been appalled by this and brought it to the committee asking what action we should take. For us the paper was describing misconduct of a high order—actively infecting patients and putting them at risk. The committee took a very different view, pointing out that at that time the vast majority of people in China would have no access to the drugs used to treat HIV. It was thus legitimate to consider any treatment that might be beneficial, and it is within the living memory of older doctors in Britain that infecting patients—'fever therapy'—was used as a treatment for various conditions.

The committee was very helpful in the case of a paper from a medical student and others describing how medical students were performing intimate examinations (vaginal and rectal examinations) on anaesthetized patients without consent—an illegal act. The *BMJ* had been about to publish the paper, together with a critical commentary, when one of the authors, a dean, suddenly asked for the paper not to be published without further revision. We agreed, reluctantly. The paper was resubmitted with the message much diluted and a new set of authors. The guarantor of the paper (the person who accepts full responsibility for the integrity of the paper) had not even been an author on the original paper. It was hard for us to understand how anybody could be a guarantor for a paper that he or she had nothing to do with during the research. And what had happened to the original guarantor? Why had she been downgraded? Ironically, the new guarantor was a professor of medical ethics.

We were advised by the committee to persist with publishing something close to the original paper, make sure that we provided support for the medical student author (who might otherwise be mangled in the process), praise the medical school for being willing to share an embarrassing finding (because it was probably happening in other medical schools), and publish an editorial with the paper that emphasized the way forward. We might have done some of these things anyway, but the committee's advice was very useful.

The committee helped us not just with particular cases. It has devised for us a policy on getting consent for publication of material on patients. We had tried to devise a policy that meant that we could in some circumstances publish information on patients without consent—for example, when the encounter between patient and doctor took place a long time ago and the patient was highly likely to be dead. The committee devised a policy based on firm philosophical principles. The committee also reviewed our guidance to contributors and made suggestions for improving it, particularly in relation to material from the developing world.

The *Lancet*'s ombudsman and the *BMJ* ethics committee work in different ways and have different remits, but they are both concerned to raise the quality of ethical thinking within the journals, make editors more accountable, and allow the outside world into the often closed world of journals. Neither initiative has been much copied. Indeed, as far as I know, the *BMJ* is still the only journal to have an ethics committee. Is this because it's a bad idea or because other editors don't feel the need for improving their ethical thinking? Or is just a matter of time?

I've already described in chapter 12 how COPE is trying to develop a system of self-regulation for editors, but we are as far away as ever from the international medical scientific press council envisaged in the early 1990s by Altman, Chalmers and Herxheimer.[239] Yet I hope that readers of this book will agree that there is a strong need for higher ethical standards and better accountability for journals and editors. How can it happen? The answer, I think, is small initiatives like the ones described in this chapter. At some stage outrage might make the rest happen. Scandal, as I keep discovering, is a powerful motor for change.

▶20

Libel and medical journals: proper constraint or against the public interest?

Some *BMJ* authors imagine that the law of libel doesn't cover medical journals. They think that libel applies to tabloid newspapers and that they can surely say what they want within a medical journal, 'especially when it's true'. The law of libel does, of course, apply to medical journals, and the *BMJ* was involved in one of the longest running libel cases in British legal history.[393] An editor can bankrupt a journal through a libellous statement, and the threat of a libel action can be used to silence a journal. There is a difficult path that editors must try to follow between committing libel and being so scared of an action and its dire consequences that right and proper criticism is muted.

The *BMJ* stumbled into its long running case. It published an article in May 1969 that showed that patients given an intravenous drug called methohexitone as an anaesthetic suffered various abnormal physiological responses.[394] The abnormal responses seen in these patients may have explained why some patients in routine practice had died while being anaesthetized for dental surgery. The message was that the technique was dangerous and should not be used. Intravenous anaesthesia in dental surgeries has long been a controversial business. If something goes wrong, as things always may with anaesthesia, then the facilities for resuscitation are inadequate. The *BMJ* had peer reviewed the study in the normal way and decided to accompany it with an editorial (and editorials in those days were anonymous) underlining the importance of the message.[395]

This all sounds like the routine fare of medical journals. The safety of patients is traditionally the first concern of doctors. It may be something of a scientific leap from showing abnormal physiological responses in a series of patients to suggesting that they might sometimes prove fatal, but clearly it's hard to study rare and serious side-effects.

You cannot libel a technique, but unfortunately for the *BMJ* one man—a dentist called Stanley Drummond-Jackson—was particularly associated with the technique. He was able to convince a judge, Lord Pearson, that this article was defamatory of him. Pearson said:

> 'A professional man's technique is at least relatively permanent, and it belongs to him: it may be considered to be an essential part of his professional activity and of him as a professional man. In the case of a dentist it may be said: if he uses a bad technique, he is a bad dentist and a person needing dental treatment should not go to him.'

In order to bring a libel action in England a person has to do no more than show that a defamatory statement has been published which refers to him or her. And a defamatory statement is one 'that tends to lower the person concerned in the estimation of right thinking members of society' or exposes the person to 'hatred, ridicule and contempt'. There is clearly a difference of degree between these two definitions. The *BMJ* carried many letters that suggested that I'd been writing nonsense, had completely misjudged an issue or had been hopelessly biased. Were these defamatory? People who read them might think less of me, but they probably wouldn't stimulate 'hatred, ridicule and contempt'. There is, unsurprisingly, lots of room for arguing about what is defamatory. One famous English case—famous for its absurdity—concerned remarks about the size of an actress's bottom.

Five days after the two articles were published in the *BMJ*, the journal received a letter from Drummond-Jackson's lawyers alleging grave defamation and that his general professional reputation was severely damaged. The lawyers wanted the *BMJ* to unreservedly withdraw all imputations, make an agreed statement in open court and undertake not to publish any similar statements in future.

Drummond-Jackson and his lawyers were very fast out of the blocks. I wasn't at the *BMJ* at the time—although my predecessor and mentor, Stephen Lock (then an assistant editor), was and dealt with the case, spending 11 weeks in court—but my strong instinct would have been to resist such a 'bully boy' attack.

People—including a former chief medical officer for England—occasionally ask my advice on whether or not they should take a libel action. My usual advice is no. It can be a long drawn out, draining and hugely expensive process that takes over your life. If your aim is to clear your reputation you will rarely succeed because of the universal feeling that 'there is no smoke without fire'. What's more, allegations that have been read by few people and forgotten by most may suddenly be covered in extensive and lubricious detail in the daily papers. And once you are in the witness box it's war. The opposition's barristers will do everything they can to make you look a fool, a charlatan or both—and they are very good at it.

A British cardiologist, Peter Nixon, took a libel action against Channel 4, a British television channel that had broadcast a programme accusing him of scientific misconduct. After 23 days of the trial and four days in the witness box, he was forced to admit that errors made by him in papers he'd published 'were more than an honest slip of the pen', that he didn't seek ethical approval for diagnostic tests that could be fatal, and that he hadn't informed his patients of the risks.[396] His insurers picked up a bill for £2m, and he had to remove himself from the medical register.

Another fundamental problem with libel is that the side with the deepest pockets—or the strongest nerve—can win. It's like a poker game. The stakes rise. This naturally favours an organization over an individual, but it isn't always like that. A Dr Gee, for example, took an action against the BBC, which had alleged that a slimming treatment of Gee's could kill people. The case went on for 92 days, and the BBC had not even had a chance to make its case. It capitulated—largely, I believe, to avoid spending public money on such a never-ending case.

Lawyers may be inclined to advise you to take an action—because they 'win' whatever. (This would be a libellous statement if made against a particular lawyer.)

Lawyers will also tell you that your case is 'strong' when it isn't, perhaps because the whole process is so uncertain. The wise say that the only reason to take a libel action is for money in an open and shut case. The case won't get to court, and you'll receive a substantial payment.

The *BMJ* tried to persuade Drummond-Jackson that the way to sort out a complex and important scientific dispute was not through the courts but rather through debate in the journal. The editors offered to consider a letter for publication. He declined and issued a writ.

The *BMJ* applied in October 1969 to have the case struck out because Drummond-Jackson had disclosed no cause for action.[393] It lost and appealed. The Court of Appeal heard the appeal in February 1970 and dismissed it.[397] Lord Denning, the Master of the Rolls, who would have struck out the case, made some interesting points. First, he predicted—rightly, as it turned out—that the time to prepare for the trial and the length of the trial could be enormous. Then he drew a distinction between libel and lawful criticism: 'Lawful criticism,' he was reported as saying, 'was impersonal and objective: it was criticism of goods, of a design, a system or a technique. It pointed out defects and deficiencies without attacks on the man himself.'[397]

Pointing out 'defects and deficiencies' is at the very heart of science and the very stuff of medical journals. When we send out even the very best studies for review we expect to receive detailed critiques of their 'defects and deficiencies'. If we get back simple approvals then we think that the reviewers have not done their jobs. The letters published in the *BMJ* are mostly about 'defects and deficiencies'. Most scientific theories eventually need to be replaced because they are full of 'defects and deficiencies'. Newtonian physics was eventually replaced, but that doesn't stop Newton being one of the greatest scientists ever.

Denning continued: 'It would be a sorry day if scientists were to be deterred from publishing their findings for fear of libel actions. So long as they refrain from personal attacks, they should be free to criticize the systems and techniques of others. It is in the interest of truth itself. Were it otherwise no scientific journal would be safe.'[397]

The case began in the High Court in June 1972, more than three years after the articles were published.[398] The case was against the British Medical Association (BMA), the owners and publishers of the *BMJ*, and the four authors of the study. One of Drummond-Jackson's central points was that the authors said they had used his technique but hadn't.

There are three main defences to a charge of libel: privilege, justification and fair comment. Privilege defines circumstances where for the greater public good people should be able to communicate without fear of libel. This applies in Parliament and to the reporting of Parliament, the courts, and lesser tribunals like the General Medical Council so long as the reports are fair and accurate and give all sides of the story. If, for example, you report on the prosecution's case you must report that the defendant denied the charges and later report the defendant's case and the verdict.

The *BMJ* argued that qualified privilege applied in the Drummond-Jackson case.[399] If qualified privilege applies then 'a man behaving honestly may make statements about another which are defamatory and in fact untrue without being liable for so doing'. A 19th century judge explained the reasoning: 'It is better for the general good that individuals should occasionally suffer than that freedom of communication between persons in certain relations should be in any way impeded.' Scientific journals might seem like a case where qualified privilege should apply, but this has never happened. The *BMJ* never got to advance its argument in the Drummond-Jackson case because it was settled after 35 days in court before Drummond-Jackson had finished making his case.

The second defence against libel is justification—that what is written is 'true'. But the crucial point to understand is that what matters is not whether or not a statement *is* true but whether or not it can be *proved* to be true—and the onus is on the defendants to prove that what they have published is true.

What this means in practical terms is that if somebody sends a journal an article that is defamatory but, the editors judge, very much in the public interest, then before the journal can publish it has to assemble enough evidence to convince a court of its truth. This is usually a time consuming and expensive business, which puts it beyond the means of most medical journals. Plus it is impossible to eradicate all risk. Judgements of the quality of the evidence are necessary. Uncertainties remain. Some 15 years ago the *BMJ* published an article where we spent £10,000 assembling evidence. After publication we were still sued, and the case went on for years. There was really no chance of us losing but despite 'winning' we still had costs of £107,000.[400]

It's impossible for me to argue that journals should be free to go ahead and publish what they like without fear of libel, but I think that the effect of Britain's libel laws are to keep poor behaviour hidden. Robert Maxwell, a rich rogue, kept the press out of his nefarious affairs for years through repeatedly threatening and taking libel actions. (I attack him as well in chapter 17 on the ethics of the business of scientific publishing. You can't libel the dead, at least not in Britain.) What Britain needs, I believe, is a better balance between the public interest and damage to individuals, particularly as only the rich can sue for libel: you can't get state support for an action and the costs are enormous, not least because you need to employ a specialist lawyer.

In the Drummond-Jackson case the defendants would have had to prove everything to be true to establish a defence of justification. As Lord Denning said before in the appeal to have the case struck out: 'The defendants must be prepared to prove the correctness of all their tests and experiments and to justify all their conclusions…Just imagine the time required to prepare for trial; and the length of the trial.'[397] The *BMJ* published a weekly account of the trial,[398,401-410] and—even though the *BMJ* hadn't begun its defence—there was a strong sense of the case becoming so complex that it might never end.

The third defence to a charge of libel is fair comment, but the comment must be based on facts. You cannot simply say that X has behaved scandalously. You must give true facts to prove that he or she has behaved scandalously. As a report on the Drummond-Jackson case written by the *BMJ*'s legal correspondent says:[398]

'The law of defamation gives considerable latitude to the authors of defamatory comment so long as at the same time they do not make defamatory and untrue statements of fact. The test…is to ask, Would any fair man, however prejudiced he may be, however exaggerated or obstinate his views, have said what had been published?'

A defence of fair comment is, however, undermined if the plaintiff can demonstrate malice, which in libel means 'not simply spite but also the existence of an ulterior motive'. Drummond-Jackson alleged this not against the *BMJ* but against the authors of the study. Then he discovered the identity of the author of the leading article and produced evidence that he was malicious. A previous case involving the *Times Literary Supplement* seemed to establish that the publishers of anonymous pieces became responsible for the malice alleged against the author.

Justification—correctly—is not undermined by malice. As the *BMJ* legal correspondent put it: 'The truth may always be published no matter by what disgraceful motives the defendant is actuated.'[398]

The Drummond-Jackson case took a heavy toll on both parties. The costs were enormous. The cost to the *BMJ* was around one-quarter of a million pounds (equal to several million pounds in 2003), plus the time spent preparing the case and in court. Stephen Lock has described to me how he would spend all day in court and then return to do his day's work. Understandably, it made him very cautious—probably too cautious—about running the risk of another such case.

In his postscript to the history of the *BMJ* he wrote: 'Above all, I envy Wakley and Hart [19th century editors of the *Lancet* and *BMJ*] their radical journals relatively unfettered by the libel laws; what medicine needs today perhaps more than anything else is its own *Private Eye* [a satirical magazine that exposes corruption]…All professions need to be reminded of "how things really are"—the deceits, the shabby compromises, and the true reasons for particular decisions.'[411]

The *BMJ* has not had another Drummond-Jackson case, but we received plenty of threats and lawyers' letters. The one case that cost us a lot of money—£107,000—we won.[401] We were sued—together with the BBC and the *New Statesman*—by Dr James Sharp, a doctor, and Jabar Sultan, a vet. They were pedalling a bogus treatment for AIDS, and were exposed by Duncan Campbell, an investigative journalist, who went to see Sultan pretending he had AIDS and with a tape recorder strapped to his leg. Sharp was eventually struck off for serious professional misconduct.

Campbell's interview with Sharp was broadcast on the BBC, and he wrote an article for the *New Statesman*. I wrote an article for the *BMJ* off the back of Campbell's investigation in which I concentrated on the point that a great many doctors knew about this bogus treatment and yet did nothing.[412] This was the article I mentioned earlier in this chapter where we spent a great deal of money before publication making sure that we could prove everything.

Ironically we were sued not over this article but over the news story that reported Sharp being struck off.[413] Sharp sued us not for libel but for 'malicious falsehood', a more serious offence where the plaintiff has to have experienced financial loss and has to prove malice. A great advantage of suing for malicious falsehood is that you can be given legal aid (government financial support). Sharp was given legal aid, but then it was withdrawn on his own barrister's advice. Sultan sued for libel and represented himself. The case, which was defended primarily by the BBC, dragged on for seven years until it collapsed completely. Sultan had no money, and so we had to meet our own costs.

Since I wrote the first draft of this chapter I have found myself involved in a prolonged wrangle over whether or not an article we published in 2002 was defamatory. The article, which I discussed in chapter 8, told a simple story. A surgeon, Anjan Banerjee, produced fraudulent research in the early 1990s but the research was not retracted and Banerjee was not referred to the General Medical Council for 10 years—despite many people knowing the work to be fraudulent.[146] Nobody disputes these broad facts. The point of the article was not to attack individuals but institutions, where nobody seemed to be responsible for taking action. We judged that the article made broad important points and thought it important to publish. We spent thousands on legal fees in preparing the article for publication. Since publication we spent some £20,000 fending off accusations of libel. In one case we had to apologize and make a payment, the only case I lost in my time as editor. Ironically, the main accusation of those suing us was that they had no responsibility to do anything—exactly the point of the article. It felt very much to me as if England's libel laws were impeding an important debate on the way that medicine has failed to protect patients. The laws are acting against the public interest. I recognize that those suing us have a very different view.

The *BMJ* was much more at risk of libel than the BMJ Publishing Group's specialist journals, but a throwaway remark could kill a journal with few resources. This nearly happened, ironically, with the *Journal of Medical Ethics*. An editorial on an academic dispute included an injudicious clause, and angry academics threatened action. After prolonged discussion and wrangling everything was settled, but the journal could have been destroyed financially by fighting a case and losing. Even winning the case would have harmed the journal. The group's insurance policy said that it must pay the first £20,000 of any action. This was affordable to the *BMJ*, but is a destabilizing sum for smaller journals.

Another of the group's journals—*Tobacco Control*—was almost put out of business by British libel laws without an action being taken against it. The journal, as the title implies, is concerned with the harm caused by tobacco and measures taken to reduce the harm. This makes it unpopular with tobacco companies, and the journal contains lots of material critical of them. Our insurers decided that the risk of being sued by them was too large and declined to insure the journal. This presented a great problem to the treasurer of the BMA, the ultimate owners of the journal. He was being asked to pick up the risk of what could be a £2m action on a journal that at the time was losing money and probably would never make much. It made no commercial sense. Did the BMA care enough about the cause to pick up the risk?

While he was considering the problem, we tried to persuade the insurers. There was no case, as far as we knew, of a company taking an action against an academic journal, and it probably wouldn't do so because the adverse publicity would be huge and the gain minimal. And, we argued (a risky argument), if the companies were ever to take an action it was more likely to be against the *BMJ* than against *Tobacco Control*. Eventually the insurers agreed to insure the journal on the condition that every issue was read before publication by a libel lawyer. This led to some bizarre conversations with the editor, an American, who found himself perplexed by the concerns of the lawyer—particularly as he was often not allowed to print material that had appeared widely in the American media. (As I explain below, Britain has much more restrictive libel laws than the United States, and it is no defence against an accusation of libel to say that the libel has been published elsewhere.) Ten years later the journal had not been sued, and the insurers have dropped the condition that the journal has to be read by a libel lawyer.

It became like all our other journals. We consulted the lawyer, only if we are worried. This was often several times a week with the *BMJ*, and I learnt to negotiate with the lawyers. Like anybody else lawyers have different feelings about risk, and I tried to recalibrate our lawyers to be less risk averse. They would advise on whether or not something was defamatory, which was not so difficult, and on our chances of defending the statement, which was a harder judgement. They also advised us on revising the words to make a successful action less likely, which was very useful. They didn't advise, however, on the chances of somebody bringing an action. We had to judge that, and, as I said earlier, it's usually smarter for people not to sue. So, in a sense, we were constantly straining against England's restrictive libel laws.

England seems to have some of the most restrictive libel laws in the world, although New South Wales is said by some to be the 'libel capital of the world'. My American friends tell me that it's because we in England are subjects, whereas Americans are citizens. We are encouraged to be deferential to the rich and powerful. Our lawyers favour the governors rather than the governed. England has no equivalent of the first amendment, which says that 'Congress shall make no law…abridging the freedom of speech, or of the press.'

Certainly it is much harder to bring a successful libel action in the United States, particularly if you are a public figure. The onus is on the plaintiff to prove defamation and fault. If you are a public figure—and this includes people involved in specific public controversies—proving fault means proving 'actual malice'. This means the defendant knew his or her statement was false or recklessly disregarded the truth or falsity of his or her statement. These things are very hard to prove, and public figures rarely try to. Private individuals must show not only that the defendant was negligent but also that he or she failed to act with due care in the situation.

My belief is that Britain has the balance between public good and the harm to individuals wrong. Public debate and the accountability of the governors and the powerful would be strengthened by moving closer to the Americans. We in Britain should be less subjects and more citizens—and this may be more true in medicine with its hierarchical, paternalistic culture than almost anywhere else.

►21

The case that concern with ethical issues in publishing medical research is overdone

Three of us from the Committee on Publication Ethics (COPE) were giving a press conference on research fraud when Sir Richard Peto—a fellow of the Royal Society, one of Britain's leading researchers, and somebody far more distinguished than any of us giving the press conference—stood up in the audience and said: 'I want to put the case for fraud.' It was a perplexing moment for the journalists, none of whom chose to write a story entitled 'Top boffin favours fraud.' Peto, an intensely clever man, has a taste for the theatrical, but he had a serious point to make—and any book on the ethics of medical journals would be incomplete if it didn't include and examine his case.

His argument in essence is that clinical trials, which are extremely important, are hard to do and that anything that makes them harder to do is working against the public interest. The result of creating a fuss about research misconduct is that it increases the bureaucracy around trials and makes them more difficult and expensive to do. The 'solution' is then worse than the 'problem'. Misconduct, he believes, is rare, and the apparatus being constructed to deal with it is disproportionate.

Peto—together with 20 other researchers, including Sir Richard Doll, perhaps Britain's most famous researcher—has laid out his arguments most clearly in a paper on the case of Bernard Fisher, a researcher who, Peto and others believe, was unjustly dismissed.[414] These researchers emphasize repeatedly the need for large, simple randomized trials.[415] They are the only 'scientifically serious' way of telling whether treatments work. They need to be large in order to avoid the play of chance and because the benefits from medical treatments are often so small, and they need to be simple so that it's easy for doctors to enter large numbers of people into the trials.

Fisher was the chairman of the National Surgical Adjuvant Breast and Bowel Project (NSABP), 'one of the biggest, and hence the best, cancer trial organizations in the world'.[414] It included several hundred hospitals, had randomized about 50,000 patients and conducted several dozen trials. One of the project's most important trials was to show that 'lumpectomy' together with radiotherapy is as safe as mastectomy.

It's perhaps important to the story that this result felt uncomfortable to some surgeons and 'counterintuitive' to many journalists and members of the public who felt that the more of the cancer and the breast you removed the better the results. Indeed, surgeons in America invented and regularly performed 'radical mastectomies', where not only was the breast removed but also many surrounding tissues including the muscles on the front of the chest and lymph nodes from the armpit. This was a disabling operation that was disfiguring and often led to intractable swelling of the arm. But some surgeons—and particularly American surgeons, replete perhaps with the pioneering spirit—have always been attracted to radical surgery. Interestingly Geoffrey Keynes—a surgeon in London and brother of Maynard Keynes, the economist—performed lumpectomies in the early part of the 20th century.

In 1991 it was discovered that a doctor in Montreal, Roger Poisson, had entered about 100 patients into these trials who were ineligible. In order to make them seem eligible he had falsified patient details. These problems were picked up by the project and reported to the National Institutes of Health. After two years of deliberation it said that trial results should be republished without data on any of the 1500 patients from Montreal. The project was unhappy about excluding data from 1400 patients as these were real patients who had been properly included in the trials. (As I explained in chapter 6, it is poor scientific practice to leave out such data.)

There was thus a dispute over re-analysing and republishing the data. The argument of Peto and others was that this was a non-issue scientifically. The results could not be materially changed by re-analysis. 'It needs to be understood,' they write (in bold), 'that randomization of a few slightly ineligible patients into a large clinical trial is a type of change that *cannot* [bold italic] introduce any material bias into the main results of that trial.' In other words, the anxiety was misplaced—and Bernard Fisher and others had much more useful things to do scientifically.

Then the media became involved. Poisson had been reported to the Office of Scientific Integrity, a federal office, when the problems were first discovered, but it wasn't until 1993 that he was found formally guilty of research misconduct. The finding was published in various federal publications, but—illustrating how few people read federal publications (why do they bother?)—the mass media didn't notice until the following March. Then there was a tremendous hullabaloo. The press suggested that none of the results could be trusted. Women who had been in the trials felt abused and let down. Women who had had breast cancer worried that they may have been wrongly advised on treatment. The editors of the *New England Journal of Medicine*, which published the initial results, were offended that nobody had thought fit to inform them of problems with a study they'd published.[416]

The world of cancer trials was shaken to its foundations—despite the fact, as Peto and others later argued correctly, that the whole thing was scientifically unimportant in that the results could not be wrong. There were two congressional subcommittee hearings on the case, and these and other congressional hearings had the feeling of a political witch hunt to many scientists. Bernard Fisher and a statistical colleague were then investigated for scientific misconduct. They were of course the ones who had 'blown the whistle' on the false data. Their 'crime' was to be too slow in correcting the scientific record.

In addition, the project was audited and other problems were identified—'inevitably' in the view of Peto and others. Clearly if you have data on 50,000 people over decades there will be problems. The project trials were stopped, and—worst of all from the point of view of Peto and others—a Clinical Trials Monitoring Branch—was instigated 'to supervise the aggressive auditing of trials'.

To Peto and others 'this whole Kafkaesque episode seems absurd but also nasty...From a scientific viewpoint, none of the data alterations or errors that have been found in Montreal (or, subsequently, elsewhere) could have materially affected the scientific reliability of any NSABP studies, so the senior NSABP staff did not deserve any serious censure (let alone suspension) for giving low priority to the republication of various trials with the Montreal data deleted.'

Perhaps from a scientific and utilitarian point of view Peto and others are right. Poisson has been found guilty of research misconduct, but conceivably his behaviour could be explained by naïve zeal. He was so convinced by the arguments for big trials—which means recruiting as many patients as possible—that he got carried away. The falsification, however, is very difficult to excuse. The falsified data can be excluded without materially affecting the results, but purity of data is very important in science. Yes, data are full of imperfections—measurement error, for example—but once you add in falsification the whole enterprise begins to totter. Can we be sure that only 100 cases were falsified?

The scientific defence of Fisher and his colleagues at the centre is much stronger. They did alert the relevant authorities as soon as they identified the problem. They knew that re-analysing the data was not scientifically very important. They were simply slow.

From a utilitarian point of view no great harm was done. The patients that Poisson entered into the trial received good treatment within the context of a trial. The results of the trials still stand. Whatever harm was done was the fuss made by the media, which must have made some women anxious and undermined confidence in science unnecessarily. Plus harm will be done through the extra bureaucracy piled onto trials.

It was, I think, no accident that the paper by Peto and others was published in a journal called *Controlled Clinical Trials*. They were preaching to the converted. They should have tried advancing these arguments in the press or on live television. They would, I think, have found it more difficult.

The scale of the error is not what's important to many people. The fact that the ends are the same doesn't justify dubious means. The magic word is trust. As Drummond Rennie, a former Himalayan climber as well as inventor of the phrase 'publication ethics', says 'trust is an on–off switch'. If you trust somebody 60% you don't trust them. Trust in Poisson was destroyed by him falsifying data. Trust in Fisher and colleagues was damaged by them seeming to hide the problem. They did of course report it to the relevant authorities, and they presumably thought that was enough. They should probably have notified the *New England Journal of Medicine* and other journals where they had published. They should probably have quickly re-analysed the data and then held a press conference explaining the problem and reassuring people that the problem did not change the results of their studies. Instead, they were 'found out' and had to explain not only the changes to the results but also why they were offering these explanations four years after the event. People were inevitably suspicious, thinking that they must have something to hide.

Their error was in a sense tactical—and they paid a very heavy price for a tactical error. But there's also a question of accountability. Who are these researchers accountable to? They were legally accountable to their employers, funders and various federal agencies. But aren't they also accountable to the broader public and to the patients in their trials? Don't they have a duty to spell out to them just what has happened, what it means and how they will change their practice?

The paper in *Controlled Clinical Trials*—published in 1997—has an elitist, 'scientist (rather than doctor) knows best' feel that is very out of step with the times. The scientists might be saying: 'This is a lot of fuss about nothing. Don't worry your pretty heads. Relax and leave us to get on with our important work, which is all, by the way, for your benefit.' The paper doesn't propose solutions. It simply argues that there wasn't a serious problem. The public might respond: 'Wait a minute. How can you excuse falsifying data and keeping us in the dark for all those years? What else are you up to?' There has to be a better dialogue, and the onus is on the researchers to explain what they are doing.

They do need, for example, to get over the importance of large well done trials and just how hard they are to do. Because they are right that we could end up with 'solutions' to research misconduct that are worse than the problem. Some scientists—perhaps including Peto at our press conference—are tempted to argue that misconduct is on a small scale and could be safely ignored. Ironically, it might, however, be the common, lesser forms of misconduct—like publishing material more than once and not declaring conflicts of interest—that cause the problem. I write ironically because an epidemiologist like Peto recognizes that most strokes happen in people with moderately raised blood pressure rather than people with very high blood pressure—simply because there are so many more of them.

If the amount of bureaucracy attached to trials becomes excessive then fewer will be done, and we will be left not knowing whether or not many of the treatments doctors use every day work. The one group who might benefit from trials becoming more elaborate is the pharmaceutical industry. They benefit because as the cost of a trial rises higher it becomes harder for anybody apart from a major company to bring drugs to market. Biotech companies that develop new drugs may have to join with a large company. So one result of editors making a fuss about research misconduct might be that we'll end up with more trials in our journals from drug companies and fewer that address health problems that matter most to the public.

Peto, along with many other researchers, is not keen on people who describe themselves as 'ethicists'. These are the people who have instituted the elaborate, malfunctioning bureaucracy of research ethics committees. Then they've got excited about informed consent, making it ever harder to get people into trials. The Declaration of Helsinki—driven by the World Medical Association, which is infested with ethicists—is getting completely out of hand, potentially stopping important work in the developing world. Now they are bothering themselves with conflict of interest, research misconduct and a whole lot of issues that make research more difficult. Why can't they spend their time doing something more useful?

A middle way is needed. These ethical concerns will not all disappear, but people must be helped to understand that too much bureaucracy and audit will be counterproductive. Researchers and editors have a role here, and there must be a continuing dialogue among researchers, the public, ethicists, practitioners and editors. Such a dialogue needs an institution, and many countries don't have one. They should.

Section 7: The future

22. **Ethical manifestos for four different futures for medical publishing**

► 22

Ethical manifestos for four different futures for medical journals*

Lord Kelvin, a great physicist and president of the Royal Society from 1890 to 1895, predicted that radio had no future, X-rays would prove to be a hoax, and that heavier than air flying machines were impossible. Nobody predicted the explosion of the internet, the end of communism in the Soviet Union, or the attacks on New York and Washington of 11 September 2001, whereas many people, including me, have predicted things such as the paperless office, leisure society and the death of the book. It's very easy to get the future wrong, which is perhaps why Sam Goldwyn Mayer wisely said: 'I never make predictions, especially about the future.'

Why bother then looking to the future—because many organizations and governments spend much time and money doing just that? One answer comes from the business guru Charles Handy quoting George Bernard Shaw: 'The future belongs to the unreasonable ones, the ones who look forward not backward, who are certain of only uncertainty, and who have the confidence and the ability to think completely differently.'

It is probably important how you think about the future. Rather than make predictions it seems to be a better method to imagine several different but plausible futures, a process called 'scenario planning'. As with so many such processes the valuable part may be the interactions and conversations that go on during the process rather than the result, but the scenarios created may be useful for others. The point of scenario planning is then to look at features that are common to the different futures and to think about how you might prepare your organization (or yourself) for each of those futures.

As difficult as getting the future right is to get the speed of change right. Ian Morrison, a friend and once president of the Institute for the Future in California, told me that people persistently overestimate the speed and extent of short-term change but underestimate the effect of long-term change. I think we've seen some of this confusion over the speed and extent of change within scientific publishing. It was 30 years ago that people began to talk about the electronic revolution in publishing, but nothing happened for a long time—leading some to think that perhaps it never would happen. Then came the explosion of the internet and the dot.com revolution, and many of us, including me, expected radical change fast. The arrival of the internet was as

---

*This chapter overlaps considerably with the article on four futures for scientific and medical publishing published in the BMJ.[417] I don't feel that this is too terrible as I wrote the first draft of the BMJ paper and what was published was very close to that draft.

significant as the invention of fire or printing. It was a 'disruptive' technology that would change everything. Then came dot.bomb, and senior publishers began to think that the present forms of publishing science would at least 'see them out'. They could be right, but I think—and I could of course be wrong—that we are still at the beginning of the electronic revolution.

At the *BMJ* we tried to get ourselves thinking about the future by doing some scenario planning.[417] We began by identifying 'drivers of change' and then imagined four futures where those drivers might take us. These scenarios—which we named after four characters from the American cartoon, the Simpsons—are not, I repeat, predictions of the future. We didn't expect any of them to happen as described. Rather they are aids for thinking about the future.

One issue that always arises with scenario planning is how much you inject value judgements. You are supposed to create futures that you think might happen rather than you would like to happen. You mustn't therefore think: 'I don't like the sound of this future. Let's forget it or change it to something nicer.' Nevertheless, there is an inevitable tendency when looking to the future as to the past to see what you want to see. 'Myself creating what I saw', wrote the English poet William Cowper.

Here I want not only to describe the drivers of the change and the four scenarios of the future but also to inject some ethical considerations and to say how I think editors, journals and their owners should respond if these scenarios were to come to pass. And as I'm writing this final draft four years after the scenarios were first created I can make some judgement on their likelihood. This concluding chapter might present some sort of ethical manifesto for each of the futures, promoting remedies for the many deficiencies in medical journals that I've described in this book. I've resisted the temptation to prescribe my 'treatment' for the problems of medical journals. It's always easier to identify problems, and doctors have always cared more about diagnosis than treatment.

The strongest driver of change in the publishing of science and medical research is the appearance and spread of the World Wide Web, opening up the possibilities that authors might communicate directly with readers and that many intermediaries—publishers, librarians or editors—may not be needed. This is accompanied by increasing resentment in the academic community that it is having to pay ever more for information that it effectively produces itself, as I discussed in chapter 17.

The rise of evidence-based medicine and systematic reviews in particular has helped us understand how medical information is disorganized and 'Balkanized', and that finding information is expensive and difficult. In this way publishers have created rather than solved problems, enabling the creation of too many journals—often for financial rather than scientific benefit. The excessive number of journals together with the many free newspapers created by publishers to harvest profits from the advertising of the pharmaceutical industry has helped compound the 'information paradox', whereby doctors are overwhelmed with information and yet cannot find the information they need when they need it. Most of the studies included in these journals are of low quality and of limited relevance to clinicians.

The globalization of medical publishing is exposing weak local products to strong international competitors, but it also means that those in the developing world can increasingly get access to the latest information. The challenge now is to try and ensure that more research is undertaken in the developing world, that it is widely disseminated and that something emerges—it might be local journals—that will make a useful connection between the research and clinicians. Those in the developing world might if we are not careful move quickly from famine to feast and find themselves caught in the same information paradox as doctors in the rich world.

As the world changes, many 'new players' are emerging—such as HighWire Press, BioMed Central, the Public Library of Science and PubMed Central—to try and capture value (or should I say income and profits?) that currently resides with publishers and is transferred to their shareholders and owners. The 'old players' will try to keep the money to themselves—and might well succeed, at least for a while.

Doctors are under increasing pressure to base their management of patients on evidence, but we know there is a substantial gap—the Institute of Medicine in the United States called it a 'chasm'—between what the evidence says should be done and what is done. So leaders in healthcare are very interested to find ways to encourage change, but we understand much better than we did that information alone does not change practice. The old idea that doctors read about something new in a journal on a Friday morning and then change their practice is now known to be a myth, but like most myths it has remarkable staying power. It's still believed by some editors. We now know that improved healthcare comes not from exhorting individuals but by improving systems, but we are still not clear of the best ways to improve systems.

Another important driver of change is the rise of patient power and the doctor–patient partnership means that an increasing number of patients expect access to the same information as doctors and that 'patients' evidence' is just as important as doctors' or research-based evidence.

There is growing acceptance that doctors cannot work unaided. It is, as John Fox, head of the Advanced Computing Laboratory and one of the world's leading medical informaticists, puts it 'an inhuman activity'. Nobody expects travel agents to know the times of trains from Venice to Bologna without consulting guides. Similarly doctors and other healthcare workers need support from information and decision-making tools. Doctors need machines to help them, and the spread of palm pilots, Blackberries and mobile phones opens up new possibilities of delivering 'just in time' information to doctors, many of whom are 'nomadic'—that is do not practise at a desk.

The idea that doctors and other health workers could be trained and then trusted to stay up to date is dead, and they will now have to be regularly revalidated or recertificated. Their performance will be counted and audited as is that of researchers, but those doing applied research are becoming increasingly impatient with systems that reward basic researchers but not them—systems like impact factors. The applied researchers are proposing new evaluation systems that place more value on change in the real world and less on scientific originality. This might upset the traditional hierarchy of journals with those with the highest impact factors at the top.

The falling price of information is also driving change. Many organizations—such as pharmaceutical companies, big hospitals and the National Health Service (NHS)—make information available for free on the internet. The marginal price (letting one more customer or reader have access) of electronic information is effectively zero, and so is the real price of long distance telephone calls. These developments mean that information can be shifted around the world immediately and almost for free in a way that was completely impossible in the paper world.

This is probably not a complete list of drivers operating to change journals and the publishing of medical research, and even if it were new drivers will soon be recognized. Nevertheless, we at the *BMJ* used this list of drivers and imagined four possible futures that might result from their interplay. Two of the scenarios are fairly familiar, and in both publishers still exist. The other two scenarios describe very different worlds where scientific publishers as we know them now may be gone, and it is possible to see the beginnings of both in our present world. Interestingly the world that is the least changed from now—the world of Homer, which I want to describe first—already begins to seem the most implausible.

Homer is the fat, lazy, rather gormless father in the Simpsons. His large belly often hangs out, and my daughter thinks I resemble him. His philosophy of the world of medical publishing is: 'It ain't that broke, so there's no great need to fix it.'

This is a scenario where—despite the drivers of change—the world doesn't change that much. Researchers continue to publish in the same old way because it's familiar and doesn't demand big—and therefore unpredictable—changes in the academic reward system. All journals have both paper and electronic versions. Peer review is still largely closed in that authors don't know who has reviewed their papers. Homer, a professor in neurology, is nervous that he might lose out in a new system. He reads the journals he's always read and prefers them in paper form. They come to him through his membership of various societies, and he can't see the point in subscribing to a journal. He has more than enough to read. He's uncomfortable with computers and keyboards, and his secretary looks after his email. Although he sometimes uses the web to find material, he always reads on paper.

Homer is, however, finding it increasingly difficult to keep up with all the material that is published, which he finds tiresome because he has now to revalidate every five years and show he's up to date. He's thus grateful for the distilled information he receives. Some of it is sent to him free (paid for by advertising, he assumes), and the rest is provided either by his society or by his hospital, which has recognized its responsibility to keep him up to date. The arrangement used to be that the hospital provided the space and the support, but the doctors were responsible for the quality of care. Now the board of the hospital is responsible not only for the budget but the quality of care. One consequence is that it must provide Homer and the other doctors with information and learning materials.

This is a familiar world for publishers. They have increased the value they add to information through filtering, distilling and organizing it better. And they have broken out of the bad old model of 'less for more' (where subscriptions fall and so prices are raised to make up for the loss, meaning that librarians are getting less material for more money) to a world of 'more for more' (electronic access to much more material for slightly more money, based on the marginal cost of electronic material being zero).

Although I was a publisher, I was ethically uncomfortable with this world. I think that research, most of which is funded with public money, should be available for free. Ideas breed ideas, and ideas create wealth. It's in the interest of all of us to make ideas free—so society should underwrite the costs. A closed peer review system is, as I've argued in chapter 7, wrong. The system of rewarding academics in relation to the journals in which they publish is, ironically, scientifically unsound. The impact factor of the journal is used as a surrogate for the quality of the individual study performed by the academic, but there is actually very little correlation between the citations of individual articles in a journal and the impact factor of the journal—because the impact factor is driven by a few articles that are very highly cited.[418] Plus the point of the research published in medical journals is to improve people's health. That is thus what should be rewarded—otherwise, academics will concentrate on work that will be cited rather than work that will improve health. I'm not arguing that we don't need basic science. We do. But we also need unglamorous research—on, for example, incontinence—and we therefore need different systems for measuring the worthiness of the research.

Much of the distilled information that Homer receives will still be supported by advertising from pharmaceutical companies. I'm not against advertising or pharmaceutical companies, but it seems wrong to me that so much of the information and education supplied to doctors—particularly in the United States—should be supported with pharmaceutical company money. Isn't it a bit like handing over the training of teachers to Walt Disney? I've also found it very odd that doctors' employers should not provide information and learning materials for them—and that instead they have come to depend on being supported by pharmaceutical companies.

I spoke once in the postgraduate centre attached to Worcester Royal Infirmary. A huge new hospital was being built with money from the private finance initiative, but the doctors were having to raise the money for the postgraduate centre. You might think that in a modern health service facilities for training and updating staff would be at the centre of the enterprise, not left out altogether. But things are changing, and it may well be that pharmaceutical companies have a smaller role in the education of doctors in the future—at least in Britain.

Marge is the wise mother in the Simpsons who sorts out everybody's problems. Hers is a world of academic innovation, where the academic community has won out in its battle with publishers. All original research is made available for free through the web—either through something like PubMed Central or the Public Library of Science, or on sites owned by universities, research institutions, companies or the NHS. The sites are all linked and can be searched simultaneously. Peer review is entirely open. The whole world can watch if it is interested.

As a practising geriatrician, Marge rarely accesses original research. Instead, she is sent magazines that summarize for her the small amount of research that matters for her practice. Some come on paper, but increasingly she reads them on the screen that she carries in her purse: the resolution is marvellous. The magazines contain news and gossip about her specialty and the rest of medicine. They also include educational material, most of it linked to material on the web. All the magazines are free to her, paid for by advertising, the associations she belongs to or her hospital. It is the hospital that pays for her to access the educational material on the web. She has to show that she's used it in order to get revalidated.

Marge's consultant colleague, Philip, who has an academic appointment, is electronically alerted to the small amount of research that is directly related to his research interest. His academic status is based partly on the number of hits received by his research on the web, partly on how much his research is mentioned in the magazines all doctors receive, but mostly on whether or not his research improves patient outcomes.

Marge has several decision support systems to help her in her clinical work. These are portable, linked to a constantly updated evidence base, and extremely easy to use. They prompt her gently. Her patients and their carers have access to exactly the same information sources and decision support systems.

Publishers have given up on publishing science. They produce the magazines and must add a great deal of value in order to stay ahead of their competitors. The added value is expensive, and the publishers are profitable only because they sell large numbers of paper and electronic copies at low unit price to purchasers like governments, healthcare plans or hospitals.

As I've described, about a dozen of us produced these scenarios, but Marge is a world that seems much better to me than what we have now or Homer. We should be sceptical about utopias, and I wonder if I've succeeded in projecting my ethical fantasies into the world of Marge.

It's good that doctors are not being sent a whole lot of material that is not useful to them and that the worlds of academics and practitioners relate more logically than now. The system of rewarding academics makes much more sense than now. Publishers far from subtracting value will have to add a lot of value to survive in this world. Peer review is open. Everybody can get all research for free. These are both things I advocate. Employers accept responsibility for providing doctors and others with high-quality learning materials. Pharmaceutical companies are less prominent. Doctors have accepted that they need decision support systems to practise effectively, and patients are equals in the process.

The world of Lisa—the smart, sassy, well informed daughter—is a world of scientific communication that is very different from now, and yet it's a world that we can see here now in the streets of London or Venice, where every third person is using a mobile phone. It's a world of global conversations. Information exchange occurs predominantly not through 'published' information but through conversation (much of it over the telephone), email, texting, list serves, bulletin boards and informal websites.

When we created this scenario blogging, let alone vlogging, did not exist. Nor had any of us heard of MSN messenger, which my teenage daughter uses all the time, or Blackberries. The Wikipedia had not started, and we had no idea that you could take and send a photo—or even a short video—with your phone. I have a sense now that Lisa's world is arriving very fast. It's a world that with my populist, anarchic, iconoclastic instincts I find very attractive but which traditional publishers find appalling and threatening: 'It's nothing more than writing on toilet walls.'

Lisa is a paediatric surgeon with a specialist interest in liver surgery. She's interested in cricket, romantic poetry and camels and is connected to a series of electronic communities that keep her up to date with her interests. She keeps electronic copies of some of the material. An advanced search engine allows her to find whatever she wants within her own database. (Again when we wrote this Google, which has astonishing search power, did not exist and nor did Google Desktop, which allows you to apply the power of Google to your own disorganized cairn of information.)

The research Lisa is conducting is part of a project that is proceeding in many centres. The data are kept centrally, and a constant electronic and sometimes voice conversation goes on among all those involved in the research. Once a week there is a conference call that many of the participants join. In some ways publication of the research is unimportant because everybody who needs to know is part of the research, but the research is archived on an academically sponsored website. Conversation about the research circulates around related communities, and sometimes but rarely clinicians and researchers from other parts of medicine will access the archive. Lisa's academic credit comes from the 'buzz' in the community. Everybody knows who is thinking originally and doing highly innovative work.

Sometimes Lisa needs information from beyond her special interests. She then either uses a search engine to direct her to the relevant electronic community or she asks somebody within her communities she thinks will know where to go. 'I don't know, but I know a man who does', is the mantra; and, even though the world has six billion inhabitants, we are all only five links from each other.

Lisa picks up general information from the mass media, blogs and from chat in her communities. The conversation is not all about the special interests. When something interesting happens in medicine or healthcare it spreads very quickly, like gossip, through the linked communities.

Companies producing hardware are making money in Lisa's world, but there's little role for publishers. The communities are self-generating and contain the information they need. Information is a side product of their professional and leisure activities. People keep their own databases. There is a Wikipedia specifically for medicine with Wikipedias appearing all the time for the different branches of medicine. The 'wisdom of the many' far exceeds the wisdom of the old time expert who sat down to write the definitive textbook.

Although this world might sound far fetched, it exists already—and is much closer in 2006 than we could imagine in 2002. Doctors, we know, get most of their information from each other, not from published material. The information from colleagues is directly relevant to them, is more credible than what is published, can be understood and internalized through conversation, and may be directly actionable in a way that is unusual with published material. Many doctors belong to groups, often international, related to their special interests. And most research that is published is already known to the 'invisible college' of people interested in that area of research.

BioMed Central is trying to create a business for this world by providing infrastructure (even electronic journals) for the communities. It is perhaps doubtful, however, whether communities need much more infrastructure than is easily and cheaply available through Yahoo and the like. It's the quality of the conversation that matters, not the technology or infrastructure. As I write in 2006 I know that open source software is being produced that will make available to everybody for free the technology necessary to transport a scientific manuscript through the entire publishing process. The software will also allow enrichment of the process through commentary, debate at all stages and the addition of multimedia.

This is a world that makes me feel old—not least because I can't text message and don't have a mobile phone (I have an ambition to be the last person in Britain to have a mobile phone, and I sometimes think I may have achieved it.) My children live in this world, constantly in conversation with friends and bored by objects like journals. But even though largely 'past it' I also live in this world: much of the information that is most important to me comes through conversation. This has probably always been true.

(I wrote the previous paragraph in 2003, but in 2006 through some magical reversal of the ageing process I find that the 'new media' make me feel young. I not only have a mobile phone but also a Blackberry, and I can text and send pictures via the phone. I'm an enthusiastic blogger, contribute to the Wikipedia, and am flattered to have an entry in the Wikipedia—albeit considerably shorter than my brother's.)

Perhaps the most worrying aspect of this world is that it may have no history. Solid artefacts—books, sculptures, pictures—have proved vital to historians. Conversations disappear. The conversations of Dr Johnson are remembered only because Boswell put them in a book. The world of Lisa is short on artefacts, and electronic archives seem to fade fast. There have been great difficulties accessing the records of the Manhattan project, which were some of the first to be kept electronically, whereas anybody can read the *Domesday Book* from the 11th century. Presumably somebody would find a way to create an archive, but a world without history seems frightening to me. 'Those who forget the past will be forced to repeat it', as it reminds us in the Holocaust Museum in Washington.

Reading the previous paragraph, which I wrote in 2003, it seems unnecessarily anxious. The big libraries of the world are busy with projects to keep several copies of everything, and Google is busy copying all the old books in these libraries. They are copying 10,000 books a week from the Bodleian in Oxford. Far from material disappearing much material that was effectively unavailable is appearing.

The world of Bart, the streetwise son, is perhaps the scariest for some. It's a world where the big guys, the big corporations, have taken over. Scientific and medical information is provided by large organizations, mostly companies—Microsoft, Tesco, Walt Disney, UnitedHealth Group, the World Health Organization, Merck and the like—as a side product of their usual business. Traditional scientific, technical and medical (STM) publishers have gone. Editors now work for the large companies, and their job is not to think for themselves but to promote the mission of their employers.

Most research is funded by the large organizations. Many academics are now employed by the companies, but even those remaining in academia tend to have their research funded by the organizations. Academic success is measured primarily by ability to raise money from the organizations. Teaching and research have been separated, and most universities are now teaching factories

Bart, a general practitioner, receives his information from his employer, Healthcare Plus, and from those organizations—such as Merck—that provide him with the products he needs to treat his patients. His patients have access to the same information. Nobody worries about the independence of information. The whole idea that information might be neutral is seen as naïve and old fashioned.

The market in ideas and the money markets are now tied closely together, which ensures that good ideas are quickly exploited. There is none of the delay that was so common in the old world, when academics and business were suspicious of each other. Bart sometimes amuses himself late at night by accessing the rabble-rousing website run by the 80-year-old Tony Delamothe that attacks the big companies. Nobody needs to stop such inflammatory material because nobody much pays attention.

This is a world that is ethically scary to those who have read George Orwell's *1984*. Individuals don't seem to matter much, and independent thought is not valued unless it's in the service of the company. It's a world where those inside the organizations, most people, might feel more secure, and maybe security might come to seem steadily more important. But those outside the organizations may be lost.

As I've written, one of the ideas of preparing different scenarios of the future is to allow people and organizations to prepare for them. There are some things that are common to all the worlds or at least to more than one.

Community information (gossip) will be important in all of these worlds. It has been important in all communities that have existed so far. Talking and gossiping are profoundly human. All the worlds are 'global', and patients are a growing audience in all of the worlds. The concept that doctors have one set of information and patients another set seems increasingly unsustainable. Patients' evidence may become as important as doctors' evidence.

For publishers, editors and journals a strategy that depends on publishing original research will work in only one of these futures—Homer. In contrast, producing distilled, value added material will be important in three of the worlds; it's not important in Lisa's world, where information is gained through conversation, probably an electronic one.

Educational material will be important in three of the worlds, but doctors don't pay for the material in any of the worlds. The money comes from large organizations or advertisers. A hundred even 30 years ago doctors did expect to pay for the information that kept them up to date. The advertising market was much less developed, and doctors were suspicious of information supplied by the government. Doctors set great store by being independent. Perhaps we were too cynical to imagine such a world returning, and maybe it will.

The web is important in all the worlds, and so potentially are other means of delivery (mobile phones, palm pilots, digital television and means not yet invented), emphasizing the importance of producing information that can be used in different media. Paper survives in three of the worlds, which is not surprising in that new media don't usually replace the old—just as radio didn't displace newspapers and television didn't replace radio. Rather the media find a new place in the ecology of information. In all the worlds there is ample room for innovation in delivering information. There will be many new ways that we haven't thought of yet.

In all the worlds there will be increasing competition for doctors' attention as there is for everybody's attention. I feel that I should thus thank anybody who has taken the trouble to read this book. Will these worlds have books? Homer, Marge and Bart will have books, although it will be the company manual in Bart's world. Books will perhaps be thought of not as pages between a cover but as electronic databases that will be constantly updated. I can't be bothered with such a database. I've found it very pleasurable to sit down every day for eight weeks in my palazzo and sketch the world of medical journals as I see it. It's a picture at a moment in time. I hope that you, reader, might capture some of the pleasure.

One of the beauties of both reading and writing books is that they surprise you. Writing this book has surprised me. I knew that I was frustrated by many aspects of medical journals, but this book has turned out to be much more negative than I expected. Perhaps I shouldn't be surprised—as I know that I have a strong iconoclastic streak. Sitting every day and writing the book has perhaps allowed me to indulge my iconoclasm. But more importantly I have also had time to read widely, to assemble studies, data and stories that previously were scattered. The picture that I assembled may have surprised me somewhat, but I believe it to be a realistic picture. I want to end by quoting the 150-word summary that the publishers asked me to write. (I cheated a little—it's 158 words.)

'Medical journals have many problems and need reform. They are overinfluenced by the pharmaceutical industry, too fond of the mass media, and yet neglectful of patients. The research they contain is hard to interpret and prone to bias, and peer review, the process at the heart of journals and all of science, is deeply flawed. It's increasingly apparent that many of the studies journals contain are fraudulent, and yet the scientific community has not responded adequately to the problem of fraud. Editors themselves also misbehave. The authors of the studies in journals have often had little do with the work they are reporting and many have conflicts of interest that are not declared. And the whole business of medical journals is corrupt because owners are making money from restricting access to important research, most of it funded by public money. All this matters to everybody because medical journals have a strong influence on their healthcare and lives.'

References

1   Wakefield AJ, Murch SH, Linnell AAJ *et al*. Ileal-lymphoid-nodular hyperplasia, non-specific colitis and pervasive developmental disorder in children. *Lancet* 1998;**351**:637–41.
2   Laumann E, Paik A, Rosen R. Sexual dysfunction in the United States: prevalence and predictors. *JAMA* 1999;**281**:537–44 (published erratum appears in *JAMA* 1999;**281**:1174).
3   Moynihan R. The making of a disease: female sexual dysfunction. *BMJ* 2003;**326**:45–7.
4   Hudson A, McLellan F. *Ethical issues in biomedical publication*. Baltimore: Johns Hopkins University Press, 2000.
5   Sackett DL, Haynes RB, Guyatt GH, Tugwell P. *Clinical epidemiology: a basic science for clinical medicine*. London: Little, Brown, 1991.
6   Haynes RB. Where's the meat in clinical journals? *ACP Journal Club* 1993;**119**:A23–4.
7   Altman DG. The scandal of poor medical research. *BMJ* 1994;**308**:283–4.
8   Shaughnessy AF, Slawson DC, Bennett JH. Becoming an information master: a guidebook to the medical information jungle. *J Fam Pract* 1994;**39**:489–99.
9   Bartrip P. *Mirror of medicine: a history of the* BMJ. Oxford: British Medical Journal and Oxford University Press, 1990.
10 Chen RT, DeStefano F. Vaccine adverse events: causal or coincidental? *Lancet* 1998;**351**:611–12.
11 Pobel D, Viel JF. Case-control study of leukaemia among young people near La Hague nuclear reprocessing plant: the environmental hypothesis revisited. *BMJ* 1997;**314**:101.
12 Horton R. A statement by the editors of the *Lancet*. *Lancet* 2004;**363**:820–1.
13 Murch SH, Anthony A, Casson DH *et al*. Retraction of an interpretation. *Lancet* 2004;**363**:750.
14 Smith R. The discomfort of patient power. *BMJ* 2002;**324**:497–8.
15 Antithrombotic Trialists' Collaboration. Collaborative meta-analysis of randomised trials of antiplatelet therapy for prevention of death, myocardial infarction and stroke in high risk patients. *BMJ* 2002;**324**.71–86.
16 Cleland JGF. For debate: Preventing atherosclerotic events with aspirin. *BMJ* 2002;**324**:103–5.
17 Bagenal FS, Easton DF, Harris E et al. Survival of patients with breast cancer attending Bristol Cancer Help Centre. *Lancet* 1990;**336**:606–10.
18 Fox R. Quoted in: Smith R. Charity Commission censures British cancer charities. *BMJ* 1994;**308**:155–6.
19 Richards T. Death from complementary medicine. *BMJ* 1990;**301**:510.
20 Goodare H. The scandal of poor medical research: sloppy use of literature often to blame. *BMJ* 1994;**308**:593.
21 Bodmer W. Bristol Cancer Help Centre. *Lancet* 1990;**336**:1188.
22 Budd JM, Sievert ME, Schultz TR. Phenomena of retraction. Reasons for retraction and citations to the publications. *JAMA* 1998;**280**:296–7.
23 McVie G. Quoted in: Smith R. Charity Commission censures British cancer charities. *BMJ* 1994;**308**:155–6.
24 Smith R. Charity Commission censures British cancer charities. *BMJ* 1994;**308**:155–6.
25 Feachem RGA, Sekhri NK, White KL. Getting more for their dollar: a comparison of the NHS with California's Kaiser Permanente. *BMJ* 2002;**324**:135–41.

26 Himmelstein DU, Woolhandler S, David DS *et al.* Getting more for their dollar: Kaiser v the NHS. *BMJ* 2002;**324**:1332.

27 Talbot-Smith A, Gnani S, Pollock A, Pereira Gray D. Questioning the claims from Kaiser. *Br J Gen Pract* 2004;**54**:415–21.

28 Ham C, York N, Sutch S, Shaw R. Hospital bed utilisation in the NHS, Kaiser Permanente, and the US Medicare programme: analysis of routine data. *BMJ* 2003;**327**:1257–61.

29 Sanders SA, Reinisch JM. Would you say you 'had sex' if...? *JAMA* 1999;**281**:275–7.

30 Anonymous. It's over, Debbie. *JAMA* 1988;**259**:272.

31 Lundberg G. 'It's over, Debbie,' and the euthanasia debate. *JAMA* 1988;**259**:2142–3.

32 Smith R. Euthanasia: time for a royal commission. *BMJ* 1992;**305**:728–9.

33 Doyal L, Doyal L. Why active euthanasia and physician assisted suicide should be legalised. *BMJ* 2001;**323**:1079–80.

34 Emanuel EJ. Euthanasia: where The Netherlands leads will the world follow? *BMJ* 2001;**322**:1376–7.

35 Angell M. The Supreme Court and physician-assisted suicide—the ultimate right. *N Engl J Med* 1997;**336**:50–3.

36 Marshall VM. It's almost over—more letters on Debbie. *JAMA* 1988;**260**:787.

37 Smith R. Cheating at medical school. *BMJ* 2000;**321**:398.

38 Davies S. Cheating at medical school. Summary of rapid responses. *BMJ* 2001;**322**:299.

39 Ewen SWB, Pusztai A. Effects of diets containing genetically modified potatoes expressing Galanthus nivalis lectin on rat small intestine. *Lancet* 1999;**354**:1353–4.

40 Horton R. Genetically modified foods: 'absurd' concern or welcome dialogue? *Lancet* 1999;**354**:1314–15.

41 Kuiper HA, Noteborn HPJM, Peijnenburg AACM. Adequacy of methods for testing the safety of genetically modified foods. *Lancet* 1999;**354**:1315.

42 Bombardier C, Laine L, Reicin A *et al.* Comparison of upper gastrointestinal toxicity of rofecoxib and naproxen in patients with rheumatoid arthritis. *N Engl J Med* 2000;**343**:1520–8.

43 Curfman GD, Morrissey S, Drazen JM. Expression of concern: Bombardier *et al.*, 'Comparison of Upper Gastrointestinal Toxicity of Rofecoxib and Naproxen in Patients with Rheumatoid Arthritis.' *N Engl J Med* 2000;**343**:1520–8. *N Engl J Med* 2005;**353**:2813–4.

44 Curfman GD, Morrissey S, Drazen JM. Expression of concern reaffirmed. *N Engl J Med* 2006;**354**:1193.

45 Laumann E, Paik A, Rosen R. Sexual dysfunction in the United States: prevalence and predictors. *JAMA* 1999;**281**:537–44 (published erratum appears in *JAMA* 1999;**281**:1174).

46 Smith R. In search of 'non-disease.' *BMJ* 2002;**324**:883–5.

47 Hughes C. *BMJ* admits 'lapses' after article wiped £30m off Scotia shares. *Independent* 10 June 2000.

48 Hettiaratchy S, Clarke J, Taubel J, Besa C. Burns after photodynamic therapy. *BMJ* 2000;**320**:1245.

49 Bryce R. Burns after photodynamic therapy. Drug point gives misleading impression of incidence of burns with temoporfin (Foscan). *BMJ* 2000;**320**:1731.

50 Richmond C. David Horrobin. *BMJ* 2003;**326**:885.

51 Enstrom JE, Kabat GC. Environmental tobacco smoke and tobacco related mortality in a prospective study of Californians, 1960–98. *BMJ* 2003;**326**:1057–60.

52 Roberts J, Smith R. Publishing research supported by the tobacco industry. *BMJ* 1996;**312**:133–4.

53 Lefanu WR. *British periodicals of medicine 1640–1899.* London: Wellcome Unit for the History of Medicine, 1984.

54 Squire Sprigge S. *The life and times of Thomas Wakley.* London: Longmans, 1897.

55 Bartrip PWJ. *Themselves writ large: the BMA 1832–1966.* London: BMJ Books, 1996.

56 Delamothe T. How political should a general medical journal be? *BMJ* 2002;**325**:1431–2.

57 Gedalia A. Political motivation of a medical journal [electronic response to Halileh and

Hartling. Israeli–Palestinian conflict]. *BMJ* 2002. http://bmj.com/cgi/eletters/324/7333/361#20289 (accessed 10 Dec 2002).

58 Marchetti P. How political should a general medical journal be? Medical journal is no place for politics. *BMJ* 2003;**326**:1431–32.

59 Roberts I. The second gasoline war and how we can prevent the third. *BMJ* 2003;**326**:171.

60 Roberts IG. How political should a general medical journal be? Medical journals may have had role in justifying war. *BMJ* 2003;**326**:820.

61 Institute of Medicine. *Crossing the quality chasm. A new health system for the 21st century.* Washington: National Academy Press, 2001.

62 Oxman AD, Thomson MA, Davis DA, Haynes RB. No magic bullets: a systematic review of 102 trials of interventions to improve professional practice. *Can Med Assoc J* 1995;**153**:1423–31.

63 Grimshaw JM, Russell IT. Effect of clinical guidelines on medical practice: a systematic review of rigorous evaluations. *Lancet* 1993;**342**:1317–22.

64 Grol R. Beliefs and evidence in changing clinical practice. *BMJ* 1997;**315**:418–21.

65 Smith R. What clinical information do doctors need? *BMJ* 1996;**313**:1062–8.

66 Godlee F, Smith R, Goldman D. Clinical evidence. *BMJ* 1999;**318**:1570–1.

67 Smith R. The *BMJ*: moving on. *BMJ* 2002;**324**:5–6.

68 Milton J. *Aeropagitica.* World Wide Web: Amazon Press (digital download), 2003.

69 Coulter A. *The autonomous patient ending paternalism in medical care.* London: Stationery Office Books, 2002.

70 Muir Gray JA. *The resourceful patient.* Oxford: Rosetta Press, 2001.

71 World Health Organization. *Macroeconomics and health: investing in health for economic development.* Report of the commission on macroeconomics and health. Geneva: WHO, 2001.

72 Müllner M, Groves T. Making research papers in the *BMJ* more accessible. *BMJ* 2002;**325**:456.

73 Godlee F, Jefferson T, eds. *Peer review in health sciences*, 2nd edn. London: BMJ Books, 2003.

74 Relman AS. Dealing with conflicts of interest. *N Engl J Med* 1984;**310**:1182–3.

75 Hall D. Child protection: lessons from Victoria Climbié. *BMJ* 2003;**326**:293–4.

76 McCombs ME, Shaw DL. The agenda setting function of mass media. *Public Opin Q* 1972;**36**:176–87.

77 McCombs ME, Shaw DL. The evolution of agenda-setting research: twenty five years in the marketplace of ideas. *J Commun* 1993;**43**:58–67.

78 Edelstein L. *The Hippocratic oath: text, translation, and interpretation.* Baltimore: Johns Hopkins Press, 1943.

79 www.pbs.org/wgbh/nova/doctors/oath_modern.html (accessed 8 June 2003).

80 Weatherall DJ. The inhumanity of medicine. *BMJ* 1994;**309**:1671–2.

81 Smith R. Publishing information about patients. *BMJ* 1995;**311**:1240–1.

82 Smith R. Informed consent: edging forwards (and backwards). *BMJ* 1998;**316**:949–51.

83 Calman K. The profession of medicine. *BMJ* 1994;**309**:1140–3.

84 Smith R. Medicine's core values. *BMJ* 1994;**309**:1247–8.

85 Smith R. Misconduct in research: editors respond. *BMJ* 1997;**315**:201–2.

86 McCall Smith A, Tonks A, Smith R. An ethics committee for the *BMJ*. *BMJ* 2000;**321**:720.

87 Smith R. Medical editor lambasts journals and editors. *BMJ* 2001;**323**:651.

88 Smith R, Rennie D. And now, evidence based editing. *BMJ* 1995;**311**:826.

89 Weeks WB, Wallace AE. Readability of British and American medical prose at the start of the 21st century. *BMJ* 2002;**325**:1451–2.

90 O'Donnell M. Evidence-based illiteracy: time to rescue 'the literature'. *Lancet* 2000;**355**:489–91.

91 O'Donnell M. The toxic effect of language on medicine. *J R Coll Physicians Lond* 1995;**29**:525–9.

92   Berwick D, Davidoff F, Hiatt H, Smith R. Refining and implementing the Tavistock principles for everybody in health care. *BMJ* 2001;**323**:616–20.
93   Gaylin W. Faulty diagnosis. Why Clinton's health-care plan won't cure what ails us. *Harpers* 1993;**October**:57–64.
94   Davidoff F, Reinecke RD. The 28th Amendment. *Ann Intern Med* 1999;**130**:692–4.
95   Davies S. Obituary for David Horrobin: summary of rapid responses. *BMJ* 2003;**326**: 1089.
96   Butler D. Medical journal under attack as dissenters seize AIDS platform. *Nature* 2003;**426**:215.
97   Smith R. Milton and Galileo would back *BMJ* on free speech. *Nature* 2004;**427**:287.
98   Carr EH. *What is history?* Harmondsworth: Penguin, 1990.
99   Popper K. *The logic of scientific discovery.* London: Routledge, 2002.
100 Kuhn T. *The structure of scientific revolutions.* London: Routledge, 1996.
101 www.guardian.co.uk/newsroom/story/0,11718,850815,00.html (accessed 14 June 2003).
102 Davies S, Delamothe T. Revitalising rapid responses. *BMJ* 2005;**330**:1284.
103 Morton V, Torgerson DJ. Effect of regression to the mean on decision making in health care. *BMJ* 2003;**326**:1083–4.
104 Horton R. Surgical research or comic opera: questions, but few answers. *Lancet* 1996;**347**:984–5.
105 Pitches D, Burls A, Fry-Smith A. How to make a silk purse from a sow's ear—a comprehensive review of strategies to optimise data for corrupt managers and incompetent clinicians. *BMJ* 2003;**327**:1436–9.
106 Poloniecki J. Half of all doctors are below average. *BMJ* 1998;**316**:1734–6.
107 Writing group for the Women's Health Initiative Investigators. Risks and benefits of estrogen plus progestin in healthy postmenopausal women. *JAMA* 2002;**288**:321–33.
108 Shumaker SA, Legault C, Thal L *et al.* Estrogen plus progestin and the incidence of dementia and mild cognitive impairment in postmenopausal women: the Women's Health Initiative Memory Study: a randomized controlled trial. *JAMA* 2003;**289**:2651–62.
109 Yusuf S, Collins R, Peto R. Why do we need some large, simple randomized trials? *Stat Med* 1984;**3**:409–22.
110 Leibovici L. Effects of remote, retroactive intercessory prayer on outcomes in patients with bloodstream infection: randomised controlled trial. *BMJ* 2001;**323**:1450–1.
111 Haynes RB, McKibbon A, Kanani R. Systematic review of randomised trials of interventions to assist patients to follow prescriptions for medications. *Lancet* 1996;**348**:383–6.
112 Schulz KF, Chalmers I, Hayes RJ, Altman DG. Empirical evidence of bias. Dimensions of methodological quality associated with estimates of treatment effects in controlled trials. *JAMA* 1995;**273**:408–12.
113 Altman DG, Schulz KF, Moher D *et al.*, for the CONSORT Group. The revised CONSORT statement for reporting randomized trials: explanation and elaboration. *Ann Intern Med* 2001;**134**:663–94.
114 Moher D, Jones A, Lepage L; CONSORT Group (Consolitdated Standards for Reporting of Trials). Use of the CONSORT statement and quality of reports of randomized trials: a comparative before-and-after evaluation. *JAMA* 2001;**285**:1992–5.
115 Garattini S, Bertele V, Li Bassi L. How can research ethics committees protect patients better? *BMJ* 2003;**326**:1199–201.
116 Sackett DL, Oxman AD. HARLOT plc: an amalgamation of the world's two oldest professions. *BMJ* 2003;**327**:1442–5.
117 Ioannidis JPA. Why most published research findings are false. *PLoS Med* 2005;**2**:e124.
118 Greenhalgh T. *How to read a paper.* London: BMJ Books, 1997.
119 Sterne JAC, Davey Smith G. Sifting the evidence: what's wrong with significance tests? *BMJ* 2001;**322**:226–31.
120 le Fanu J. *The rise and fall of modern medicine.* New York: Little, Brown, 1999.
121 Lock S. *A difficult balance: editorial peer review in medicine.* London: Nuffield Provincials Hospital Trust, 1985.

122 Rennie D. Guarding the guardians: a conference on editorial peer review. *JAMA* l986;**256**:2391–2.

123 Martyn C. Slow tracking for *BMJ* papers. *BMJ* 2005;**331**:1551–2.

124 Hwang WS, Roh SI, Lee BC *et al*. Patient-specific embryonic stem cells derived from human SCNT blastocysts. *Science* 2005;**308**:1777–83.

125 Normile D, Vogel G, Holden C. Stem cells: cloning researcher says work is flawed but claims results stand. *Science* 2005;**310**:1886–7.

126 Jefferson T, Alderson P, Wager E, Davidoff F. Effects of editorial peer review: a systematic review. *JAMA* 2002;**287**:2784–6.

127 Godlee F, Gale CR, Martyn CN. Effect on the quality of peer review of blinding reviewers and asking them to sign their reports: a randomized controlled trial. *JAMA* 1998;**280**:237–40.

128 Schroter S, Black N, Evans S *et al*. Effects of training on quality of peer review: randomised controlled trial. *BMJ* 2004;**328**:673.

129 Peters D, Ceci S. Peer-review practices of psychological journals: the fate of submitted articles, submitted again. *Behav Brain Sci* 1982;**5**:187–255.

130 McIntyre N, Popper K. The critical attitude in medicine: the need for a new ethics. *BMJ* 1983;**287**:1919–23.

131 Horton R. Pardonable revisions and protocol reviews. *Lancet* 1997;**349**:6.

132 Rennie D. Misconduct and journal peer review. In: Godlee F, Jefferson T, eds. *Peer review in health sciences*. London: BMJ Books, 1999.

133 McNutt RA, Evans AT, Fletcher RH, Fletcher SW. The effects of blinding on the quality of peer review. A randomized trial. *JAMA* 1990;**263**:1371–6.

134 Justice AC, Cho MK, Winker MA, Berlin JA, Rennie D, the PEER investigators. Does masking author identity improve peer review quality: a randomized controlled trial. *JAMA* 1998;**280**:240–2.

135 van Rooyen S, Godlee F, Evans S *et al*. Effect of blinding and unmasking on the quality of peer review: a randomized trial. *JAMA* 1998;**280**:234–7.

136 Fabiato A. Anonymity of reviewers. *Cardiovasc Res* 1994;**28**:1134–9.

137 Fletcher RH, Fletcher SW, Fox R *et al*. Anonymity of reviewers. *Cardiovasc Res* 1994;**28**:1340–5.

138 van Rooyen S, Godlee F, Evans S *et al*. Effect of open peer review on quality of reviews and on reviewers' recommendations: a randomised trial. *BMJ* 1999;**18**:23–7.

139 Lock S. Research misconduct 1974–1990: an imperfect history. In: Lock S, Wells F, Farthing M, eds. *Fraud and misconduct in biomedical research*, 3rd edn. London: BMJ Books, 2001.

140 Rennie D, Gunsalus CK. Regulations on scientific misconduct: lessons from the US experience. In: Lock S, Wells F, Farthing M, eds. *Fraud and misconduct in biomedical research*, 3rd edn. London: BMJ Books, 2001.

141 Royal College of Obstetricians and Gynaecologists. *Report of the independent committee of inquiry into the circumstances surrounding the publication of two articles in the* British Journal of Obstetrics and Gynaecology *in August 1994*. London: RCOG, 1995.

142 Lock S. Lessons from the Pearce affair: handling scientific fraud. *BMJ* 1995;**310**:1547.

143 Pearce JM, Manyonda IT, Chamberlain GVP. Term delivery after intrauterine relocation of an ectopic pregnancy. *Br J Obstet Gynaecol* 1994;**101**:716–17.

144 Pearce JM, Hamid RI. Randomised controlled trial of the use of human chorionic gonadotrophin in recurrent miscarriage associated with polycystic ovaries. *Br J Obstet Gynaecol* 1994;**101**:685–8.

145 Wilmshurst P. Institutional corruption in medicine. *BMJ* 2002;**325**:1232–5.

146 Smith R. What is research misconduct? In: Nimmo WS, ed. *Joint Consensus Conference on Research Misconduct in Biomedical Research*. *J R Coll Phys Edin* 2000;**30** (Suppl 7): 4–8

147 *Integrity and misconduct in research*. Report of the Commission on Research Integrity to the Secretary of Health and Human Services, the House Committee on Commerce, and the Senate Committee on Labor and Human resources. 3 November 1995. gopher.faseb.org/opar/cri.html (accessed 10 July 2003).

148 Office of Science and Technology Policy, Executive office of the President. *Federal policy on*

research misconduct. Federal Register 6 December 2000, pp 76260–4. frwebgate.access.gpo.gov/cgi-bin/getdoc.cgi?dbname=2000_register&docid=00-30852-filed (accessed 10 July 2003).

149 Nylenna M, Andersen D, Dahlquist G *et al.* on behalf of the National Committees on Scientific Dishonesty in the Nordic Countries. Handling of scientific dishonesty in the Nordic countries. *Lancet* 1999;**354**:57–61.

150 Joint Consensus Conference on Misconduct in Biomedical Research. Consensus statement. 28 and 29 October 1999. www.rcpe.ac.uk/esd/consensus/misconduct_99.html (accessed 10 July 2003).

151 Zuckerman H. *Scientific elite: Nobel laureates in the United States.* New York: Free Press, 1977.

152 Rennie SC, Crosby JR. Are 'tomorrow's doctors' honest? Questionnaire study exploring medical students' attitudes and reported behaviour on academic misconduct. *BMJ* 2001;**322**:274–5.

153 Lock S. Misconduct in medical research: does it exist in Britain? *BMJ* 1988;**297**:1531–5.

154 Smith R. Draft code of conduct for medical editors. *BMJ* 2003;**327**:1010.

155 Stoa-Birketvedt G. Effect of cimetidine suspension on appetite and weight in overweight subjects. *BMJ* 1993;**306**:1091–3.

156 Rasmussen MH, Andersen T, Breum L *et al.* Cimetidine suspension as adjuvant to energy restricted diet in treating obesity. *BMJ* 1993;**306**:1093–6.

157 Garrow J. Does cimetidine cause weight loss? *BMJ* 1993;**306**:1084.

158 White C. Suspected research fraud: difficulties of getting at the truth. *BMJ* 2005;**331**:281–8.

159 Smith R. Investigating the other studies of a possibly fraudulent author. *BMJ* 2005;**331**:288–91.

160 Chandra RK. Effect of vitamin and trace-element supplementation on cognitive function in elderly subjects. *Nutrition* 2001;**17**:709–12.

161 Chandra RK. Effect of vitamin and trace-element supplementation on immune responses and infection in elderly subjects. *Lancet* 1992;**340**:1124–7.

162 Meguid M. Retraction of: Chandra RK. *Nutrition* 2001;**17**:709–12. *Nutrition* 2005;**21**:286.

163 Carpenter RK, Roberts S, Sternberg S. Nutrition and immune function: a 1992 report. *Lancet* 2003;**361**:2247.

164 Shapiro DW, Wenger WS, Shapiro MF. The contributions of authors to multiauthored biomedical research papers. *JAMA* 1994;**271**:438–42.

165 Goodman N. Survey of fulfilment of criteria of authorship in published medical research. *BMJ* 1994;**309**:1482.

166 Flanagin A, Carey LA, Fontanarosa PB *et al.* Prevalence of articles with honorary authors and ghost authors in peer-reviewed medical journals. *JAMA* 1998;**280**:222–4.

167 Horton R. The signature of responsibility. *Lancet* 1997;**350**:5–6.

168 International Committee of Medical Journal Editors. Uniform requirements for manuscripts submitted to biomedical journals: writing and editing for biomedical publication. www.icmje.org/ (accessed 15 April 2006).

169 Bhopal R, Rankin J, McColl E *et al.* The vexed question of authorship: views of researchers in a British medical faculty. *BMJ* 1997;**314**:1009.

170 Wilcox LJ. Authorship. The coin of the realm. The source of complaints. *JAMA* 1998;**280**:216–17.

171 Eysenbach G. Medical students and scientific misconduct: survey among 229 students. www.bmj.com/cgi/eletters/322/7281/074#12443, 3 February 2001.

172 Rennie D, Yank V, Emanuel L. When authorship fails: a proposal to make contributors accountable. *JAMA* 1997;**278**:579–85.

173 Horton R. The hidden research paper. *JAMA* 2002;**287**:2775–8.

174 MAST-I Group. Randomised controlled trial of streptokinase, aspirin, and combination of both in treatment of acute ischaemic stroke. *Lancet* 1995;**346**:1509–14.

175 Tognoni G, Roncaglioni MC. Dissent: an alternative interpretation of MAST-I. *Lancet* 1995;**346**:1515.

176 Docherty M, Smith R. The case for structuring the discussion of scientific papers. *BMJ* 1999;**318**:1224–5.
177 Gøtzsche PC. Multiple publication of reports of drug trials. *Eur J Clin Pharmacol* 1989;**36**:429–32.
178 Waldron T. Is duplicate publishing on the increase? *BMJ* 1992;**304**:1029.
179 Tramèr MR, Reynolds DJM, Moore RA, McQuay HJ. Impact of covert duplicate publication on meta-analysis: a case study. *BMJ* 1997;**315**:635–40.
180 Melander H, Ahlqvist-Rastad J, Meijer G, Beermann B. Evidence b(i)ased medicine—selective reporting from studies sponsored by pharmaceutical industry: review of studies in new drug applications. *BMJ* 2003;**326**:1171–3.
181 Chalmers I. Underreporting research is scientific misconduct. *JAMA* 1990;**263**:1405–8.
182 Dickersin K. The existence of publication bias and risk factors for its occurrence. *JAMA* 1990;**263**:1385–9.
183 Dickersin K, Min YI. Publication bias: the problem that won't go away. *Ann N Y Acad Sci* 1993;**703**:135–46; discussion 146–8.
184 Egger M, Davey Smith G, Schneider M, Minder C. Bias in meta-analysis detected by a simple, graphical test. *BMJ* 1997;**315**:629–34.
185 Olson CM, Rennie D, Cook D *et al.* Publication bias in editorial decision making. *JAMA* 2002;**287**:2825–8.
186 Egger M, Bartlett C, Jüni P. Are randomised controlled trials in the *BMJ* different? *BMJ* 2001;**323**:1253.
187 Lexchin J, Bero LA, Djulbegovic B, Clark O. Pharmaceutical industry sponsorship and research outcome and quality: systematic review. *BMJ* 2003;**326**:1167–70.
188 Kjaergard LL, Als-Nielsen B. Association between competing interests and authors' conclusions: epidemiological study of randomised clinical trials published in the *BMJ*. *BMJ* 2002;**325**:249.
189 Saunders MC, Dick JS, Brown IM *et al.* The effects of hospital admission for bed rest on duration of twin pregnancy: a randomised trial. *Lancet* 1985;**ii**:793–5.
190 Smith R, Roberts I. An amnesty for unpublished trials. *BMJ* 1997;**315**:622.
191 De Angelis C, Drazen JM, Frizelle FA *et al.* Is this clinical trial fully registered? A statement from the International Committee of Medical Journal Editors. www.icmje.org/clin_trialup.htm.
192 Bekelman JE, Li Y, Gross CP. Scope and impact of financial conflicts of interest in biomedical research. A systematic review. *JAMA* 2003;**289**:454–65.
193 Thompson DF. Understanding financial conflicts of interest. *N Engl J Med* 1993;**329**:573–6.
194 Smith R. Animal research: the need for a middle ground. *BMJ* 2001;**322**:248–9.
195 Campbell EG, Louis KS, Blumenthal D. Looking a gift horse in the mouth: corporate gifts supporting life sciences research. *JAMA* 1998;**279**:995–9.
196 Krimsky S, Rothenberg LS, Stott P, Kyle G. Scientific journals and their authors' financial interests: a pilot study. *Sci Eng Ethics* 1996;**2**:395–410.
197 Stelfox HT, Chua G, O'Rourke K, Detsky AS. Conflict of interest in the debate over calcium channel antagonists. *N Engl J Med* 1998;**338**:101–5.
198 International Committee of Medical Journal Editors. Conflict of interest. *Lancet* 1993;**341**:742–3.
199 Hussain A, Smith R. Declaring financial competing interests: survey of five general medical journals. *BMJ* 2001;**323**:263–4.
200 Davidoff F, DeAngelis CD, Drazen JM *et al.* Sponsorship, authorship, and accountability. *N Engl J Med* 2001;**345**:825–6.
201 Smith R. Journals fail to adhere to guidelines on conflicts of interest. *BMJ* 2001;**323**:651.
202 Gross CP, Gupta AR, Krumholz HM. Disclosure of financial competing interests in randomised controlled trials: cross sectional review. *BMJ* 2003;**326**:526–7.
203 Fontanarosa PB, Flanagin A, DeAngelis CD. Reporting conflicts of interest, financial aspects of research, and role of sponsors in funded studies. *JAMA* 2005;**294**:110–11.
204 Rothman KJ, Evans S. Extra scrutiny for industry funded trials. *BMJ* 2005;**331**:1350–1.

205 Fontanarosa PB, DeAngelis CD. Conflicts of interest and independent data analysis in industry-funded studies—reply. *JAMA* 2005;**294**:2576–7.

206 Haivas I, Schroter S, Waechter F, Smith R. Editors' declaration of their own conflicts of interest. *Can Med Assoc J* 2004;**171**:475–6.

207 Wilkinson P. 'Self referral': a potential conflict of interest. *BMJ* 1993;**306**:1083–4.

208 Hillman BJ, Joseph CA, Mabel MR *et al*. Frequency and costs of diagnostic imaging in office practice: a comparison of self referring and radiologist referring physicians. *N Engl J Med* 1990;**323**:1504–8.

209 Hillman AI, Pauly MV, Kerslein B. How do financial incentives affect physicians' clinical decisions and the financial performance of health maintenance organizations. *N Engl J Med* 1989;**321**:86–92.

210 Chren MM, Landefeld CS. Physicians' behaviour and their interactions with drug companies. *JAMA* 1994;**271**:684–9.

211 Murray SF. Relation between private health insurance and high rates of Caesarean section in Chile: qualitative and quantitative study. *BMJ* 2000;**321**:1501–5.

212 Roberts CL, Tracy S, Peat B. Rates for obstetric intervention among private and public patients in Australia: population based descriptive study. *BMJ* 2000;**321**:137–41.

213 Rochon PA, Gurwitz JH, Simms RW *et al*. A study of manufacturer supported trials of non-steroidal anti-inflammatory drugs in the treatment of arthritis. *Arch Intern Med* 1994;**154**:157–63.

214 Lilford RJ. Ethics of clinical trials from a bayesian and decision analytic perspective: whose equipoise is it anyway? *BMJ* 2003;**326**:980–1.

215 Barnes DE, Bero LA. Why review articles on the health effects of passive smoking reach different conclusions. *JAMA* 1998;**279**:1566–70.

216 Barnes DE, Bero LA. Industry funded research and conflict of interest: an analysis of research sponsored by the tobacco industry through the Center for Indoor Air Research. *J Health Policy Law* 1996;**21**:515–42.

217 Hope S. 12% of women stopped taking their pill immediately they heard CSM's warning. *BMJ* 1996;**312**:576.

218 Vandenbroucke JP. Competing interests and controversy about third generation oral contraceptives. *BMJ* 2000;**320**:381.

219 Sheldon T. Research on third generation pill remains unpublished. *BMJ* 2001;**322**:1086.

220 Kemmeren JM, Algra A, Grobbee DE. Third generation oral contraceptives and risk of venous thrombosis: meta-analysis. *BMJ* 2001;**323**:131.

221 Skegg DCG. Oral contraceptives, venous thromboembolism, and the courts. *BMJ* 2002;**325**:504–5.

222 Spitzer WO, Lewis MA, Heinemann LAJ *et al*. Third generation oral contraceptives and risk of venous thromboembolic disorders: an international case-control study. *BMJ* 1996;**312**:83–8.

223 Lewis MA, MacRae KD, Kuhl-Habich D *et al*. The differential risk of oral contraceptives: the impact of full exposure history. *Hum Reprod* 1999;**14**:1493–9.

224 Wright J. Kenneth David MacRae. *BMJ* 2002;**324**:1041.

225 Abbasi K, Smith R. No more free lunches. *BMJ* 2003;**326**:1155–6.

226 Wilkes MS, Doblin BH, Shapiro MF. Pharmaceutical advertisements in leading medical journals: experts' assessments. *Ann Intern Med* 1992;**116**:912–19.

227 Chaudhry S, Schroter S, Smith R, Morris J. Does declaration of competing interests affect reader perceptions? A randomised trial. *BMJ* 2002;**325**:1391–2.

228 Schroter S, Morris J, Chaudhry S *et al*. Does the type of competing interest statement affect readers' perceptions of the credibility of research? Randomised trial. *BMJ* 2004;**328**:742–3.

229 Monmaney T. Medical journals may have flouted own ethics 8 times. *Los Angeles Times* 21 October 1999.

230 Drazen JM, Curfman GD. Financial associations of editors. *N Engl J Med* 2002;**346**:1901–2.

231 World Medical Association. *Declaration of Helsinki. Ethical principles for medical research involving human subjects*. http://www.wma.net/e/policy/b3.htm (accessed 25 June 2006).

232 Smith R. Beyond conflict of interest. *BMJ* 1998;**317**:291–2.

233 Smith R. Conflict of interest and the *BMJ*. *BMJ* 1994;**308**:4.

234 Smith R. Making progress with competing interests. *BMJ* 2002;**325**:1375–6.

235 Smith R, Roberts I. Patient safety requires a new way of publishing trials. PLoS Clinical Trials 2006; 1: e6 DOI: 10.1371/journal.pctr.0010006.

236 Pelosi AJ, Appleby L. Psychological influences on cancer and ischaemic heart disease. *BMJ* 1992;**304**:1295–8.

237 Altman DG, Chalmers I, Herxheimer A. Is there a case for an international medical scientific press council? *JAMA* 1994;**272**:166–7.

238 Herxheimer A, Chalmers I, Altman D. *Have we made progress in exposing and dealing with editorial misconduct?* www.publicationethics.org.uk/reports/2003/ (accessed 16 April 2006).

239 Shashok K. Pitfalls of editorial miscommunication. *BMJ* 2003;**326**:1262–4.

240 Arnaiz-Villena A, Elaiwa N, Silvera C *et al*. The origin of Palestinians and their genetic relatedness with other Mediterranean populations. *Hum Immunol* 2001;**62**:889–900. (retracted in *Hum Immunol* 2001;**62**:1063).

241 Godlee F. Dealing with editorial misconduct. *BMJ* 2004;**329**:1301–2.

242 Committee on Publication Ethics. *Who ensures the integrity of the editor? The COPE report 2000*. London: COPE, 2000.

243 Committee on Publication Ethics. *Editorial compliance with duplicate publication. The COPE report 2000*. London: COPE, 2000.

244 Committee on Publication Ethics. *Publication bias arising from an editor's activities. The COPE report 2000*. London: COPE, 2000.

245 Smith R. A fierce and independent editor: Hugh Clegg. *BMJ* 1982;**ii**:32–4.

246 Anonymous. The gold-headed cane. *BMJ* 1956;**i**:791–3.

247 Hoey J, Caplan CE, Elmslie T *et al*. Science, sex and semantics: the firing of George Lundberg. *Can Med Assoc J* 1999;**160**:507–8.

248 Davies HT, Rennie D. Independence, governance, and trust: redefining the relationship between *JAMA* and the AMA. *JAMA* 1999;**281**:2344–6.

249 www.publicationethics.org.uk/reports/2005/code/ (accessed 22 April 2006).

250 www.pcc.org.uk/ (Accessed 22 April 2006)

251 Lord Wakeham. www.pcc.org.uk/10YearBook/introduction.html (accessed 17 July 2003).

252 Sen A. *Food and freedom*. www.worldbank.org/html/cgiar/publications/crawford/craw3.pdf (accessed 17 July 2003).

253 McGoldrick S. Obituary for David Horrobin: original mind will be missed. *BMJ* 2003;**326**.1089.

254 Kane P. Obituary for David Horrobin: work inspired and continues to nurture positive clinical outcomes. *BMJ* 2003;**326**:1089.

255 Charlton BG. Obituary for David Horrobin: medicine has lost something unique and irreplaceable. *BMJ* 2003;**326**:1088.

256 Coldicott Y, Pope C, Roberts C. The ethics of intimate examinations—teaching tomorrow's doctors. *BMJ* 2003;**326**:97–101.

257 Will RG, Ironside JW, Zeidler M *et al*. A new variant of Creutzfeldt–Jakob disease in the UK. *Lancet* 1996;**347**:921–5.

258 Parkin JR, Eagles JM. Blood-letting in bulimia nervosa. *Br J Psychiatry* 1993;**162**:246–8.

259 Court C. GMC finds doctors not guilty in consent case. *BMJ* 1995;**311**:1245.

260 International Committee of Medical Journal Editors. Protection of patients' rights to privacy. *BMJ* 1995;**311**:1272.

261 General Medical Council. *Guidance from the General Medical Council: confidentiality*. London: General Medical Council, 1995.

262 Committee on Publication Ethics. *An unethical ethics committee? The COPE Report 2002*. London: COPE, 2002.

263 Smith R. Informed consent: the intricacies. *BMJ* 1997;**314**:1059.

264 Dennis M, O'Rourke S, Slattery J *et al.* Evaluation of a stroke family care worker: results of a randomised controlled trial. *BMJ* 1997;**314**:1071–6.

265 Dennis M, O'Rourke S, Slattery J *et al.* Commentary: evaluation of a stroke family care worker: why we didn't ask patients for their consent to be randomised. *BMJ* 1997;**314**:1077.

266 McLean S. Commentary: not seeking consent means not treating the patient with respect. *BMJ* 1997;**314**:1076.

267 Bhagwanjee S, Muckart D, Jenna PM, Moodley P. HIV status does not influence outcomes of patients admitted to a surgical intensive care unit. *BMJ* 1997;**314**:1077–81.

268 Bhagwanjee S, Muckart D, Jenna PM, Moodley P. Commentary: why we did not seek informed consent before testing patients for HIV. *BMJ* 1997;**314**:1082–3.

269 Seedat YK. Commentary: no simple and absolute ethical rule exists for every conceivable situation. *BMJ* 1997;**314**:1083–4.

270 Kale R. Commentary: failing to seek patients' consent to research is always wrong. *BMJ* 1997;**314**:1081–2.

271 Doyal L. Journals should not publish research to which patients have not given fully informed research—with three exceptions. *BMJ* 1997;**314**:1107–11.

272 Tobias JS. *BMJ*'s present policy (sometimes approving research in which patients have not given fully informed consent) is wholly correct. *BMJ* 1997;**314**:1111–14.

273 Bratt DE, Soutter P, Bland M *et al.* Informed consent in medical research. *BMJ* 1997;**314**:1477.

274 Doyal L, Tobias JS, eds. *Informed consent in medical research*. London: BMJ Books, 2001.

275 Declaration of Helsinki. *BMJ* 1996;**313**:1448–9.

276 Anonymous. All treatments and trials must have informed consent. *BMJ* 1997;**314**:1134–5.

277 Doyal L, Tobias JS, Warnock M *et al.* Ethical debate: informed consent in medical research. Informed consent a response to recent correspondence. Changing the *BMJ*'s position on informed consent would be counterproductive. Informed consent a publisher's duty. Trial subjects must be fully involved in design and approval of trials. Studies that do not have informed consent from participants should not be published. *BMJ* 1998;**316**:1000–5.

278 Thornton H. Informed consent in medical research. *BMJ* 1997;**314**:1477.

279 *Declaration of Helsinki*. www.wma.net/e/policy/b3.htm (accessed 22 April 2006).

280 Smith R, Chalmers I. Britain's gift: a 'Medline' of synthesised evidence. *BMJ* 2001;**323**:1437–8.

281 Relman AS. The Ingelfinger rule. *N Engl J Med* 1981;**305**:824–6.

282 Gough A, Chapman S, Wagstaff K *et al.* Minocycline induced autoimmune hepatitis and systemic lupus erythematosus-like syndrome. *BMJ* 1996;**312**:169–72.

283 Ferner RE, Moss C. Minocycline for acne. *BMJ* 1996;**312**:138.

284 Ferguson JJ, Jenkins MGV, Field J. Paper in *BMJ* influenced prescribing of minocycline. *BMJ* 1998;**316**:72–3.

285 Phillips DP, Kanter EJ, Bednarczyk B, Tastad PL. Importance of the lay press in the transmission of medical knowledge to the scientific community. *N Engl J Med* 1991;**325**:1180–3.

286 Davey Smith G, Frankel S, Yarnell J. Sex and death: are they related? Findings from the Caerphilly cohort study. *BMJ* 1997;**315**:1641–4.

287 Karpf A. *Doctoring the media: the reporting of health and medicine*. London: Routledge, 1988.

288 Horton R. Medical journals: evidence of bias against the diseases of poverty. *Lancet* 2003;**361**·712–13.

289 Obuaya C-C. Reporting of research and health issues relevant to resource-poor countries in high-impact medical journals. *Euro Sci Edit* 2002;**28**:72–7.

290 Raja AJ, Singer P. Transatlantic divide in publication of content relevant to developing countries. *BMJ* 2004;**329**:1429–30.

291 Sahni P, Reddy PP, Kiran R *et al.* Indian medical journals. *Lancet* 1992;**339**:1589–91.

292 Global Forum for Health Research. *The 10/90 report on health research 2000*. Geneva: GFHR, 2000. www.globalforumhealth.org/pages/index.asp (accessed 26 July 2003).

293   Horton R. North and South: bridging the information gap. *Lancet* 2000;**355**:2231–6.

294   Bhopal R. Racism in medicine. *BMJ* 2001;**322**:1503–4.

295   Saxena S, Levav I, Maulik P, Saraceno B. How international are the editorial boards of leading psychiatry journals? *Lancet* 2003;**361**:609.

296   Angell M. The ethics of clinical research in the third world. *N Engl J Med* 1997;**337**:847–9.

297   Lurie P, Wolf SM. Unethical trials of interventions to reduce perinatal transmission of the human immunodeficiency virus in developing countries. *N Engl J Med* 1997;**337**:853–6.

298   Halsey NA, Sommer A, Henderson DA, Black RE. Ethics and international research. *BMJ* 1997;**315**:965–6.

299   Varmus H, Satcher D. Ethical complexities of conducting research in developing countries. *N Engl J Med* 1997;**337**:1003–5.

300   Whitworth J. Quoted in: Ferriman A. World Medical Association clarifies rules on placebo controlled trials. *BMJ* 2001;**323**:825.

301   www.globalforumhealth.org/Site/000__Home.php (accessed 23 April 2006).

302   www.wame.org/ (accessed 1 August 2003).

303   Tan-Torres Edejer T. Disseminating health information in developing countries: the role of the internet. *BMJ* 2000;**321**:797–800.

304   www.who.int/hinari/en/ (accessed 23 April 2006).

305   Smith R. Closing the digital divide. *BMJ* 2003;**326**:238.

306   Godlee F, Horton R, Smith R. Global information flow. *BMJ* 2000;**321**:776–7.

307   Bhutta Z, Nundy S, Abbasi K. Is there hope for South Asia? *BMJ* 2004;**328**:777–8.

308   bmj.bmjjournals.com/content/vol328/issue7443/ (accessed 23 April 2006).

309   Clark J. Open your eyes to Africa. *BMJ* 2005; 331: 0 ; doi:10.1136/bmj.331.7519.0-g.

310   bmj.bmjjournals.com/content/vol331/issue7519/ (accessed 23 April 2006).

311   Smith R. Medical journals and pharmaceutical companies: uneasy bedfellows. *BMJ* 2003;**326**:1202–5.

312   Smith R. Medical journals are an extension of the marketing arm of pharmaceutical companies. *PLoS Med* 2005;**2**:e138.

313   Taggart HM, Alderdice JM. Fatal cholestatic jaundice in elderly patients taking benoxaprofen. *BMJ* 1982;**284**:1372.

314   Halsey JP, Cardoe N. Benoxaprofen: side-effect profile in 300 patients. *BMJ* 1982;**284**:1365–8.

315   Hindson C, Daymond T, Diffey B, Lawlor F. Side effects of benoxaprofen. *BMJ* 1982;**284**:1368–9.

316   Horton R. The dawn of McScience. *N York Rev Books* 2004:**51**, March 11.

317   Angell M. *The truth about drug companies: how they deceive us and what to do about it.* New York: Random House, 2004.

318   Kassirer JP. *On the take: how medicine's complicity with big business can endanger your health.* New York: Oxford University Press, 2004.

319   Payer L. *Disease-mongers: How doctors, drug companies, and insurers are making you feel sick.* New York: John Wiley & Sons, 1992.

320   Moynihan R. *Too much medicine.* Sydney: ABC Books, 1998.

321   Moynihan R, Heath I, Henry D. Selling sickness: the pharmaceutical industry and disease-mongering. *BMJ* 2002;**324**:886–91.

322   Moynihan R, Cassels A. *Selling sickness: how the worlds biggest pharmaceutical companies are turning us all into patients.* New York: Nation Books, 2005.

323   Moynihan R, Henry D. The fight against disease mongering: generating knowledge for action. *PLoS Med* 2006;**3**:e191.

324   Gottlieb S. Congress criticises drugs industry for misleading advertising. *BMJ* 2002;**325**:137.

325   Villanueva P, Peiro S, Librero J, Pereiro I. Accuracy of pharmaceutical advertisements in medical journals. *Lancet* 2003;**361**:27–32.

326   Gitanjali B, Shashindran CH, Tripathi KD, Sethuraman KR. Are drug advertisements in Indian edition of *BMJ* unethical? *BMJ* 1997;**315**:459.

327   Christo GG, Balasubramaniam R. Commentary: advertising adversities. *BMJ* 1997;**315**:460.

328 Macdonald R. Should there be drug advertising? *studentBMJ* 2001;**9**:207.

329 Smith R. Should there be drug advertising? *studentBMJ* 2001;**9**:206.

330 Garattini S, Bertele V. Adjusting Europe's drug regulation to public health needs. *Lancet* 2001;**358**:64–7.

331 Garattini S, Bertele V, Bassi LL. How can research ethics committees protect patients better? *BMJ* 2003;**326**:1199–201.

332 Geddes J, Freemantle N, Harrison P, Bebbington P. Atypical antipsychotics in the treatment of schizophrenia: systematic overview and meta-regression analysis. *BMJ* 2000;**321**:1371–6.

333 Yank V, Rennie D, Bero LA. Are authors' financial ties with pharmaceutical companies associated with positive results or conclusions in meta-analyses on antihypertensive medications? *Abstract presented at Fifth International Congress on Peer Review and Biomedical Publication*, Chicago, 2005. www.ama-assn.org/public/peer/abstracts.html# meta.

334 Bell CM, Urbach DR, Ray JG *et al*. Is everything in health care cost-effective? Reported cost-effectiveness ratios in published studies? *Abstract presented at Fifth International Congress on Peer Review and Biomedical Publication*, Chicago, 2005. www.ama-assn.org/public/peer/abstracts.html#effective.

335 Thompson J, Baird P, Downie J. *The Olivieri report. The complete text of the independent inquiry commissioned by the Canadian Association of University Teachers*. Toronto: James Lorimer and Company, 2001.

336 Le Carre J. *The constant gardener*. London: Sceptre, 2002.

337 Dogherty P, Einarson T, Koren G, Sher G. The effectiveness of deferiprone in thalassemia. *Blood* 1997;**90**:894.

338 Olivieri NF, Brittenham GM, McLaren CE *et al*. Long-term safety and effectiveness of iron-chelation therapy with deferiprone for thalassemia major. *N Engl J Med* 1998;**339**: 417–23.

339 Rennie D. Thyroid storm. *JAMA* 1997;**277**:1238–43.

340 Dong BJ, Hauck WW, Gambertoglio JG *et al*. Bioequivalence of generic and brand-name levothyroxine products in the treatment of hypothyroidism. *JAMA* 1997;**277**:1205–13.

341 Mayor GH, Orlando T, Kurtz NM. Limitations of the levothyroxine bioequivalence evaluation: analysis of an attempted study. *Am J Ther* 1995;**2**:417–32.

342 King R. Bitter pill: how a drug company paid for university study, then undermined it. *Wall Street Journal* 25 April 1996.

343 Eckert C. Bioequivalence of levothyroxine preparations: industry sponsorship and academic freedom. *JAMA* 1997;**277**:1200.

344 Bodenheimer T. Uneasy alliance–clinical investigators and the pharamecutical industry. *N Engl J Med* 2000;**342**:1539–44.

345 Davidoff F, DeAngelis CD, Drazen JM *et al*. Sponsorship, authorship, and accountability. *Lancet* 2001;**358**:854–6.

346 Rochon PA, Gurwitz JH, Cheung M *et al*. Evaluating the quality of articles published in journal supplements compared with the quality of those published in the parent journal. *JAMA* 1994;**272**:108–13.

347 Cho MK, Bero LA. The quality of drug studies published in symposium proceedings. *Ann Intern Med* 1996;**124**:485–9.

348 Brody BA. A historical introduction to the requirement of obtaining informed consent from research participants. In; Doyal I , Tobias JS, edc. *Informed consent in medical research*. London: BMJ Books, 2001.

349 Blunt J. The role of research ethics committees. In: Lock S, Wells F, Farthing M, eds. *Fraud and misconduct in biomedical research*, 3rd edn. London: BMJ Books, 2001.

350 Saunders J. Research ethics committees—time for change? *Clin Med* 2002;**2**:534–8.

351 Foster CM. International regulation, informed consent and medical research. The UK perspective. In: Doyal L, Tobias JS, eds. *Informed consent in medical research*. London: BMJ Books, 2001.

352 Meslin EM. International regulation, informed consent and medical research. A perspective from the USA and Canada. In: Doyal L, Tobias JS, eds. *Informed consent in medical research*. London: BMJ Books, 2001.

353 Bradford Hill A. Medical ethics and controlled trials. Marc Daniels Lecture. *BMJ* 1963;**ii**:1043–5.

354 Anonymous. Ethics of human experimentation. *BMJ* 1963;**ii**:1-2.

355 Pappworth MH. *Human guinea pigs: experimentation on man*. London: Routledge and Kegan Paul, 1967.

356 Beecher HK. Ethics and clinical research. *N Engl J Med* 1966;**274**:1354–60.

357 Rosenheim ML. Supervision of the ethics of clinical investigations in institutions. Report of the committee appointed by the Royal College of Physicians of London. *BMJ* 1967;**iii**:429–30.

358 Anonymous. Experiments on man. *BMJ* 1967;**iii**:385–6.

359 Alberti KGMM. Local research ethics committees. *BMJ* 1995;**311**:639–40.

360 Ashcroft RE, Newson AJ, Benn PMW. Reforming research ethics committees. *BMJ* 2005;**331**:587–8.

361 Baeyens AJ. Impact of the European Clinical Trials Directive on academic clinical research. *Med Law* 2004;**23**:103–1.

362 Hearnshaw H. Comparison of requirements of research ethics committees in 11 European countries for a non-invasive interventional study. *BMJ* 2004;**328**:140–1.

363 Middle C, Johnson A, Petty T, Sims L, Macfarlane A. Ethics approval for a national postal survey: recent experience. *BMJ* 1995;**311**:659 60.

364 Alberti KGMM. Multicentre research ethics committees: has the cure been worse than the disease? *BMJ* 2000;**320**:1157–8.

365 Smith R. My last choice. *BMJ* 2004;**329**:1077.

366 Savulescu J. Two deaths and two lessons: is it time to review the structure and function of research ethics committees? *J Med Ethics* 2002;**28**:1–2.

367 Institute of Medicine. *Responsible research: A systems approach to protecting research participants*. Washington: National Academy of Sciences, 2002.

368 Department of Health. *Report of the ad hoc advisory group on the operation of NHS research ethics committees*. London: DoH, 2005. www.dh.gov.uk/assetRoot/ 04/11/24/17/04112417.pdf.

369 Amdur RJ, Biddle C. Institutional review board approval and publication of human research results. *JAMA* 1997;**277**:909–14.

370 Rennie D, Yank V. Disclosure to the reader of institutional review board approval and informed consent. *JAMA* 1997;**277**:922–3.

371 Wade DT. Ethics, audit, and research: all shades of grey. *BMJ* 2005;**330**:468–71.

372 Parkins KJ, Poets CF, O'Brien LM et al. Effect of exposure to 15% oxygen on breathing patterns and oxygen saturation in infants: interventional study. *BMJ* 1998;**316**:887–91.

373 Savulescu J. Commentary: Safety of participants in non-therapeutic research must be ensured. *BMJ* 1998;**316**:891–2.

374 Hughes V. Commentary: Ethical approval of study was warranted. *BMJ* 1998;**316**:892–3.

375 Parkins KJ, Poets CF, O'Brien LM et al. Authors' reply. *BMJ* 1998;**316**:887–94.

376 Horton R. The journal ombudsperson: a step toward scientific press oversight. *JAMA* 1998;**280**:298–9.

377 Horton R. The *Lancet*'s ombudsman. *Lancet* 1996;**348**:6.

378 Sherwood T. Ombudsman's fourth report. *Lancet* 2000;**356**:8.

379 *The Parliamentary Ombudsman*. London: Central Office of Information for the Office of the Parliamentary Commissioner for Administration, 1996.

380 Sherwod T. Lancet ombudsman's first report. *Lancet* 1997;**350**:4.

381 Sherwood T. Ombudsman's second report, and tobacco. *Lancet* 1998;**352**:7.

382 Sherwood T. Ombudsman's third report. *Lancet* 1999;**354**:91.

383 Carter R. Ombudsman's fifth report. *Lancet* 2001;**358**:350.

384 Carter R. Ombudsman's sixth report. *Lancet* 2002;**360**:272.

385 Carter R. Ombudsman's seventh report. *Lancet* 2003;**362**:94.

386 Carter R. Ombudsman's eighth report. *Lancet* 2004;**364**:402.

387 Olsen O, Gotzsche PC. Cochrane review on screening for breast cancer with mammography. *Lancet* 2001;**358**:1340–2.

388 Horton R. Screening mammography—an overview revisited. *Lancet* 2001;**358**:1284–5.

389 Hawkes N. Tobacco firm had secret army of scientists in some battle. www.mapinc.org/drugnews/v98/n358/a12.html?2110 (accessed 11 August 2003).

390 Skrabanek P. Smoking and statistical overkill. *Lancet* 1992;**340**:1208–9.

391 Tonks A, McCall Smith A, Smith R. The *BMJ* 's ethics committee is open for business. *BMJ* 2001;**322**:1263–4.

392 Wager E. Experiences of the *BMJ* ethics committee. *BMJ* 2004;**329**:510–12.

393 Anonymous. Freedom of the medical press. *BMJ* 1972;**iv**:313–14.

394 Wise CC, Robinson JS, Heath MJ, Tomlin PJ. Physiological responses to intermittent methohexitone for conservative dentistry. *BMJ* 1969;**ii**:540–3.

395 Anonymous. Intermittent intravenous methohexitone. *BMJ* 1969;**ii**:525–6.

396 Dyer C. Cardiologist admits research misconduct. *BMJ* 1997;**314**:1501.

397 Legal correspondent. Libel action to proceed. *BMJ* 1970;**i**:509–10.

398 Legal correspondent. Dentist's libel action against the BMA. *BMJ* 1972;**ii**:774–5.

399 Legal correspondent. Some legal implications of the Drummond-Jackson action. *BMJ* 1972;**iv**:373–4.

400 Dyer C. BMJ faces £107000 bill over libel case. *BMJ* 1996;**313**:897a.

401 Legal correspondent. Dentist's libel action continues. *BMJ* 1972;**iii**:60–2.

402 Legal correspondent. Dentist's libel action continues. *BMJ* 1972;**iii**:122–4.

403 Legal correspondent. Dentist's libel action continues. *BMJ* 1972;**iii**:184–6.

404 Legal correspondent. Dentist's libel action continues. *BMJ* 1972;**iii**:245–7.

405 Legal correspondent. Dentist's libel action continues. *BMJ* 1972;**iii**:300–3.

406 Legal correspondent. Dentist's libel action continues. *BMJ* 1972;**iii**:360–3.

407 Legal correspondent. Dentist's libel action: end of term. *BMJ* 1972;**iii**:423–5.

408 Legal correspondent. Dentist's libel action resumed. *BMJ* 1972;**iv**:246.

409 Legal correspondent. Dentist's libel action continues. *BMJ* 1972;**iv**:308–11.

410 Legal correspondent. End of dentist's libel action. *BMJ* 1972;**iv**:372–3.

411 Lock S. Postscript. In: Bartrip PWJ. *Mirror of medicine: a history of the* BMJ. Oxford: Clarendon Press, 1990.

412 Smith R. Doctors, unethical treatments, and turning a blind eye. *BMJ* 1989;**298**:1125–6.

413 Dyer C. Sharp struck off. *BMJ* 1989;**299**:1418–19.

414 Peto R, Collins R, Sackett D *et al.* The trials of Dr Bernard Fisher: a European persepective on an American episode. *Controlled Clin Trials* 1997;**18**:1–13.

415 Peto R, Baigent C. Trials: the next 50 years. *BMJ* 1998;**317**:1170–1.

416 Angell M, Kassirer JP. Setting the record straight in the breast-cancer trials. *N Engl J Med* 1994;**330**:1448–50.

417 Abbasi K, Butterfield M, Connor J et al. Four futures for scientific and medical publishing. *BMJ* 2002;**325**:1472–5.

418 Seglen PO. Why the impact factor of journals should not be used for evaluating research. *BMJ* 1997;**314**:498–502.

Index